RJ399.C6O355 2009

Obesity in youth

D0742561

Cosumnes River College Library
8401 Center Parkway
Sacramento, CA 95823

OBESITY
IN YOUTH

. . . . . . River College . . .
. . . Center Park . . .
. . . . . . , CA 95 . . .

OBESITY IN YOUTH

CAUSES, CONSEQUENCES, AND CURES

EDITED BY LESLIE J. HEINBERG AND J. KEVIN THOMPSON

American Psychological Association • Washington, DC

Copyright © 2009 by the American Psychological Association. All rights reserved. Except as permitted under the United States Copyright Act of 1976, no part of this publication may be reproduced or distributed in any form or by any means, including, but not limited to, the process of scanning and digitization, or stored in a database or retrieval system, without the prior written permission of the publisher.

Published by
American Psychological Association
750 First Street, NE
Washington, DC 20002
www.apa.org

To order
APA Order Department
P.O. Box 92984
Washington, DC 20090-2984
Tel: (800) 374-2721; Direct: (202) 336-5510
Fax: (202) 336-5502; TDD/TTY: (202) 336-6123
Online: www.apa.org/books/
E-mail: order@apa.org

In the U.K., Europe, Africa, and the Middle East, copies may be ordered from
American Psychological Association
3 Henrietta Street
Covent Garden, London
WC2E 8LU England

Typeset in Goudy by Circle Graphics, Columbia, MD

Printer: Data Reproductions, Auburn Hills, MI
Cover Designer: Naylor Design, Washington, DC
Technical/Production Editor: Harriet Kaplan

The opinions and statements published are the responsibility of the authors, and such opinions and statements do not necessarily represent the policies of the American Psychological Association.

Library of Congress Cataloging-in-Publication Data

Obesity in youth : causes, consequences, and cures / edited by Leslie J. Heinberg and J. Kevin Thompson. — 1st ed.
    p. ; cm.
  Includes bibliographical references and index.
  ISBN-13: 978-1-4338-0427-4
  ISBN-10: 1-4338-0427-1
  1. Obesity in adolescence—United States. I. Heinberg, Leslie J. II. Thompson, J. Kevin. III. American Psychological Association.
  [DNLM: 1. Obesity—prevention & control—United States. 2. Obesity—psychology—United States. 3. Adolescent—United States. 4. Child—United States. WD 210 O1123 2009]
  RJ399.C6O355 2009
  618.92'398—dc22
                                2008030291

British Library Cataloguing-in-Publication Data

A CIP record is available from the British Library.

Printed in the United States of America
First Edition

CONTENTS

Contributors .... *vii*

Preface .... *ix*

Acknowledgments .... *xi*

Introduction: The Obesity Epidemic in Children and Adolescents 3
Leslie J. Heinberg and J. Kevin Thompson

**I. Formative Influences: Risk for Obesity in
Childhood and Adolescence** **15**

Chapter 1.   Biological and Genetic Influences 17
              *Nathan J. Markward, Martha J. Markward,
              and Catherine A. Peterson*

Chapter 2.   Early Physical Activity, Sedentary Behavior,
              and Dietary Patterns 37
              James F. Sallis, Dori Rosenberg, and Jacqueline Kerr

Chapter 3.   Social and Interpersonal Influences on Obesity
               in Youth: Family, Peers, Society.................................... 59
               Alison E. Field and Nicole R. Kitos

II. Psychosocial, Interpersonal, and Intrapersonal
   Effects of Obesity 77

Chapter 4.   Psychosocial Consequences of Obesity and
               Weight Bias: Implications for Interventions.................. 79
               Jess Haines and Dianne Neumark-Sztainer

Chapter 5.   Body Image in Pediatric Obesity 99
               Sylvia Herbozo and J. Kevin Thompson

Chapter 6.   Psychological Comorbidity and
               Childhood Overweight 115
               *Rebecca M. Ringham, Michele D. Levine,
               and Marsha D. Marcus*

III. Assessment, Intervention, and Prevention.................................... 135

Chapter 7.   Assessment of Overweight Children
               and Adolescents 137
               Lindsay Varkula and Leslie J. Heinberg

Chapter 8.   Intervention: Strategies Designed to Affect
               Activity Level, Intake Patterns, and Behavior 159
               Myles S. Faith and Brian H. Wrotniak

Chapter 9.   Prevention: Changing Children's Diet
               and Physical Activity Patterns via Schools,
               Families, and the Environment.................................... 183
               *Russell Jago, Debbe Thompson, Sharon O'Donnell,
               Karen Cullen, and Tom Baranowski*

Chapter 10.   Future Directions in Pediatric Obesity.......................... 203
               J. Kevin Thompson and Leslie J. Heinberg

Author Index   209

Subject Index   229

About the Editors 243

CONTRIBUTORS

Tom Baranowski, Baylor College of Medicine, Houston, TX

Karen Cullen, Baylor College of Medicine, Houston, TX

Myles S. Faith, University of Pennsylvania School of Medicine, Philadelphia, PA; Children's Hospital of Philadelphia, Philadelphia, PA

Alison E. Field, Brigham and Women's Hospital and Harvard Medical School, Boston, MA

Jess Haines, Harvard Medical School/Harvard Pilgrim Health Care, Boston, MA

Leslie J. Heinberg, Cleveland Clinic Lerner College of Medicine of Case Western University, Cleveland, OH

Sylvia Herbozo, Yale University, New Haven, CT

Russell Jago, University of Bristol, Bristol, England

Jacqueline Kerr, San Diego State University, San Diego, CA

Nicole R. Kitos, Harvard Medical School, Boston, MA

Michele D. Levine, University of Pittsburgh School of Medicine, Pittsburgh, PA

Marsha D. Marcus, University of Pittsburgh School of Medicine, Pittsburgh, PA

Martha J. Markward, University of Missouri—Columbia

Nathan J. Markward, Pennington Biomedical Research Center, Baton Rouge, LA

Dianne Neumark-Sztainer, University of Minnesota, Minneapolis

Sharon O'Donnell, Baylor College of Medicine, Houston, TX

Catherine A. Peterson, University of Missouri—Columbia

Rebecca M. Ringham, University of Pittsburgh, School of Medicine, Pittsburgh, PA

Dori Rosenberg, SDSU/UCSD Joint Doctoral Program in Clinical Psychology, San Diego, CA

James F. Sallis, San Diego State University, San Diego, CA

Debbe Thompson, Baylor College of Medicine, Houston, TX

J. Kevin Thompson, University of South Florida, Tampa

Lindsay Varkula, Cleveland State University, Cleveland, OH

Brian H. Wrotniak, Children's Hospital of Philadelphia, Philadelphia, PA

PREFACE

The topic of childhood and adolescent obesity has received an extraordinary degree of attention in recent years from psychological and medical professionals and the popular media. As we completed our final edits for this book, *TIME* magazine devoted a special issue to "our super-sized kids." A variety of medical and psychological journals have also devoted special issues to the topic, and there has been an explosion of research articles in the past few years dealing with obesity in youth. Many of the media and research studies have focused on the physical health problems, such as diabetes, associated with an overweight or obese condition. However, the most widespread and immediate sequelae are psychological and social in nature. Unfortunately, these issues, and especially the psychosocial hazards of obesity, have received far less attention than research related to physical problems and medical morbidity. Our book fills the gap by focusing on the psychological aspects of obesity in youth. Although this book was written with psychologists and other mental health professionals in mind, the importance of psychological factors and the psychosocial effects of obesity should be a concern for all who work in pediatric obesity and anyone involved in finding solutions to the obesity epidemic facing children and adolescents in the United States and throughout the world.

Our interest in editing a book on this topic flows mainly from our clinical endeavors and professional research in the area of psychological factors and obesity (in particular, our work on body image) and the need to bring together experts who could provide a distillation of recent findings in this rapidly emerging field. However, we also have a personal interest—we each have two young children and deal on a day-to-day basis with many of the challenges that confront families. Some of our experiences inform our research whereas others sober us to the realities of raising young children in an environment that seems to promote obesity, yet at the same time rejects the young child who has a weight problem.

Leslie's sons (ages 8 and 11) have had to endure countless mind-numbing lectures on media literacy, nutrition, viral marketing, and weight discrimination in response to their comments and questions (e.g., "Will you buy me PowerAde so I can be a better soccer player?" "I had the best cereal at the sleepover—Reese's Peanut Butter Crunch!" "Can we go to Burger King? They have Indiana Jones toys." "Can we rent *Norbert?*"). Most recently, her older son had to suffer the embarrassment of his mother bringing healthy snacks to the baseball game, resulting in complaints from several teammates. Yet, she also struggles with the issue of "How much is too much?" How do you encourage nutrition without encouraging obsession? (There was a bit too much focus on macronutrients after a nutrition unit in her younger son's first-grade classroom; e.g., "How many fat grams does this cheese have?"; "Am I allowed to have protein?") How do we model moderation and enjoyment of good food without using food as a reward ("Of course we'll join the team for ice cream after the game")? Given her difficulty with finding the right balance, it is hard to imagine that other families negotiate these issues easily.

Kevin's son, who is now 12, has always been an active athlete, playing competitive soccer for 5 years as well as team lacrosse and basketball. Yet, he has always been a bit heavier than his friends, and when he was 10, the school nurse sent home a note about his body mass index (BMI; a common practice in schools), saying he was above the 90th percentile. Kevin remembers that Jared had tears in his eyes as he handed him the note, and it took a long conversation to calm him down and frame the issue (BMI is only one measure of overweight and not necessarily accurate for someone who is physically active, etc.) so that he did not take it personally.

We hope this book will provide not only a review of the recent work that is accessible for the researcher and clinician but also a framework for future research activity and a guide for everyone interested in working with youth, their families, and their environments to prevent and treat pediatric obesity.

ACKNOWLEDGMENTS

Our first thanks must go to the many parents, adolescents, and children who struggle with eating and weight issues. In working as a clinical director of a pediatric obesity program, Leslie Heinberg has seen the frustration and the pain, yet also the hope, evidenced by these remarkable families. Today, working with a severely obese population, she sees the challenges of growing up obese faced by her patients; she sees their strengths as well. It is our hope that this volume will lead to better care for these individuals and stimulate even more research designed to prevent and treat pediatric obesity.

Our thanks also go to the contributors to this text. We are acutely aware of the hard work, tedious edits, and quest for excellence that they each engaged in. We also thank the American Psychological Association for its continued interest and support of our work in obesity and other topics.

Leslie acknowledges the support of the National Cancer Institute (U54 CA116867) and the principal investigator, Nathan Berger, whose salary support was beneficial in preparing this volume.

Finally, we thank the people who have been particularly supportive of our work. Leslie thanks two individuals who have provided unfailing support, guidance, and mentorship in her career: Jennifer Haythornthwaite and Sarah McCue Horwitz. She also thanks her coeditor. Kevin Thompson has been a mentor; colleague; collaborator; and most important, good friend. Finally, she thanks her husband, Tony Inskeep, and sons, Aaron and Alex. Their support, good humor, love, and ability to endure her diatribes with minimal eye-rolling are forever appreciated.

Kevin thanks his wife, Veronica; his two children, Jared and Carly; and numerous research colleagues, including graduate students and collaborators from many different institutions, for their encouragement and input in the research process.

OBESITY
IN YOUTH

INTRODUCTION: THE OBESITY EPIDEMIC IN CHILDREN AND ADOLESCENTS

LESLIE J. HEINBERG AND J. KEVIN THOMPSON

The prevalence of pediatric overweight and obesity in the United States has more than quadrupled over the past 40 years (Y. Wang & Beydoun, 2007), resulting in a public health crisis for America's youth. U.S. Surgeon General Richard Carmona called obesity the greatest threat to public health today (American Medical Association [AMA], n.d.), and obesity is second only to smoking in frequency of causes of death in the United States (Mokdad, Marks, Stroup, & Gerberding, 2004). It is also a condition riddled with untoward medical, social, and psychological consequences.

To examine overweight in children and adolescents, it must first be defined. Unfortunately, this is not clear-cut in pediatric populations. Because ideal ranges for body mass index (BMI) vary considerably in children and adolescents on the basis of age and sex, age- and sex-specific BMI percentiles are frequently used to define overweight. Many clinicians and researchers use z-scores, which are standardized scores where the mean is set to 0 and the standard deviation is set to 1. These standardized scores are informative because at greater degrees of obesity, percentiles are not descriptive. Because the terminology used varies by researcher, z-scores, BMI percentiles, excess body weight, and other metrics may be discussed.

A lack of consistency on what is considered overweight may also lead to confusion. Most researchers have used the Centers for Disease Control and Prevention (CDC) cut-off criteria to categorize children and adolescents as "overweight" or "at risk for overweight." Children and adolescents above the 95th percentile for age and sex are deemed overweight whereas those between the 85th and 95th percentile for age and sex are considered at risk for overweight (National Center for Health Statistics, n.d.). Recently, an expert committee of the AMA has strongly suggested replacing the terms *overweight* with *obese* and *at risk for overweight* with *overweight* (AMA, n.d.). This shift in terminology is controversial because *obese* as a diagnostic label is considered pejorative. However, phrases such as *at risk for overweight* are unlikely to motivate behavior change. Another problem with the change in criteria is that the extant literature uses the CDC distinctions. Readers should be aware of the controversy and potential shift in terminology. Generally, we use the AMA terminology in our discussions, but the CDC criteria (e.g., at risk for overweight) may be used for consistency in describing reported results. The criteria used for labels (e.g., *overweight*) will be stated (e.g., 85th–95th percentile for age and gender).

Between 2003 and 2006, based on the most recent National Health and Nutrition Examination Survey (NHANES), Ogden, Carroll, and Flegal (2008) reported that 11.3% of children and adolescents were at or above the 97th percentile for age and sex growth charts, 16.3% were at or above the 95th percentile, and an additional 31.9% were at or above the 85th percentile. More than one third of 6- to 11-year-old boys and 35% of 12- to 19-year-old boys were overweight or obese and 32.6% of 6- to 11-year-old girls and 33.3% of 12- to 19-year-old girls were overweight or obese (Ogden et al., 2008). This represents more than a 700% increase for both age groups since the 1960s and an increase of 250% since the 1990s (Ogden, Flegal, Carroll, & Johnson, 2002). However, the most recent data suggest some plateauing of prevalence rates (Ogden et al., 2008). Between the 1976–1980 and 2003–2004 NHANES surveys, the average annual rate of increase was approximately 0.5 percentage points for children and adolescents (Y. Wang & Beydoun, 2007). Figure 1 shows these trends by age group and gender. The data are more striking when examining children by gender, ethnicity (see Figure 2), and socioeconomic status (SES; Mei et al., 1998; Mirza et al., 2004). The obesity epidemic has disproportionately affected certain ethnic and racial groups such as African Americans, Latinos, and Native Americans (Barlow & the Expert Committee, 2007). Poverty is also a potent risk factor (Barlow & the Expert Committee, 2007), and epidemiological data suggest that minority children from lower SES households have an almost 1 in 2 chance of being overweight or obese (Mei et al., 1998; National Center for Health Statistics, n.d.). Unfortunately, this suggests that children who are already at high risk for poor health outcomes are further compromised by high rates of overweight and obesity.

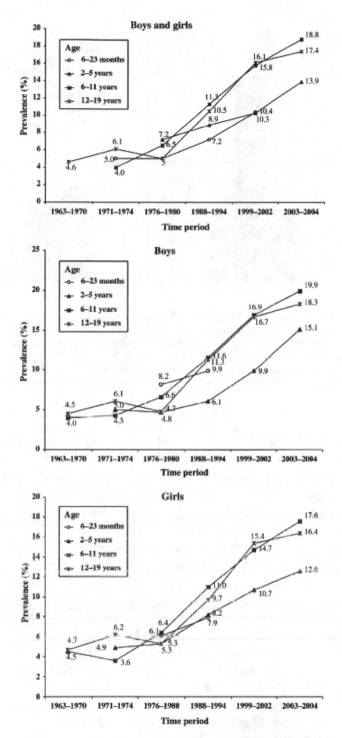

Figure 1. Trends in prevalence of obesity (BMI ≥ 95th percentile) in U.S. children and adolescents by gender. From "The Obesity Epidemic in the United States—Gender, Age, Socioeconomic, Racial/Ethnic, and Geographic Characteristics: A Systematic Review and Meta-Regression Analysis," by Y. Wang and M. A. Beydoun, 2007, *Epidemiologic Reviews, 29,* p. 17. Copyright 2007 by Oxford University Press. Reprinted with permission.

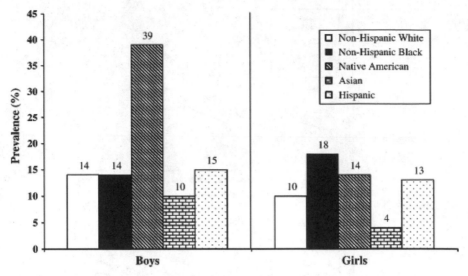

Figure 2. Prevalence of obesity (BMI ≥ 30 kg/m²) among U.S. adolescents by ethnicity. From "The Obesity Epidemic in the United States—Gender, Age, Socio-economic, Racial/Ethnic, and Geographic Characteristics: A Systematic Review and Meta-Regression Analysis," by Y. Wang and M. A. Beydoun, 2007, *Epidemiologic Reviews, 29,* p. 17. Copyright 2007 by Oxford University Press. Reprinted with permission.

PEDIATRIC OBESITY AND MEDICAL MORBIDITY

Although the focus of this book is on the psychological and social hazards and causes of pediatric obesity, pediatric obesity also has alarming effects on physical health. A brief overview is given here to alert the reader to the importance of prevention and early treatment.

The increase in pediatric obesity is alarming because of its association with health and as a critical early risk factor for adult morbidity and mortality (American Academy of Pediatrics, 2003; Freedman, Khan, Dietz, Srinivasan, & Berenson, 2002; Must, Jacques, Dallal, Bajema, & Dietz, 1992). The effect of obesity on medical sequelae, including death, has been known for more than 2,000 years—Hippocrates recognized that death was more common in those who were fat versus those who were lean (Bray, 2004). Adiposity in children is associated with numerous cardiovascular risk factors such as total cholesterol, low-density and high-density lipoprotein cholesterol, triglycerides, fasting insulin, and systolic blood pressure (Freedman et al., 2002; Higgins, Gower, Hunter, & Goran, 2001). Other adverse health effects include increased rates and severity of asthma, sleep apnea, and early puberty. Hyperinsulinism, insulin resistance, impaired glucose tolerance, metabolic syndrome, liver abnormalities, and Type 2 diabetes mellitus are strongly associated with degree of adiposity (American Academy of Pediatrics, 2003; Aye & Levitsky, 2003; Daniels, 2006; Sinha et al., 2002). Although the economic burden of obesity in adults is well studied and may account for more than 9% of annual U.S. medical spending (Daniels, 2006), little work has examined the economic burden of childhood obesity. One study examining data from 1979 to 1999 found that the proportion of hospital discharges with obesity-associated diseases increased dramatically over those 2 decades with a threefold increase in costs (from $35 million to $127 million; G. Wang & Dietz, 2002). Given that these data are almost a decade old, the current economic burden is likely to be considerably larger.

When obesity continues into adulthood, individuals are at greater risk for all-cause mortality (Jeffreys, McCarron, Gunnell, McEwen, & Smith, 2003; Peeters et al., 2003). Very high adolescent BMI has been associated with 30% to 40% higher adult mortality than medium BMI (Engeland, Brorge, Tverdal, & Sogaard, 2004). Similarly, when obesity persists into adulthood, individuals are at greater risk for a variety of medical complications. Early targeting of obesity (i.e., while still in childhood) may be a key factor in the control and prevention of many prevalent, high-cost diseases such as cancer, diabetes, and cardiovascular disease (Abu-Abid, Szold, & Klausner, 2002; Aye & Levitsky, 2003; Dyer, Stamler, Garside, & Greenland, 2004). The potential future health care costs associated with pediatric obesity and its comorbidities are staggering (American Academy of Pediatrics, 2003), and preventable morbidity and mortality associated with obesity may soon exceed the rates associated with cigarette smoking (U.S. Department of Health and Human Services, 2001; Wolf & Colditz, 1998).

Preventing or targeting pediatric obesity is imperative given the strong link between pediatric and adult obesity. The odds of being obese as an adult are 1.3 times greater for children who are obese at 2 years of age and 17.5 times greater for children who are obese at 15 to 17 years of age compared with normal weight peers (Whitaker, Wright, Pepe, Seidel, & Dietz, 1997). A more recent longitudinal study based in Louisiana (The Bogalusa Heart Study) found an even stronger association that occurred at very young ages. Among toddlers who were obese (≥ 95th percentile), 93% of boys became obese men and 73% of girls became obese women (Freedman, Khan, Serdula, Dietz, Srinivasan, & Berenson, 2005). Even infants who are at the highest end of the distribution for BMI or who may be growing more rapidly during their 1st year are at an increased risk for later obesity (Fisher et al., 2006). Associations also occur at lower levels of pediatric overweight. In a longitudinal study of children aged 8 to 15, children between the 50th and 84th percentiles for BMI were approximately 5 times as likely to be overweight or obese young adults compared with children below the 50th percentile (Field, Cook, & Gillman, 2005). In addition to genetic and biological factors, patterns of diet and physical activity are largely established in childhood (Telama,

Yang, Laakso, & Viikari, 1997), and the likelihood that early patterns persist into adulthood may help explain the strong link between child and adult obesity and overweight.

PSYCHOLOGICAL AND PSYCHOSOCIAL MORBIDITY

Obesity is one of the most stigmatizing and least socially acceptable conditions in childhood (Schwimmer, Burwinkle, & Varni, 2003). Unfortunately, weight bias and stigma lead to stereotyping by peers, teachers, and even family members and health professionals (Puhl & Latner, 2007). Such bias is pervasive and has been documented across diverse samples with diverse research methods (Puhl & Latner, 2007). Overweight children are at risk for school performance deficits and increased victimization by bullies (Janssen, Craig, Boyce, & Pickett, 2004); reduced social and psychological functioning (Gortmaker, Must, Perrin, Sobol, & Dietz, 1993; Schwimmer et al., 2003); depression, low self-esteem, and body image disturbances (Banis et al., 1988; Strauss, 2000; Thompson et al., 2007); and negatively altered life aspirations (Ball, Crawford, & Kenardy, 2004). A key aspect of weight bias and stigmatization experienced by obese children involves the receipt of negative social feedback (e.g., teasing, cruel and hurtful comments) from others (Thompson, Herbozo, Himes, & Yamamiya, 2005). This type of negative feedback is positively related to the development of body image problems, depression, and low self-esteem (Cattarin & Thompson, 1994; Thompson, Coovert, Richards, Johnson, & Cattarin, 1995; Thompson et al., 2007).

One of the most alarming findings is that children seeking obesity treatment have a 5.5-fold risk of a low health–related quality of life compared with normal-weight, same-aged peers—analogous to, and on some measures worse than, children undergoing cancer treatment (Schwimmer et al., 2003). A recent study suggests that poorer health–related quality of life seen in overweight youth is associated with peer victimization and their parents' distress (Janicke et al., 2007). Although researchers have yet to fully evaluate the role of psychological and psychosocial factors in the quality of life of overweight and obese youngsters, it is likely that future research will document the association of some of the factors discussed earlier and throughout this book (e.g., teasing, weight bias, stigmatization, family and peer issues).

Given the prevalence rates noted previously, psychologists and other mental health professionals working with youth or families probably will encounter overweight and obese children regularly. It will be imperative to assess the physical and medical aspects of each case. It will also be necessary to evaluate the etiology of weight problems from a psychological perspective, and detail such issues as diet and exercise patterns, family and peer influences, environmental factors (e.g., access to healthy food, exercise options, sedentary behaviors such as TV and video activity), and individual difference variables (e.g., low expectations for success, lack of motivation, low self-esteem). Research in many of these areas is in the formative stages but is vigorous, and new findings are occurring at a rapid pace, informing researchers' and clinicians' understanding of potential causal factors, prevention options, and treatment strategies. The time appears right for a distillation of these exciting and intriguing findings. This should help a broad array of professionals and non-professionals rise to the challenge of controlling the problem of pediatric obesity.

The chapters in this book have been written by leading experts in the field of pediatric obesity. The chapters are united by their focus on the interplay of behavioral, social, and psychological factors in the etiology, prevention, and treatment of obesity. It is our belief that an optimal awareness of the individual's unique experience of obesity is not possible without considering psychological and psychosocial factors.

A ROADMAP FOR OBESITY IN YOUTH: CAUSES, CONSEQUENCES, AND CURES

We propose a sharp focus on the psychological aspects of obesity in youth and implications of overweight and obesity for mental health practitioners. Although a few recent books have examined obesity, this volume is among the few that examines the psychological issues involved and is targeted to psychologists and other mental health professionals interested in working with overweight children and adolescents. The contributors, leading experts in the field, present up-to-date research findings and clinical guidelines.

The book is organized into three sections. Part I, "Formative Influences: Risk for Obesity in Childhood and Adolescence," examines seminal influences and addresses risk factors for obesity in childhood and adolescence. This section begins at the most elementary level with chapter 1, "Biological and Genetic Influences." This chapter will help familiarize clinicians with the latest research findings on genetic and biological influences in the development of obesity and will serve as a helpful review for researchers interested in the basic science underlying pediatric obesity. Although many of the studies are based on animal models or adult humans, findings are discussed in terms of pediatric obesity.

Although multifactorial in its etiology, obesity is ultimately the result of *energy imbalance* (i.e., when energy intake is greater than energy expenditure). Chapter 2 focuses on the two arms of energy balance—physical activity and diet. In this chapter, the authors review the literature on developmental influences on physical and sedentary activity with attention to periods of physical activity decline in children ages 4 to 12. This chapter also emphasizes behavioral influences on activity patterns, reviewing family influences on dietary patterns and eating habits. Recommendations and guidelines for families regarding physical activity, sedentary activity, and dietary intake are also included. Although the primary focus of the review is the behavioral literature, this chapter will likely be of great interest to dietitians and exercise physiologists as well as mental health professionals. Part I concludes with chapter 3, "Social and Interpersonal Influences on Obesity in Youth: Family, Peers, Society," in which the authors review the influence of the family environment and the effects of modeling on dietary and activity patterns; studies on peer influences on diet and activity—particularly in adolescents; and finally, the influence of the greater "toxic environment" on children's and adolescents' diet and activity. They also discuss the effects of television, advertising, changes in school curriculum, sociohistorical changes in dietary patterns, and changes in the built environment as well as treatment recommendations for working with families and strategies for helping children and adolescents address positive and negative peer relationships. This chapter should be of interest to a wide variety of professionals interested in families, public health, and public policy.

Part II, "Psychosocial, Interpersonal, and Intrapersonal Effects of Obesity," begins with chapter 4, "Psychosocial Consequences of Obesity and Weight Bias: Implications for Interventions." The authors address the common psychosocial stressors and difficulties to which overweight and obese children may be exposed and the psychosocial consequences of weight bias within a society that values thinness. This chapter concludes with discussion of the implications for working toward the prevention of obesity and weight bias and their associated psychosocial consequences. Chapter 5, "Body Image in Pediatric Obesity," addresses body image development, dissatisfaction, and disturbance in children and adolescents who are overweight or obese. Discussion of sociocultural thin ideals and media exposure to such ideals is included, along with assessment and treatment recommendations. Although the chapter includes many practical recommendations, it will also appeal to body image researchers. Chapter 6, "Psychological Comorbidity and Childhood Overweight," concludes the section. The authors review the literature on the co-occurrence of overweight and obesity and *Diagnostic and Statistical Manual of Mental Disorders* (4th ed., text revision; American Psychiatric Association, 2000) disorders. Particular focus is given to binge eating disorder and the challenges in correctly assessing this disorder in younger populations. Guidelines are provided for addressing lifestyle change in children with psychological comorbidities.

The third and final section of the book is "Assessment, Intervention, and Prevention." Chapter 7, "Assessment of Overweight Children and Adolescents," reviews clinical interview and psychometric assessment techniques commonly used by psychologists and mental health professionals in assessing the weight history, family history, dietary patterns, physical and sedentary activities, self-esteem, peer difficulties, self-efficacy, and body image of overweight and obese youth. In addition, the authors include practical information that will appeal to various members of multidisciplinary teams working with pediatric obesity (e.g., pediatricians, nurses, dietitians, exercise physiologists, and health educators) as well as recommendations for screening measures for psychopathology. In chapter 8, "Intervention: Strategies Designed to Affect Activity Level, Intake Patterns, and Behavior," the authors review the extant literature focusing on behavioral interventions designed to help youth and their families develop healthier lifestyles and implement the skills to change dietary behavior and activity patterns. The focus of much of the review is on family-based interventions and addresses the need for lifelong lifestyle changes rather than specific diet plans. Although this chapter reviews the research literature, specific strategies that may be used by clinicians with individual families is emphasized. In the final chapter in this section, "Prevention: Changing Children's Diet and Physical Activity Patterns via Schools, Families, and the Environment," the authors outline the findings of the literature examining obesity prevention efforts in children and adolescents. Family-based and school-based prevention efforts are addressed. Community-based, environmental, and health policy prevention efforts are also reviewed. Specific recommendations that clinicians can give to concerned families are included but should also appeal to public health and education researchers. The book concludes with a brief chapter discussing future directions in the field. The focus is on understudied areas within the literature and the need for better assessment and intervention strategies.

Given the prevalence of pediatric overweight and obesity, psychologists and other mental health professionals working with children, adolescents, and their families need to be familiar with the causes, consequences, and cures discussed in this book. A wealth of information is offered in these pages that summarizes the current state of research in specific areas and provides concrete directions for future research and clinical intervention. This information should resonate with the concerns and questions of a variety of professionals, including psychologists, psychiatrists, dieticians, pediatricians, teachers, coaches, and many others. It is our hope that this volume will offer guidance and direction to the many individuals who have chosen to devote their energies to understanding and reversing the public health conundrum that is pediatric obesity.

REFERENCES

Abu-Abid, S., Szold, A., & Klausner, J. (2002). Obesity and cancer. *Journal of Medicine*, *33*, 73–86.

American Academy of Pediatrics. (2003). Policy statement: Prevention of pediatric overweight and obesity. *Pediatrics, 112*, 424–430.

American Medical Association. (n.d.). *Obesity*. Retrieved August 9, 2007, from http://www.ama-assn.org/ama/pub/category/11759.html

American Psychiatric Association. (2000). *Diagnostic and statistical manual of mental disorders* (4th ed., text revision). Washington, DC: Author.

Aye, T., & Levitsky, L. L. (2003). Type 2 diabetes: An epidemic disease in childhood. *Current Opinions in Pediatrics, 15,* 411–415.

Ball, K., Crawford, D., & Kenardy, J. (2004). Longitudinal relationships among overweight, life satisfaction, and aspirations in young women. *Obesity Research, 12,* 1019–1030.

Banis, H. T., Varni, J. W., Wallander, J. L., Korsch, B. M., Jay, S. M., Adler, R., et al. (1988). Psychological and social adjustment of obese children and their families. *Child: Care, Health, and Development, 14,* 197–212.

Barlow, S. E., & the Expert Committee. (2007). Expert committee recommendations regarding the prevention, assessment and treatment of child and adolescent overweight and obesity: Summary report. *Pediatrics, 120,* S164–S192.

Bray, G. A. (2004). Medical consequences of obesity. *Journal of Clinical Endocrinology and Metabolism, 89,* 2583–2589.

Cattarin, J., & Thompson, J. K. (1994). A three-year longitudinal study of body image and eating disturbance in adolescent females. *Eating Disorders, 2,* 114–125.

Daniels, S. R. (2006). The consequences of childhood overweight and obesity. *Future Child, 16,* 47–67.

Dyer, A. R., Stamler, J., Garside, D. B., & Greenland, P. (2004). Long-term consequences of body mass index for cardiovascular mortality: The Chicago Heart Association Detection Project in Industry study. *Annals of Epidemiology, 14,* 101–108.

Engeland, A., Brorge, B., Tverdal, A., & Sogaard, A. J. (2004). Obesity in adolescence and adulthood and the risk of adult mortality. *Epidemiology, 15,* 79–85.

Field, A. E., Cook, N. R., & Gillman, M. W. (2005). Weight status in childhood as a predictor of becoming overweight or hypertensive in early adulthood. *Obesity Research, 13,* 163–169.

Fisher, D., Baird, J., Payne, L., Lucas, P., Kleijnen, J., Roberts, H., & Law, C. (2006). Are infant size and growth related to burden of disease in adulthood? A systematic review of literature. *International Journal of Epidemiology, 35,* 1196–1210.

Freedman, D. S., Khan, L. K., Dietz, W. H., Srinivasan, S. R., & Berenson, G. S. (2002). The relation of overweight to cardiovascular risk factors among children and adolescents: The Bogalusa heart study. *Pediatrics, 103,* 1175–1182.

Freedman, D. S., Khan, L. K., Serdula, M. K., Dietz, W. H., Srinivasan, S. R., & Berenson, G. S. (2005). Racial differences in the tracking of childhood BMI to adulthood. *Obesity Research, 13,* 928–935.

Gortmaker, S. L., Must, A., Perrin, J. M., Sobol, A. M., & Dietz, W. H. (1993). Social and economic consequences of overweight in adolescence and young adulthood. *New England Journal of Medicine, 329,* 1008–1012.

Higgins, D. B., Gower, B. A., Hunter, G. R., & Goran, M. I. (2001). Defining health-related obesity in pre-pubertal children. *Obesity Research, 9,* 233–240.

Janicke, D. M., Marciel, K. K., Ingerski, L. M., Novoa, W., Lowry, K. W., Sallinen, B. J., & Silverstein, J. H. (2007). Impact of psychosocial factors on quality of life in overweight youth. *Obesity, 15,* 1799–1807.

Janssen, I., Craig, W. M., Boyce, W. F., & Pickett, W. (2004). Associations between overweight and obesity with bullying behaviors in school-aged children. *Pediatrics, 113,* 1187–1194.

Jeffreys, M., McCarron, P., Gunnell, D., McEwen, J., & Smith, G. D. (2003). Body mass index in early and mid-adulthood, and subsequent mortality: A historical cohort study. *International Journal of Obesity and Related Metabolic Disorders, 27,* 1391–1397.

Mei, Z., Scanlon, K. S., Grummer-Strawn, L. M., Freedman, D. S., Yip, R., & Trowbridge, F. L. (1998). Increasing prevalence of overweight among US low-income preschool children: The Centers for Disease Control and Prevention Pediatric Nutrition Surveillance, 1983 to 1995. *Pediatrics, 101,* E12.

Mirza, N. M., Kadow, K., Palmer, M., Solano, H., Rosche, C., & Yanovski, J. A. (2004). Prevalence of overweight among inner city Hispanic-American children and adolescents. *Obesity Research, 12*(8), 1298–1310.

Mokdad, A. H., Marks, J. S., Stroup, D. F., & Gerberding, J. L. (2004). Actual causes of death in the United States, 2000. *JAMA, 291*(10), 1238–1245.

Must, A., Jacques, P. F., Dallal, G. E., Bajema, C. J., & Dietz, W. H. (1992). Long-term morbidity and mortality of overweight adolescents: A follow-up of the Harvard Growth Study of 1922–1935. *New England Journal of Medicine, 327,* 1350–1355.

National Center for Health Statistics. (n.d.). *Prevalence of overweight among children and adolescents: United States, 1999–2002.* Retrieved August 9, 2007, from http://www.cdc.gov/nchs/products/pubs/pubd/hestats/overwght99.htm

Ogden, C. L., Carroll, M. D., & Flegal, K. M. (2008). High body mass index for age among US children and adolescents, 2003–2006. *JAMA, 299*(20), 2401–2405.

Ogden, C. L., Flegal, K. M., Carroll, M. D., & Johnson, C. L. (2002). Prevalence and trends in overweight among US children and adolescents, 1999–2000. *JAMA, 288,* 1728–1732.

Peeters, A., Barendregt, J. J., Willekens, F., Mackenbach, J. P., Al Mamun, A., & Bonneux, L. (2003). Obesity in adulthood and its consequences for life expectancy: A life-table analysis. *Annals of Internal Medicine, 138,* 24–32.

Puhl, R. M., & Latner, J. D. (2007). Stigma, obesity, and the health of the nation's children. *Psychological Bulletin, 133,* 557–580.

Schwimmer, J. B., Burwinkle, T. M., & Varni, J. W. (2003). Health-related quality of life of severely obese children and adolescents. *JAMA, 289,* 1813–1819.

Sinha, R., Fisch, G., Teague, B., Tamborland, W. V., Banyas, B., Allen, K., et al. (2002). Prevalence of impaired glucose tolerance among children and adolescents with marked obesity. *New England Journal of Medicine, 346,* 802–810.

Strauss, R. S. (2000). Childhood obesity and self-esteem. *Pediatrics, 105,* e1–e5.

Telama, R., Yang, X., Laakso, L., & Viikari, J. (1997). Physical activity in childhood and adolescence as predictor of physical activity in young adulthood. *American Journal of Preventive Medicine, 13*(4), 317–323.

Thompson, J. K., Coovert, M., Richards, K., Johnson, S., & Cattarin, J. (1995). Development of body image, eating disturbance, and general psychological functioning in female adolescents: Covariance structure modeling and longitudinal investigations. *International Journal of Eating Disorders, 18*, 221–236.

Thompson, J. K., Herbozo, S., Himes, S., & Yamamiya, Y. (2005). Effects of weight-related teasing in adults. In K. D. Brownell, R. M. Puhl, & M. B. Schwartz (Eds.), *Weight bias: Nature, consequences and remedies* (pp. 137–149). New York: Guilford Press.

Thompson, J. K., Shroff, H., Herbozo, S., Cafri, G., Rodriguez, J., & Rodriguez, M. (2007). Relations among multiple peer influences, body dissatisfaction, eating disturbance, and self-esteem: A comparison of average weight, at risk of overweight, and overweight adolescent girls. *Journal of Pediatric Psychology, 32*, 24–29.

U.S. Department of Health and Human Services. (2001). *The Surgeon General's call to action to prevent and decrease overweight and obesity.* Rockville, MD: U.S. Department of Health and Human Services, Public Health Service, Office of the Surgeon General.

Wang, G., & Dietz, W. H. (2002). Economic burden of obesity in youths aged 6 to 17 years: 1979–1999. *Pediatrics, 109*(5), E81.

Wang, Y., & Beydoun, M. A. (2007). The obesity epidemic in the United States— Gender, age, socioeconomic, racial/ethnic, and geographic characteristics: A systematic review and meta-regression analysis. *Epidemiologic Reviews, 29*, 6–28.

Whitaker, R. C., Wright, J. A., Pepe, M. S., Seidel, K. D., & Dietz, W. H. (1997). Predicting obesity in young adulthood from childhood and parental obesity. *New England Journal of Medicine, 337*, 869–873.

Wolf, A. M., & Colditz, G. A. (1998). Current estimates of the economic cost of obesity in the United States. *Obesity Research, 6*, 97–106.

I

FORMATIVE INFLUENCES: RISK FOR OBESITY IN CHILDHOOD AND ADOLESCENCE

1

BIOLOGICAL AND
GENETIC INFLUENCES

NATHAN J. MARKWARD, MARTHA J. MARKWARD,
AND CATHERINE A. PETERSON

Obesity is a major medical and public health problem. Its stigmatizing and debilitating effects impose a heavy burden on the lives of affected individuals, their family members, and the American health care infrastructure (Ogden et al., 2006). As noted in the introduction to this volume, the rise in childhood obesity is particularly disconcerting because of the short- and long-term health risks associated with being overweight at an early age and the lack of adult treatment programs that are effective at maximizing and maintaining weight loss over time (see also Ogden et al., 2006). As such, the most promising strategy for curbing the obesity "epidemic" may be primary prevention of the disorder in children or, at the very least, strategic minimization of weight gain during the early and middle phases of life.

Recent advances in the health and genome sciences suggest that traditional approaches to obesity prevention and treatment—health education, increased physical activity, eating behavior modification, and health and social policy advocacy—might be enhanced by incorporating biological data into the risk assessment process (Subbiah, 2007). For example, twin, adoption, and family studies have demonstrated that lifetime obesity risk is moderated, in part, by genetic factors (Bouchard & Perusse, 1993; Loos & Bouchard, 2003; Rankinen & Bouchard, 2006). Moreover, genetic linkage and association studies have identified several candidate genes that may predispose individuals to gain weight when exposed to "obesigenic" lifestyle and environmental stimuli (Loos & Bouchard, 2003; Rankinen & Bouchard, 2006).

Knowledge of these interactions and their influences on biological processes could aid pediatricians and other health professionals in their efforts to (a) identify children who are more or less likely to become obese, (b) understand how children will respond to different dietary and exercise interventions over time, and (c) develop patient-centered lifestyle recommendations that better meet the unique needs of children and their families. With this possibility in mind, this chapter provides an introduction to the biological basis of weight gain for nongeneticists, summarizing key physiological and genetic factors that are known or hypothesized to influence early-onset obesity.

HORMONAL, METABOLIC, AND NEURONAL FACTORS

Constant body weight can be maintained only if energy intake and expenditure are properly balanced over long periods of time (Woods & Seeley, 2005). If the compensatory effects of metabolism and exercise do not offset the amount of energy consumed, fat mass and body weight will tend to increase or decrease as a function of the direction and magnitude of the imbalance (Woods & Seeley, 2005). This parsimonious model—*the energy balance equation*—holds that pathological weight gain is the consequence of chronic disturbances in energy regulation that promote a net positive energy balance, excess fat production, and progression to the obese state (Woods & Seeley, 2005).

Long-term disruption of energy homeostasis was historically attributed to frequent and unregulated consumption of foods that are high in fat. More recently, however, carbohydrate intake and a measure known as the glycemic index (GI) have garnered increased attention among researchers and clinicians (Ludwig et al., 1999). GI is primarily determined by carbohydrate content and gauges the rise in glucose (blood sugar) that occurs after a meal (Ludwig et al., 1999). The pragmatic importance of GI is illustrated by marked physiological changes that occur in response to the ingestion of high-GI foods (Ludwig et al., 1999). Indeed, human feeding studies have revealed significant correlations between GI and (a) levels of key metabolic fuels and regulatory molecules and (b) excessive hunger and overeating in obese subjects (Ludwig et al., 1999).

In this section, we present an annotated inventory of hormonal, metabolic, and neuronal factors that influence energy balance in humans. Our primary goal is to familiarize colleagues with prominent regulators of food intake and meal termination—peripheral hormones, gastrointestinal peptides, and neuropeptides—and their documented or hypothesized role in obesity pathogenesis. We believe the annotated summary presented in the following paragraphs accomplishes this task with reasonable proficiency, although we caution readers that our presentation is largely based on findings from the animal and adult literature. For the time being, we are comfortable with the simplistic assumptions that the rudimentary molecular basis of energy metabolism is unaffected by development and that the essential biochemical pathways involved in energy regulation are invariant across the life span. Future research will no doubt test the validity of these hypotheses, and we look forward to modifying or expanding our list as new information becomes available. We also direct readers to the review articles by Pérusse and Bouchard (2000) and Permutt, Wasson, and Cox (2005) for additional information regarding the molecular epidemiology of obesity.

Peripheral Hormones

Accurate monitoring of body fat is a key aspect of long-term weight maintenance (Woods & Seeley, 2005). Both human and animal studies have demonstrated that individuals tend to consume more energy in response to weight loss, thereby restoring body weight to baseline levels (Woods & Seeley, 2005). In contrast, overeating and weight gain tend to reduce food intake and promote weight loss (Woods & Seeley, 2005). These relationships imply that the body generates signals that accurately reflect adiposity levels, and these signals interact with the brain structures that regulate food intake and energy expenditure (Morton, Cummings, Baskin, Barsh, & Schwartz, 2006). This negative feedback system is rooted in the notion that "circulating signals inform the brain of changes in body fat mass and . . . the brain mounts adaptive adjustments of energy balance to stabilize fat stores" (Morton et al., 2006, p. 289).

Supervision of nonlocal fat depots presents a distinct challenge to the brain because adipose tissue is stored in multiple sites throughout the body (Woods & Seeley, 2005). In theory, neurons could extend directly from the central nervous system to fat production and storage sites, thus facilitating rapid and immediate communication between the brain and distant organs and tissues (Woods & Seeley, 2005). However, researchers now understand that the hypothalamus monitors fat stores by selectively "sampling" the peripheral circulation and assessing the relative concentrations of "adiposity signals" that are secreted by the pancreas and fat cells (Morton et al., 2006; see Table 1.1). These hormones bind to receptors in the hypothalamus and trigger downstream neuronal signaling cascades that lead to increases or decreases in food intake (Morton et al., 2006; Woods & Seeley, 2005).

By definition, a true adiposity signal must satisfy three criteria (Morton et al., 2006; Woods & Seeley, 2005). First, it must circulate at levels that are proportional to the amount of fat stored in the body and enter the brain at levels that reflect its relative concentration in the bloodstream. Second, it must promote weight loss by acting on brain centers that regulate energy balance.

TABLE 1.1
Summary of Obesity-Related Peripheral Hormones

Hormone	Secretor	Function	Reference
Insulin	Pancreas	Suppress hunger and appetite	Woods and Seeley (2005)
Leptin	Adipocytes (fat cells)	Suppress hunger and appetite	Morton et al. (2006)

Third, food intake and body weight must increase if the signal's actions are systematically inhibited or negated. Several molecules, cytokines, and nutrients meet at least one of these requirements, but only two hormones, insulin and leptin, fulfill all three (Morton et al., 2006; Schwartz, 2006).

Insulin is a hormone secreted by pancreatic β-cells in response to glucose load (Woods & Seeley, 2005; Wynne, Stanley, McGowan, & Bloom, 2005). Circulating insulin levels vary directly with changes in visceral fat mass and tend to increase and decrease in response to positive and negative energy balance (Wynne et al., 2005). In contrast to insulin, *leptin* is a hormone secreted by *adipocytes* (fat cells) and a principal indicator of adiposity and overall nutritional status (Woods & Seeley, 2005; Wynne et al., 2005). Circulating leptin levels are proportional to fat content and tend to be higher in overweight and obese individuals (Woods & Seeley, 2005; Wynne et al., 2005). In concert, insulin and leptin work to suppress hunger and appetite, thereby promoting negative energy balance (Morton et al., 2006).

Gastrointestinal Peptides

The ability to detect when energy stores are low and, therefore, when food intake is necessary is only one piece of the physiological puzzle (Woods & Seeley, 2005). The body also requires a reliable means of measuring how much food has been ingested after a meal has commenced and, by extension, recognizing when enough food energy (in calories) has been consumed to maintain proper energy balance (Cummings & Overduin, 2007). These tasks are accomplished by gastrointestinal peptides that originate in the stomach, proximal and distal small intestine, colon, and pancreas (Cummings & Overduin, 2007; Woods & Seeley, 2005). Such "satiation signals" promote meal termination, prevent excess food intake and incomplete digestion, and optimize nutrient digestion and absorption (Cummings & Overduin, 2007; see Table 1.2).

A genuine satiation signal must satisfy four criteria (Cummings & Overduin, 2007). First, the signal must be secreted during food ingestion. Second, exogenous administration of the signal decreases meal size in a dose-

TABLE 1.2
Summary of Obesity-Related Gastrointestinal Peptides

Peptide	Location	Function	Reference
CCK	Brain, enteric nervous system, and small intestine	Satiation signal	Wynne et al. (2005); Cummings and Overduin (2007)
GLP-1	Intestinal L cells	Inhibit food intake	Wynne et al. (2005); Druce and Bloom (2006)
Peptide YY	Distal intestine	Inhibit food intake	Wynne et al. (2005); Druce and Bloom (2006)
Ghrelin	Intestine	Promote appetite	Wynne et al. (2005); Druce and Bloom (2006)
Amylin	Pancreas	Decrease food intake	Reda, Geliebter, and Pi-Sunyer (2002)

Note. CCK = cholecystokinin; GLP-1 = glucagon-like-peptide-1.

dependent, rapid, and transient manner. Third, the signal does not cause unnatural eating behavior or illness. Fourth and finally, inhibition of the signal's activity leads to increased meal size. In contrast with adiposity signals discussed previously, many satiation peptides have been identified in humans, including cholecystokinin (CCK), glucagon-like-peptide-1 (GLP-1), and peptide YY (PYY) (Wynne et al., 2005).

CCK is secreted by the small intestine, brain, and enteric nervous system in response to ingested carbohydrates and fats (Cummings & Overduin, 2007; Wynne et al., 2005). CCK is an archetypal satiation signal, exhibiting effects on meal termination that are both potent and transitory (Cummings & Overduin, 2007; Wynne et al., 2005). CCK also induces contraction of the gallbladder, stimulates release of bile and secretion of pancreatic digestive enzymes, and may participate in long-term energy regulation by interacting with leptin (Cummings & Overduin, 2007; Wynne et al., 2005).

GLP-1 is synthesized by intestinal L cells in response to food intake (Cummings & Overduin, 2007; Neary, Goldstone, & Bloom, 2004; Wynne et al., 2005). In rodents, infusion of GLP-1 decreases food intake, whereas administration of its receptor agonist has the opposite effect (Wynne et al., 2005). In humans, GLP-1 has been shown to inhibit food intake in healthy, diabetic, and nondiabetic obese males, and secretion levels tend to be muted in obese participants (Druce & Bloom, 2006; Wynne et al., 2005). GLP-1 is also capable of stimulating insulin production in a glucose-independent manner (Cummings & Overduin, 2007).

PYY is secreted in the distal intestine and released into the circulation at levels that are proportional to the amount and source of food energy (carbohydrates, fat, protein, and other nutrients) ingested during a meal (Druce & Bloom, 2006; Wynne et al., 2005). In rodents and humans, peripheral infusion of its active form, PPY_{3-36}, inhibits food intake and prevents weight gain, although the effects in animal models may be confounded by stress (Druce & Bloom, 2006; Wynne et al., 2005). In obese participants, PYY's repressive effects are preserved, but levels are lower and tend to rise more slowly on meal termination (Druce & Bloom, 2006). PYY production may also depend on meal composition because higher levels are observed when fat, rather than carbohydrate or protein, is consumed (Wynne et al., 2005).

Ghrelin is an intestinal hormone that encourages appetite and food intake (Cummings & Overduin, 2007; Druce & Bloom, 2006; Wynne et al., 2005). In rodents, ghrelin stimulates feeding, and chronic administration induces adiposity (Druce & Bloom, 2006). In nonobese humans, circulating ghrelin levels are inversely proportional to body mass index (BMI), rise sharply after fasting and before meals, and decrease during meals or after nutrient infusion into the stomach (Cummings et al., 2002; Druce & Bloom, 2006). In obese participants, peripheral concentrations of ghrelin are higher, do not decline on food ingestion, and increase in response to weight loss (Druce & Bloom, 2006).

Amylin is a pancreatic enzyme that is cosecreted with insulin in response to food intake (Fry, Hoyda, & Ferguson, 2007). In humans and animals, amylin assists in nutrient control by inhibiting gastric emptying and glucagon secretion and, by so doing, limiting the activation of receptors in the liver that promote (a) conversion of glycogen to glucose and (b) release of glucose into the circulation (Fry et al., 2007; Lutz, 2006; Reda, Geliebter, & Pi-Sunyer, 2002). In general, amylin levels are elevated in obese humans, leading to downregulation of amylin receptors and reduced satiety and gastric emptying (Reda et al., 2002).

Neuropeptides

The neurobiological mechanisms underlying energy metabolism are highly evolved and redundant, affording humans considerable plasticity in their ability to adapt to acute changes in food availability and environmental factors (Cummings & Overduin, 2007; Morton et al., 2006; Schwartz, 2006; Woods & Seeley, 2005). Energy intake and expenditure are primarily mediated by the hypothalamus and, specifically, by neuronal circuits concentrated in and projecting from its arcuate, paraventricular, ventromedial, and dorsomedial nuclei (Cummings & Overduin, 2007; Morton et al., 2006; Schwartz, 2006; Woods & Seeley, 2005). These brain centers facilitate appetite control and moderation of food intake and maintain body weight within a range that each individual is willing and able to defend (Berridge, 2004; Woods & Seeley, 2005; see Table 1.3).

The arcuate nucleus (ARC) houses two groups of neurons that play vital roles in energy physiology (Bell, Walley, & Froguel, 2005; Druce & Bloom, 2006). One set promotes food intake and energy expenditure by producing

TABLE 1.3
Summary of Obesity-Related Neuropeptides

Peptide	Location	Function	Reference
NPY	Brain	Induce feeding	Neary et al. (2004)
AGRP	Brain	Increase appetite; decrease metabolism and energy expenditure	Neary et al. (2004)
POMC neuron	Hypothalamus	Decrease appetite	Wynne et al. (2005); Morton et al. (2006)
CART neuron	Brain	Inhibit feeding	Wynne et al. (2005)

Note. NPY = neuropeptide Y; AGRP = agouti-related protein; POMC = proopiomelanocortin; CART = cocaine- and amphetamine-related transcript.

neuropeptide Y (NPY) and agouti-related protein (AGRP), whereas the other suppresses food intake by producing proopiomelanocortin (POMC) and cocaine- and amphetamine-related transcript (CART) (Bell et al., 2005; Druce & Bloom, 2006). The NPY/AGRP neurons are inhibited by leptin, insulin, and PYY_{3-36} but they are activated by ghrelin (Bell et al., 2005, Neary et al., 2004). Reciprocally, the POMC/CART neurons are stimulated by leptin and insulin and repressed by ghrelin (Bell et al., 2005; Neary et al., 2004).

NPY/AGRP and POMC/CART neurons receive and process a wide array of neuroendocrine signals that convey information to the brain regarding adiposity levels, satiety, nutrient availability, and sensory stimuli (Cummings & Overduin, 2007; Morton et al., 2006; Schwartz, 2006; Woods & Seeley, 2005). Both neuronal clusters project to the paraventricular nucleus (PVN) and other neuronal groups that influence energy regulation, including the melanin-concentrating hormone (MCH) neurons, orexin/hypocretin neurons, thyrotrophin-releasing hormone neurons, and γ-aminobutyric acid–releasing interneurons (Bell et al., 2005). Important signals also arrive via the dopamine, serotonin, and endocannabinoid pathways (Bell et al., 2005; Schwartz, 2006).

NPY is a member of the pancreatic polypeptide (PP)-fold family of peptides that includes PYY and PP (Wynne et al., 2005). NPY is expressed in the ARC and induces feeding by activating receptors in the PVN (Wynne et al., 2005). Studies have demonstrated that administration of NPY directly to the hypothalamus causes overeating and weight gain, whereas infusion of NPY antagonists reduces food intake (Neary et al., 2004). Hypothalamic NPY levels serve as an index of overall nutrition, rise rapidly before a meal, and remain elevated as long as food is withheld (Wynne et al., 2005).

In parallel, AGRP stimulates appetite, decreases metabolism, and increases energy expenditure (Neary et al., 2004; Wynne et al., 2005). AGRP is up-regulated by fasting and leptin deficiency and exerts its effects by antagonizing melanocortin receptors 3 (MCR3) and 4 (MCR4). By so doing, AGRP negates MCR3/MCR4 inhibition of α-melanocyte-stimulating hormone (α-MSH), thus promoting food intake (Neary et al., 2004; Wynne et al., 2005). In rodents, central administration of AGRP can increase food intake for up to 1 week, whereas chronic administration causes extreme overeating and obesity (Wynne et al., 2005).

Hypothalamic POMC levels serve as an additional indicator of overall nutritional status. Activation of the POMC signaling cascade occurs when leptin and insulin bind to their respective receptors on POMC/CART neurons, leading to reduced appetite and anorexia (Morton et al., 2006; Wynne et al., 2005). Laboratory experiments have demonstrated that POMC gene expression is reduced in fasted animals and increased in response to exogenous administration of leptin (Wynne et al., 2005). Moreover, deletion of one copy of the POMC gene in mice appears to be sufficient to leave these animals susceptible to diet-induced obesity (Wynne et al., 2005).

All POMC neurons also coexpress CART, a neuropeptide that has been demonstrated to (a) inhibit feeding in normal and 24-hour fasted rats and (b) suppress the normal appetite-stimulating effects of NPY (Wynne et al., 2005). However, despite these fascinating results, the precise role of CART in human feeding behavior is debatable (Wynne et al., 2005). More than one population of CART-expressing neurons may exist in the brain, and each subgroup may affect food intake in different ways (Wynne et al., 2005). CART peptides are also involved in fear and startle responses and may mediate the actions of certain psychostimulant drugs.

GENETIC FACTORS

Twin studies suggest that genetic factors may account for as much as 50% to 90% of the observed variance in BMI, and a wide array of rare mutations and chromosomal abnormalities are now known to cause severe, early-onset obesity or multispectrum Mendelian syndromes that include obesity as a distinguishing clinical feature (Farooqi & O'Rahilly, 2000; Loos & Bouchard, 2003; Rankinen & Bouchard, 2006). More recently, family- and population-based epidemiologic studies have identified several obesity "susceptibility" loci that may predispose individuals to gain weight when they are exposed to deleterious lifestyle and environmental factors. Large-scale research projects are now underway to elucidate the nature and scope of these complex relationships and to understand their implications for obesity prevention and treatment.

In this section, we summarize recent findings from the genetic and genomic literature, focusing on discoveries pertaining to children and adolescents (see Table 1.4). Our emphasis on early-onset obesity is important because the inventory of genes influencing energy balance in children may only par-

TABLE 1.4
Summary of Obesity-Related Genomic Alterations

Type	Gene or chromosome	Reference
Monogenic	MC4R	Rankinen et al. (2006)
Syndromic		
PWS	15q (deletion, disomy)	Loos and Bouchard (2003)
AHO	20q (parental imprinting)	Loos and Bouchard (2003)
BBS	Multiple mutations	Mutch and Clément (2006)
Polygenic		
Linkage	19q, 10p11.23, 11q13	Saar et al. (2003)
	1, 5, 7, 12, 13, 18	Chen et al. (2004)
	11	Heude et al. (2004)
	18	Cai et al. (2006)
Association	POMC, CART	del Giudice, Cirillo, et al. (2001); del Giudice, Santoro, et al. (2001)
	GHRL	Korbonits et al. (2002)
	MC4R	Hinney et al. (2003)
	POMC	Santoro et al. (2004)
	ENPP1, GAD2	Meyre, Boutin, et al. (2005); Meyre, Bouatia-Naji, et al. (2005)
	PPARγ-2	Ghoussaini et al. (2005)
	MCHR1	Wermter et al. (2005); Bell, Meyre, et al. (2005)

Note. MC4R = melanocortin-4 receptor; PWS = Prader-Willi syndrome; AHO = Albright hereditary osteo-dystrophy; BBS = Bardet-Biedl syndrome; POMC = proopiomelanocortin; CART = cocaine- and amphetamine-related transcript; GHRL = ghrelin; ENPP1 = ectonucleotide pyrophosphatase/phosphodiesterase 1; GAD2 = glutamic acid decarboxylase 2; PPARγ-2 = peroxisome proliferator-activated receptor gamma 2; MCHR1 = melanin-concentrating hormone receptor 1.

tially overlap with those regulating weight in adults. Indeed, intraindividual correlations of BMI are lower between childhood and adulthood than adolescence and adulthood, indicating that different genes may be selectively activated or repressed as a normal aspect of aging and development or as plastic responses to evolving environmental conditions (Hebebrand & Theisen, 2005). As a complement to this material, we also encourage readers to consult several excellent review articles (Bell et al., 2005; Farooqi & O'Rahilly, 2000; Rankinen & Bouchard, 2006; Yang, Kelly, & He, 2007) and the Obesity Gene Map resource developed and maintained by our colleagues at Pennington Biomedical Research Center (Rankinen et al., 2006, see http://obesitygene.pbrc.edu).

The "Thrifty Genome"

The current obesity epidemic is thought to be rooted in the dynamic coevolution of the human genome and the environment (Loos & Bouchard, 2003). As first postulated by Neel (1962), humans may have evolved in "restrictive" environments where food resources were scarce and extensive physical exertion was required to acquire food (Civitarese & Ravussin, 2005). Over time, this environmental pressure resulted in selection of a "thrifty genotype" or, in modern parlance, a "thrifty genome," whose carriers were better able to maximize energy storage over time, thereby enhancing their survival and fitness during prolonged periods of starvation or famine (Civitarese & Ravussin, 2005). As a result, these individuals were more likely to reproduce and, in turn, to make a larger contribution to the modern gene pool than their energy-expending counterparts.

More than 4 decades later, Neel's (1962) basic hypothesis has retained its elegance and salience, providing a logical explanation for the recent explosion of overweight and obesity in developed nations (Civitarese & Ravussin, 2005; Loos & Bouchard, 2003). Environmental and working conditions have changed rapidly over the past 20 years, and our "hunter–gatherer" genomes have not been able to evolve at an equivalent pace. As such, the hallmarks of Western culture—abundant and available energy-dense food, sedentary lifestyles, increased reliance on motorized transportation, and the heightened pressure to consume imposed by ubiquitous advertising and marketing campaigns—may have made obesity "an 'essential' condition, and only those with fewer obesity susceptibility genes (the former non-survivors) are now apt to resist our 'obesigenic' environment and remain normal weight without conscious effort" (Civitarese & Ravussin, 2005, p. 125).

Monogenic Obesity

Approximately 200 cases of monogenic obesity are caused by point mutations in single genes (Bell et al., 2005; Farooqi & O'Rahilly, 2005; Loos & Bouchard, 2003; Mutch & Clément, 2006; Rankinen et al., 2006). These familial forms of obesity typically involve severe impairment of food intake regulation; emerge during late infancy or early childhood; and may present concomitantly with debilitating behavioral, developmental, and endocrine abnormalities (Mutch & Clément, 2006). The most common form of monogenic obesity arises from mutations in the melanocortin-4 receptor (MC4R) gene that result in partial or complete loss of MC4R signaling function (Loos & Bouchard, 2003). Deleterious alterations have been localized to genes coding for the carboxypeptidase E corticotropin releasing hormone receptors 1 and 2, G protein-coupled receptor 24, leptin, leptin receptor, melanocortin 3 receptor, neurotrophic tyrosine kinase receptor type 2, proopiomelanocortin, proprotein convertase subtilisin/kexin type 1, and several others (Rankinen et al., 2006).

Syndromic Obesity

Between 20 and 30 Mendelian syndromes include early onset obesity, mental retardation, heterogeneous dysmorphia, and a spectrum of organ system–specific developmental anomalies (Bell et al., 2005; Farooqi & O'Rahilly, 2005; Loos & Bouchard, 2003; Mutch & Clément, 2006; Rankinen et al., 2006). Prader-Willi syndrome (PWS), Albright hereditary osteodystrophy (AHO), and Bardet-Biedl syndrome (BBS) are well-known among clinical geneticists, although many others have been documented in the literature (Rankinen et al., 2006). In most instances, researchers have successfully identified the causative mutations or chromosomal rearrangements underlying the disorder, but they have not been able to establish a definitive connection between the variant gene's product and energy metabolism (Loos & Bouchard, 2003). Moreover, investigators have also struggled to associate or link the genes involved with these syndromes to "normal" obesity-related phenotypic variation observed in the general population (Loos & Bouchard, 2003).

PWS is the most common obesity syndrome, occurring at a rate of approximately 1 per 25,000 live births (Loos & Bouchard, 2003). PWS is an autosomal dominant disorder characterized by obesity, reduced fetal activity, neonatal hypotonia, short stature, hypogonadotropic hypogonadism, mental retardation, small hands and feet, and extreme hyperphagia (Loos & Bouchard, 2003; Mutch & Clément, 2006). The most frequent genetic abnormality observed in PWS is a deletion of a single or multiple genes on the proximal long arm of the paternal chromosome 15 and uniparental (maternal) disomy 15 (Loos & Bouchard, 2003).

AHO is an autosomal dominant disorder characterized by obesity, round face, short stature, brachydactyly, subcutaneous calcifications, isolated mental retardation, hypocalcemia, elevated serum parathyroid hormone, and parathyroid hyperplasia (Loos & Bouchard, 2003). AHO is caused by parental imprinting of deleterious mutations in the guanine nucleotide-binding α-stimulating polypeptide 1 gene located on chromosome 20. In like manner, BBS is a complex syndrome characterized by early onset obesity, rod–cone dystrophy, polydactyly, mental retardation, hypogonadism, and renal dysfunction (Loos & Bouchard, 2003; Mutch & Clément, 2006). Although once thought to follow an autosomal recessive mode of inheritance, BBS is now recognized as a dynamic and heterogeneous disorder with at least 11 distinct chromosome locations (Mutch & Clément, 2006).

Polygenic (Common) Obesity

The majority of obesity cases observed in the population are multifactorial in nature, stemming from the cumulative effects of multiple genes and their interactions with behavioral, nutritional, and environmental factors (Rankinen & Bouchard, 2006). Over the past 2 decades, the search for obesity-related genes has been guided primarily by two analytical frameworks: *Linkage analysis* seeks to identify genes and chromosomal regions that are systematically transmitted with a trait or disease in families, and *association analysis* relies on epidemiologic principles to identify susceptibility or protective loci that influence phenotypic variation in populations (Ziegler & König, 2006).

Linkage Studies

Saar et al. (2003) used a two-sample approach and maximum likelihood binomial linkage analysis to test for linkage between 357 microsatellite markers and childhood obesity. The study generated suggestive evidence for linkage between markers located on 1, 2, 4, 8, 9, 10, 11, 14, and 19. The strongest signals were localized to chromosomes 8p and 19q for sample 1 and 10p11.23 and 11q13 for sample 2. The authors noted that although their findings were relatively modest, several of the identified linkages coincided with chromosomal regions that have been implicated by more robust studies of adult obesity, thereby suggesting that the genetic basis of childhood and adult obesity may overlap to a substantial degree.

Chen et al. (2004) conducted heritability and variance components linkage analyses to assess the contribution of genetic factors to the long-term burden and trend of obesity traits, including BMI, from childhood to adulthood. Their study used phenotype and genotype data collected for 342 families and 782 Caucasian sibling pairs (521 full siblings, 39 half siblings) who participated in the Bogalusa Heart Study. Heritability analysis indicated that 78% of the observed variance in long-term BMI could be attributed to genetic factors. Linkage analysis generated suggestive evidence for linkage on chromosomes 1, 5, 7, 12, 13, and 18. Several of the identified regions include obesity-related candidate genes.

Heude et al. (2004) analyzed the relationship between a genetic marker located close to the insulin gene (chromosome 11) and adiposity variability in a sample of French children and adolescents. The study used data for 293 nuclear families, including 431 children and adolescents (ages 8 to 18) and their parents. Multivariate regression analysis revealed that genotype was a significant predictor of age-, gender-, and Tanner stage-adjusted BMI and waist circumference. The authors also revealed that segregation ratios were distorted for class III alleles transmitted from parents to their overweight offspring. Moreover, individuals who were homozygous for the class III allele had significantly lower BMI and waist circumference than did individuals who carried the class I allele.

Cai et al. (2006) conducted heritability and variance components linkage analyses to evaluate the influence of genetic factors on physical activity and dietary intake phenotypes. The study used data for 319 families and 1,030 children who participated in the Viva La Familia Study. Heritability was estimated to be 0.46, 0.69, and 0.18 for physical activity, dietary intake, and vigorous physical activity, respectively. Linkage analyses generated evidence for linkage between sedentary activity (percentage of time) and markers proximal to the

MC4R gene on chromosome 18. Quantitative trait loci for total activity counts, percentage time in light or in moderate activity, carbohydrate intake, and percentage of energy intake from carbohydrates were also detected on chromosome 18.

Association Studies

del Giudice, Cirillo, et al. (2001) conducted mutation screening in the POMC coding region of 87 unrelated Italian obese children and adolescents. In three patients, the authors detected G/C variations at positions 3834 and 3804 (exon 7), respectively, and a C/T mutation within the beta-endorphin peptide at codon 236. In an additional 9 participants, screening revealed an insertion variant between positions 6997 and 6998 (exon 9), and this mutation was significantly associated with BMI-, gender-, and pubertal stage-adjusted leptin levels in obese individuals. del Giudice, Santoro, et al. (2001) also screened the CART gene in 130 unrelated patients (72 girls, 58 boys), identifying two previously described silent polymorphisms in the 3' untranslated region. However, no significant associations were detected between each variant and obesity age-of-onset, BMI z scores, and leptin levels.

Korbonits et al. (2002) examined the relationship between molecular variation in the grhelin gene and obesity in 70 tall, obese children. The authors identified 10 single nucleotide polymorphism variants, one of which was significantly associated with higher BMI and decreased insulin secretion during the first phase of an oral glucose tolerance test. This marker encodes an amino acid change in the tail of the prepro-ghrelin molecule, suggesting that it may influence the functional properties of the ghrelin protein.

Hinney et al. (2003) screened for MC4R mutations in a study of 808 extremely obese children and adolescents and 327 underweight or normal-weight controls. The authors identified a total of 16 mutations in the obese study group, 5 of which had not been described previously. A significant association was detected for mutations that had been deemed functionally relevant in laboratory studies. In addition, the authors screened for MC4R mutations in 1,040 parents of 520 of the aforementioned obese patients and detected significantly distorted segregation patterns. Collectively, these results support the hypothesis that variation in the MC4R gene significantly influences childhood obesity.

Santoro et al. (2004) assessed the relationship between an insertion located in the POMC gene and insulin levels in 380 obese Italian children and adolescents. In obese patients, the authors demonstrated that the polymorphism was associated with differences in age-, sex-, and puberty-stage-adjusted fasting insulin levels. Heterozygotes had higher insulin levels than wild type homozygotes and showed a stronger relationship between insulin and BMI. These findings support the hypothesis that the melanocortin pathway may modulate glucose metabolism in obese participants and could be involved in the natural history of polygenic obesity during late adolescence and adulthood.

Meyre, Bouatia-Naji, et al. (2005) analyzed polymorphisms in the ecto-nucleotide pyrophosphatase/phosphodiesterase 1 (ENPP1) gene of 6,147 subjects, demonstrating a significant association between a three-allele haplotype and (a) childhood obesity and (b) moderate to morbid adult obesity. The authors also revealed that the ENPP1 haplotype contributes to a previously documented linkage between chromosome 6q and childhood obesity. The haplotype is associated with higher risk of glucose intolerance and Type 2 diabetes in obese children and their parents and with increased serum levels of soluble ENPP1 protein in children. In a related study, Meyre, Boutin, et al. (2005) also demonstrated that a polymorphism located in the glutamic acid decarboxylase 2 (GAD2) gene region is a significant predictor of fetal growth, insulin secretion, food intake, and risk of obesity in severely obese French Caucasian children.

Ghoussaini et al. (2005) assessed the effects of two genetic variants in the peroxisome proliferator-activated receptor gamma 2 (PPARγ-2) gene region and obesity-related type 2 diabetes in three independent case-control groups (2,126 cases, 1,124 controls) of French descent. The results indicated the first polymorphism of interest was not associated with childhood or adult obesity. However, the second variant appears to be a significant predictor of type 2 diabetes in obese subjects in which it may amplify insulin resistance and increase fasting insulin levels.

Wermter et al. (2005) detected an association between two variants located in the MCH receptor Type 1 (MCHR1) gene region and extreme obesity in German children and adolescents. The authors suggested that the association may be related to juvenile-onset obesity, conditional on a particular genetic and/or environmental background. In like manner, Bell, Meyre, et al. (2005) examined the relationship between six MCHR1 variants and weight in 557 morbidly obese adults, 552 obese children, and 1,195 nonobese nondiabetic control subjects. A polymorphism located in the MCHR1 promoter region was associated with a weight-protective effect in obese children. Similar associations were also found when children and adults were analyzed together.

IMPLICATIONS FOR RESEARCH AND CLINICAL PRACTICE

This chapter has provided an overview of the progress that molecular biologists and geneticists have made toward understanding the roots of the obesity epidemic over the past 2 decades. Researchers have unveiled ancient physiological and neurological pathways that regulate energy balance in mammals, single-gene mutations, and Mendelian syndromes that cause obesity in children and in common genetic variants that influence obesity risk in families and the general population. In the wake of these findings, the pace of obesity-related human research and discovery is rapidly accelerating, and expectations are high that findings generated by these endeavors will arm practitioners with an additional line of defense against the rising tide of overweight and obesity in the industrialized world. On the basis of these trends, we believe that expanded knowledge of molecular genetics, child- and adolescent-focused amendments to the Obesity Gene Map (Rankinen et al., 2006), and a heightened emphasis on cross-disciplinary research could aid medical and public health experts in two important ways.

First, integration of molecular and genomic information into childhood obesity risk assessment models may improve the ability to identify children who are more or less likely to become obese as adolescents and adults. For example, the clinical features and course of pathological weight gain are highly variable between and within individuals, but the large majority of prevention and treatment programs do not account for patient-specific heterogeneity in key health outcomes of interest. Improved knowledge of the molecular basis of energy regulation, especially in children, may allow further stratification of commonly used risk categories—age, gender, ethnicity, high fat diet, and physical activity level—into distinct obesity subtypes that incorporate information on each person's unique genetic makeup. Moreover, one might reasonably speculate that genome-based obesity classification may be useful for understanding the epidemiology of certain comorbidities—mental disorders, diabetes, cardiovascular disease, and certain forms of cancer—that tend to occur at a higher rate in individuals who were obese as children.

Second, detailed knowledge of gene–diet, gene–behavior, and gene–environment interactions may facilitate design of patient-centered nutritional, psychoanalytical, and pharmacological remedies that target the unique needs of children and their families. Within this domain of inquiry, the first generation of "nutritional genomic" studies has already demonstrated that certain nutrients and botanicals modify the expression of genes involved in metabolism, and high-throughput genomic technologies are now being used to identify additional gene–diet interactions that influence each individual's response to dietary interventions. In addition, pharmaceutical research has revealed that variation in certain genes significantly predicts drug efficacy, and large-scale pharmacogenomic studies are now underway to understand how genomic information can be used to streamline the development, dissemination, and prescription of novel antiobesity medications that transcend the one-size-fits-all alternatives that are currently available on the market.

Realization of this proposed model of personalized or individualized obesity risk assessment and case management will no doubt hinge on (a) the extent to which geneticists and epidemiologists are successful at advancing our knowledge of energy regulation; (b) the ability of universities and corporations to develop obesity diagnostic, prognostic, and *theragnostic* (diagnostic + treatment) tools that are safe and effective for use in children; and (c) the continued evolution of health and social policies that regulate how genomic information can be ethically and legally applied in medicine and public health. Assuming that these scientific, economic, and political challenges can be adequately addressed in the coming years, the collection, analysis, and interpretation of genomic data may become essential aspects of childhood obesity research and intervention programs.

LIMITATIONS

The primary limitation in this area of research is the paucity of physiological and genetic data available on children and adolescents at the present time. For example, because of the lack of experimental and longitudinal studies conducted to date, we based our review of mammalian energy regulation largely on evidence generated by animal and adult human studies. Although we believe this approach is warranted given the well-documented centrality of hypothalamic control of food intake and satiation, we acknowledge that future research may reveal subtle age-dependent nuances in gene expression that indirectly modify energy balance through gene–diet, gene–behavior, or gene–environment interactions. This possibility highlights the imminent need for collaborative, large-scale genetic and genomic studies that focus explicitly on understanding the etiology of the obesity phenotype and its evolution across different stages of human development.

CONCLUSIONS

Future efforts aimed at understanding the nature and long-term consequences of childhood obesity will necessitate an intimate and ongoing dialogue between molecular physiologists, human geneticists, and their colleagues in related scientific disciplines. To be sure, the effective, timely, and compassionate prevention and treatment of the disorder will require a holistic model of case management that integrates technical input and expertise from clinical geneticists, genetic counselors, nutritionists, child psychologists, and social workers. Indeed, this paradigm of multidisciplinary cooperation and its underlying ethical principles have guided the care of individuals affected with monogenic and syndromic forms of obesity for many years. Generalization of this conceptual framework to upstream research and technology development efforts may be vital to understanding more complex forms of the disorder.

REFERENCES

Bell, C. G., Meyre, D., Samson, C., Boyle, C., Lecoeur, C., Tauber, M., et al. (2005). Association of melanin-concentrating hormone receptor 15' polymorphism with early-onset extreme obesity. *Diabetes, 54*(10), 3049–3055.

Bell, C. G., Walley, A. J., & Froguel, P. (2005). The genetics of human obesity. *Nature Reviews Genetics, 6*(3), 221–234.

Berridge, K. C. (2004). Motivation concepts in behavioral neuroscience. *Physiology and Behavior, 81*(2), 179–209.

Bouchard, C., & Perusse, L. (1993). Genetic aspects of obesity. In C. L. Williams & S. Y. S. Kimm (Eds.), *Annals of the New York Academy of Sciences: Vol. 699. Prevention and treatment of childhood obesity* (pp. 26–35). New York: New York Academy of Sciences.

Cai, G., Cole, S. A., Butte, N., Bacino, C., Diego, V., Tan, K., et al. (2006). A quantitative trait locus on chromosome 18q for physical activity and dietary intake in Hispanic children. *Obesity, 14*(9), 1596–1604.

Chen, W., Li, S., Cook, N. R., Rosner, B. A., Srinivasan, S. R., Boerwinkle, E., et al. (2004). An autosomal genome scan for loci influencing longitudinal burden of body mass index from childhood to young adulthood in white sibships: The Bogalusa heart study. *International Journal of Obesity, 28*(4), 462–469.

Civitarese, A., & Ravussin, E. (2005). Obesity and gene discovery approaches. In J. Antel, N. Finer, D. Heal, & G. Krause (Eds.), *Obesity and metabolic disorders* (pp. 123–138). Amsterdam: IOS Press.

Cummings, D. E., & Overduin, J. (2007). Gastrointestinal regulation of food intake. *Journal of Clinical Investigation, 117*(1), 13–23.

Cummings, D. E., Weigle, D. S., Frayo, R. S., Breen, P. A., Ma, M. K., Dellinger, E. P., et al. (2002). Plasma ghrelin levels after diet-induced weight loss or gastric bypass surgery. *New England Journal of Medicine, 346*(21), 1623–1630.

del Giudice, E., Cirillo, G., Santoro, N., D'Urso, L., Carbone, M. T., Di Toro, R., et al. (2001). Molecular screening of the proopiomelanocortin (POMC) gene in Italian obese children: Report of three new mutations. *International Journal of Obesity, 25*(1), 61–67.

del Giudice, E. M., Santoro, N., Cirillo, G., D'Urso, L., Di Toro, R., & Perrone, L. (2001). Mutational screening of the CART gene in obese children: Identifying a mutation (Leu34Phe) associated with reduced resting energy expenditure and cosegregating with obesity phenotype in a large family. *Diabetes, 50*(9), 2157–2160.

Druce, M., & Bloom, S. R. (2006). The regulation of appetite. *Archives of Disease in Childhood, 91*(2), 183–187.

Farooqi, I. S., & O'Rahilly, S. (2000). Recent advances in the genetics of severe childhood obesity. *Archives of Disease in Childhood, 83*(1), 31–34.

Farooqi, I. S., & O'Rahilly, S. (2005). New advances in the genetics of early onset obesity. *International Journal of Obesity, 29*(10), 1149–1152.

Fry, M., Hoyda, T. D., & Ferguson, A. V. (2007). Making sense of it: Roles of the sensory circumventricular organs in feeding and regulation of energy homeostasis. *Experimental Biology and Medicine, 232*(1), 14–26.

Ghoussaini, M., Meyre, D., Lobbens, S., Charpentier, G., Clement, K., Charles, M. A., et al. (2005). Implication of the Pro12Ala polymorphism of the PPAR-gamma 2 gene in type 2 diabetes and obesity in the French population. *BMC Medical Genetics, 6*, 11.

Hebebrand, J., & Theisen, F. (2005). Genetic aspects of obesity. In J. Antel, N. Finer, D. Heal, & G. Krause (Eds.), *Obesity and metabolic disorders* (pp. 109–121). Amsterdam: IOS Press.

Heude, B., Dubois, S., Charles, M. A., Deweirder, M., Dina, C., Borys, J. M., et al. (2004). VNTR polymorphism of the insulin gene and childhood overweight in a general population. *Obesity Research, 12*(3), 499–504.

Hinney, A., Hohmann, S., Geller, F., Vogel, C., Hess, C., Wermter, A. K., et al. (2003). Melanocortin-4 receptor gene: Case-control study and transmission disequilibrium test confirm that functionally relevant mutations are compatible with a major gene effect for extreme obesity. *Journal of Clinical Endocrinology and Metabolism, 88*(9), 4258–4267.

Korbonits, M., Gueorguiev, M., O'Grady, E., Lecoeur, C., Swan, D. C., Mein, C. A., et al. (2002). A variation in the ghrelin gene increases weight and decreases insulin secretion in tall, obese children. *Journal of Clinical Endocrinology and Metabolism, 87*(8), 4005–4008.

Loos, R. J., & Bouchard, C. (2003). Obesity—Is it a genetic disorder? *Journal of Internal Medicine, 254*(5), 401–425.

Ludwig, D. S., Majzoub, J. A., Al-Zahrani, A., Dallal, G. E., Blanco, I., & Roberts, S. B. (1999). High glycemic index foods, overeating, and obesity. *Pediatrics, 103*(3), E26.

Lutz, T. A. (2006). Hunger and satiety: One brain for two? *American Journal of Physiology. Regulatory, Integrative, and Comparative Physiology, 291*(4), 900–902.

Meyre, D., Bouatia-Naji, N., Tounian, A., Samson, C., Lecoeur, C., Vatin, V., et al. (2005). Variants of ENPP1 are associated with childhood and adult obesity and increase the risk of glucose intolerance and type 2 diabetes. *Nature Genetics, 37*(8), 863–867.

Meyre, D., Boutin, P., Tounian, A., Deweirder, M., Aout, M., Jouret, B., et al. (2005). Is glutamate decarboxylase 2 (GAD2) a genetic link between low birth weight and subsequent development of obesity in children? *Journal of Clinical Endocrinology and Metabolism, 90*(4), 2384–2390.

Morton, G. J., Cummings, D. E., Baskin, D. G., Barsh, G. S., & Schwartz, M. W. (2006, September 21). Central nervous system control of food intake and body weight. *Nature, 443*(7109), 289–295.

Mutch, D. M., & Clément, K. (2006). Unraveling the genetics of human obesity. *PLoS Genetics, 2*(12), e188.

Neary, N. M., Goldstone, A. P., & Bloom, S. R. (2004). Appetite regulation: From the gut to the hypothalamus. *Clinical Endocrinology, 60*, 153–160.

Neel, J. V. (1962). Diabetes mellitus: A "thrifty" genotype rendered detrimental by "progress"? *American Journal of Human Genetics, 14*, 353–362.

Ogden, C. L., Carroll, M. D., Curtin, L. R., McDowell, M. A., Tabak, C. J., & Flegal, K. M. (2006). Prevalence of overweight and obesity in the United States, 1999–2004. *Journal of the American Medical Association, 295*(13), 1549–1555.

Permutt, M. A., Wasson, J., & Cox, N. (2005). Genetic epidemiology of diabetes. *The Journal of Clinical Investigation, 115*(6), 1431–1439.

Pérusse, L., & Bouchard, C. (2000). Gene–diet interactions in obesity. *American Journal of Clinical Nutrition, 72*, 1285S–1290S.

Rankinen, T., & Bouchard, C. (2006). Genetics of food intake and eating behavior phenotypes in humans. *Annual Reviews in Nutrition, 26*, 413–434.

Rankinen, T., Zuberi, A., Chagnon, Y. C., Weisnagel, S. J., Argyropoulos, G., Walts, B., et al. (2006). The human obesity gene map: The 2005 update. *Obesity, 14*(4), 529–644.

Reda, T. K., Geliebter, A., & Pi-Sunyer, F. X. (2002). Amylin, food intake, and obesity. *Obesity Research, 10*(10), 1087–1091.

Saar, K., Geller, F., Ruschendorf, F., Reis, A., Friedel, S., Schauble, N., et al. (2003). Genome scan for childhood and adolescent obesity in German families. *Pediatrics, 111*(2), 321–327.

Santoro, N., del Giudice, E. M., Cirillo, G., Raimondo, P., Corsi, I., Amato, A., et al. (2004). An insertional polymorphism of the proopiomelanocortin gene is associated with fasting insulin levels in childhood obesity. *Journal of Clinical Endocrinology and Metabolism, 89*(10), 4846–4849.

Schwartz, G. J. (2006). Central nervous system regulation of food intake. *Obesity, 14*(Suppl.), 1S–8S.

Subbiah, M. T. (2007). Nutrigenetics and nutraceuticals: The next wave riding on personalized medicine. *Translational Research, 149*(2), 55–61.

Wermter, A. K., Reichwald, K., Buch, T., Geller, F., Platzer, C., Huse, K., et al. (2005). Mutation analysis of the MCHR1 gene in human obesity. *European Journal of Endocrinology, 152*(6), 851–862.

Woods, S. C., & Seeley, R. J. (2005). Regulation of appetite, satiety, and energy metabolism. In J. Antel, N. Finer, D. Heal, & G. Krause (Eds.), *Obesity and metabolic disorders* (pp. 93–107). Amsterdam: IOS Press.

Wynne, K., Stanley, S., McGowan, B., & Bloom, S. (2005). Appetite control. *Journal of Endocrinology, 184*, 291–318.

Yang, W., Kelly, T., & He, J. (2007). Genetic epidemiology of obesity. *Epidemiologic Reviews, 29*, 49–61.

Ziegler, A., & Konig, I. R. (2006). *A statistical approach to genetic epidemiology: Concepts and applications.* Weinheim, Germany: Wiley-VCH.

2

EARLY PHYSICAL ACTIVITY, SEDENTARY BEHAVIOR, AND DIETARY PATTERNS

JAMES F. SALLIS, DORI ROSENBERG, AND JACQUELINE KERR

The purpose of this chapter is to examine obesity-related behaviors in children aged 4 to 12 years, highlighting developmental patterns, correlates, and measurement. Obesity-related behaviors are subject to complex influences, and multiple behavioral theories have been applied to their etiology. The laws of thermodynamics dictate that obesity occurs when energy intake exceeds expenditure, although the underlying causal mechanisms of obesity likely involve interactions among genetic, biological, psychological, cultural, economic, and environmental factors (Koplan, Liverman, & Kraak, 2005). The primary modifiable behaviors implicated in energy imbalance are physical activity, sedentary behavior, and dietary habits (Andersen & Butcher, 2006), so solutions will involve these behaviors.

Almost all studies of the correlates of children's obesity-related behaviors are cross-sectional, and although causality cannot be determined, results yield hypotheses about behavioral mediators that can be tested more rigorously in intervention studies. It is difficult to measure proposed psychological correlates in young children, who are the focus of this chapter, so most research has focused on sociodemographic, social, and physical environmental factors. For this population, psychological theories have limited value, and broader social and ecological models are used as the conceptual basis of studies (Sallis & Glanz, 2006). A comprehensive discussion of physical activity, sedentary activity, and dietary patterns without inclusion of parents would be incomplete, and the role of parents and other caregivers at home and school has been a central focus of research for obesity-related behaviors. Parents can influence children's behavior through a variety of mechanisms, and specific models of parental influence on children's obesity-related behaviors have been proposed (Sallis & Nader, 1988; see also chap. 3, this volume).

PHYSICAL ACTIVITY

Physical activity refers to "any bodily movement produced by skeletal muscles that results in energy expenditure" (Caspersen, Powell, & Christenson, 1985, p. 129). Physical activity decreases throughout childhood and adolescence (Gordon-Larsen, Nelson, & Popkin, 2004; Sallis, Prochaska, & Taylor, 2000; van Mechelen, Twisk, Post, Snel, & Kemper, 2000). Prospective studies show that physical activity protects against excessive weight gain in children from 1 year old (Gillman et al., 2000; O'Loughlin, Gray-Donald, Paradis, & Meshefedjian, 2000) to 5 years old (Salbe, Weyer, Lindsay, Ravussin, & Tataranni, 2002). Larger than average declines in physical activity during youth have been related to risk of adiposity in adulthood (Tammelin, Laitinen, & Nayha, 2004; Yang, Telama, Viikari, & Raitakari, 2006).

There is some evidence for *tracking* (i.e., tendency to maintain ranking or percentile on a variable over time) of physical activity throughout youth. In a study by McMurray, Harrell, Bangdiwala, and Hu (2003), overall physical activity tracked poorly from childhood to adulthood, but stronger associations have been demonstrated between participating in organized youth sports and being active in adulthood (Strong et al., 2005; Telama, Yang, Hirvensalo, & Raitakari, 2006; Trudeau, Laurencelle, & Shephard, 2004).

Several recent trends that affect childhood physical activity levels warrant concern. Walking and biking to school has decreased significantly over the past 30 years, and current estimates indicate that only 17% of children in the United States walk to school at least 1 day per week (Dellinger & Staunton, 2002). Yet walking and biking to school are associated with higher physical activity levels (Cooper, Whelan, Woolgar, Morrell, & Murray, 2004) and lower likelihood of overweight (Gordon-Larsen et al., 2004; Rosenberg, Sallis, Conway, Cain, & McKenzie, 2006). Participation in daily physical education in high school declined from 43% of students in 1991 to 25% in 1995 (U.S. Department of Health and Human Services, 1996). Fewer than 10% of elementary school children participate in daily physical education classes (Harper, 2006).

Physical Activity Etiology

A systematic review of more than 50 studies of correlates of physical activity in children aged 4 through 12 (Sallis et al., 2000) found that boys were consistently more active than girls, but associations with race or ethnicity and socioeconomic status were not supported. Although numerous psychological variables were studied at the upper part of the age range, only intention (positive), preference for physical activity (positive), and barriers (negative) were consistently related to physical activity. Other theoretically relevant variables, such as self-efficacy, body image, attitudes, and perceived benefits, were not consistently related to physical activity. Physical activity was consistently related to healthy diet (positive) and previous physical activity (positive) but not to sedentary behaviors. No consistent correlates were observed among social and cultural variables. Parent physical activity (i.e., modeling) was a frequently studied variable but was found to be significant in only about one third of comparisons. There was little or no evidence that parent beliefs about children's physical activity or persuasive attempts were important correlates. Whereas gatekeeper functions, such as transporting the child to a place for activity and paying fees, were not consistently related to children's physical activity, these variables were related to adolescents' activity levels (for further discussion of parent variables, see chap. 3, this volume). Sibling and peer influences were rarely studied. Among the few physical environment factors that were studied, access to facilities and programs was consistently related to children's physical activity. Among preschool children, three studies using direct observation identified being outdoors as an extremely strong correlate of physical activity.

In summary, Sallis et al. (2000) identified a few psychological correlates of physical activity in children aged 4 to 12 years but provided little empirical support for social correlates. The lack of findings for social and parental factors could result from limitations of measurement and suggests a need to improve measures of proposed social influences and to expand the range of social variables studied. The strongest evidence supported a critical role of the physical environment in shaping young children's physical activity. The implication is that when children have access to facilities and programs, preferably outdoors, they are motivated to take advantage of those opportunities. It is apparent that young children derive great pleasure from movement, so their primary need is for regular access to convenient and safe places to be active. Growing parental concerns about allowing children to be outdoors unsupervised (Lindsay, Sussner, Kim, & Gortmaker, 2006) increases the importance of providing all children with suitable places and programs for physical activity near their homes. As children move into upper elementary ages, their biological drive for physical activity will wane (Ingram, 2000), and educational and motivational strategies in combination with suitable facilities and programs will likely be needed.

Gustafson and Rhodes (2006) examined parental correlates of physical activity for children and adolescents and concluded that socioeconomic status was positively related to children's physical activity. In addition, their review confirmed the lack of support for parental modeling. Parent supportive behaviors identified as consistent correlates of children's physical activity were encouragement, involvement, and facilitation (see also chap. 3, this volume).

Measurement of Physical Activity

The challenges of measuring obesity-related behaviors in children have been recognized for many years (Baranowski & Simons-Morton, 1991). About 10 to 12 years is the youngest age at which children can reliably report physical activity behaviors (Sallis & Saelens, 2000). Children's self-report is therefore not a viable option in the target age range covered in this chapter.

Parent reports of physical activity have been found to be inaccurate; few parents are able to observe their children's activity throughout the day (Sallis & Saelens, 2000). Fortunately, objective measures from accelerometers and pedometers can assess children's physical activity over several days to provide an estimate of habitual activity (Welk, Corbin, & Dale, 2000). Accelerometers have a major advantage of providing continuous records of activity intensity levels, whereas the less expensive pedometers typically produce only cumulative step counts. Pedometers have been evaluated for use in children (Rowe, Mahar, Raedeke, & Lore, 2004; Welk et al., 2000); accelerometers have been found to be reliable and valid even with preschoolers (Pfeiffer, McIver, Dowda, Almeida, & Pate, 2006). Both instruments are insensitive to common childhood activities such as bike riding and swimming. Although the expense and effort involved in using accelerometers may be justified in specialized childhood obesity clinics, pedometers are feasible for use in primary care settings.

Direct observation is the other objective measure of children's physical activity. Several observation systems have been developed for general use as well as for assessing physical education classes and activities in recreation settings (Marshall, Biddle, Sallis, McKenzie, & Conway, 2002). Although observational measures are reliable and valid, they require extensive training, substantial staff time, and complex data processing. Thus, observational measures are recommended only for research.

SEDENTARY BEHAVIOR

Although benefits are derived by engaging in some sedentary behaviors such as reading (Thakkar, Garrison, & Christakis, 2006), the use of sedentary technology for recreation apparently contributes to the obesity epidemic (Andersen, Crespo, Bartlett, Cheskin, & Pratt, 1998; Prentice & Jebb, 1995).

Sedentary behavior has yet to be adequately defined in health behavior research. Individuals who do not participate in physical activities are often considered "sedentary" (Tudor-Locke & Meyers, 2001), and it is often assumed that individuals who are highly active engage in little sedentary behavior, but the associations between physical activity and sedentary time are weak (Biddle, Gorely, Marshall, Murdey, & Cameron, 2004). Physical activity and sedentary behavior in fact are largely independent, and children can watch high amounts of television but also be very active (Marshall, Biddle, Gorely, Cameron, & Murdey, 2004; Marshall et al., 2002; Sallis et al., 2000).

Sedentary behaviors are characterized by low energy expenditure. Television watching and other screen time (i.e., computer use, and video game playing) have been examined in relation to childhood obesity. Television viewing has decreased slightly in recent years, but total screen time appears relatively stable as other behaviors supplant television viewing (Andersen & Butcher, 2006). It has been estimated that per week children spend about 19 hours watching television, 2 hours playing video games, and 2.5 hours on the computer (Andersen & Butcher, 2006; Roberts, Foehr, Rideout, & Brodie, 1999). This translates to almost 3.5 hours daily watching a screen (Harper, 2006; Roberts et al., 1999). Television viewing increases during childhood and then declines during adolescence (Certain & Kahn, 2002; Saelens et al., 2002). Many children (72% of boys and 64% of girls in one study) have televisions in their bedrooms, and children with television sets in their room watch more than those without (Roberts, Foehr, & Rideout, 2005).

Time watching television has been consistently associated with an increased risk of obesity during youth, but a meta-analysis indicates the effect size is small (Andersen & Butcher, 2006; Marshall et al., 2004). The most convincing evidence of the importance of sedentary behaviors is intervention research showing that decreasing television watching can lower body mass index (BMI) and body fat (Gortmaker et al., 1999, Robinson, 1999). Proposed mechanisms to explain the television–obesity relationship include the following: Television viewing displaces physical activity (Biddle et al., 2004), television advertising encourages children to eat unhealthy food, snacking increases during television watching (Andersen & Butcher, 2006; Coon, Goldberg, Rogers, & Tucker, 2001; Koplan et al., 2005; Saelens et al., 2002), and metabolic rates decrease while watching television (Andersen & Butcher, 2006; Koplan et al., 2005). Sedentary behavior has effects on weight status separate from physical activity and does not solely operate by displacing physical activity (Biddle et al., 2004).

Etiology of Sedentary Behavior

Correlates of sedentary behavior have not been studied extensively. Researchers have postulated that changes in the environment have led to increases in sedentary behavior among children because there are many more options now for sedentary entertainment (e.g., computers, video games; Andersen & Butcher, 2006). Time spent sitting during school has increased as activity breaks have decreased. There has been a 25% decrease in play and a 50% decrease in outdoor activities during school (Andersen & Butcher, 2006). Time spent doing homework has increased, and time spent sitting in cars has increased because children are now driven to school or take the bus instead of walking or biking (Dora, 1999).

Patterns of television viewing were studied in a nationally representative sample of 0- to 35-month-olds over 6 years (Certain & Kahn, 2002). Correlates of higher television viewing were having Black maternal race, lower maternal education, and an unmarried mother. Over the first 3 years of life, television watching increased by about 1 hour each year and then stabilized. Low maternal education continued to predict more television viewing at 6 years of age. Greater television watching in early childhood was associated with higher television viewing at school age.

Girls appear to watch less television than boys, at least from age 11 (Brodersen, Steptoe, Williamson, & Wardle, 2005; Kann et al., 2000). A nationally representative study showed that White children between 8 and 18 years of age had less daily screen time exposure (3 hours 47 minutes) than Black children (5 hours 53 minutes) and Hispanic children (4 hours and 37 minutes; Roberts et al., 2005). Other studies have confirmed that White students have the lowest levels of sedentary behavior whereas Black students have the highest (Schmitz et al., 2002) and that White students are more likely to meet television watching recommendations (less than 2 hours per day; Kann et al., 2000). These conclusions are tempered by the potential confounding role of socioeconomic status and differential access to active behaviors. School and neighborhood poverty were associated with higher sedentary time (Kann et al., 2000).

Concern about crime in the neighborhood is thought to lead children to stay inside (Burdette & Whitaker, 2005). Research has shown that children living in unsafe neighborhoods watch more television than children in safer neighborhoods (Burdette & Whitaker, 2005). Poor weather (Brodersen et al., 2005) has been associated with higher sedentary behavior. In the home environment, eating meals in front of the television and having a television in the child's bedroom were significant correlates of television viewing time (Saelens et al., 2002).

Measurement of Sedentary Behavior

Measurement of sedentary behavior in children has relied predominantly on parent reports rather than child self-reports. Diaries, interviews, questionnaires, and logs have been used, and most focus on television viewing rather than on all sedentary behaviors (Borzekowski & Robinson, 1999; Wrotniak, Epstein, Paluch, & Roemmich, 2004). The majority of studies have used unvalidated parent reports (Gordon-Larsen et al., 2004). However, parent reports of television viewing have been consistently related to child weight status (Saelens et al., 2002), suggesting adequate construct validity. For both research and practice, it appears that parent-reported child television viewing is a useful indicator of this dominant sedentary behavior.

Objective measures of sedentary behavior have been explored. Accelerometers are being used to assess total daily minutes of sitting or of very low intensity activity (Puyau, Adolph, Vohra, & Butte, 2002). Currently, there is little agreement about which accelerometer cutoff is appropriate to identify sedentary behaviors. Appliance-monitoring devices can be used to record the on–off status of "sedentary" appliances such as televisions and computers. Such devices have been used more as intervention tools (Wrotniak et al., 2004) than as measurement tools. Television viewing has been objectively measured using observation with video cameras (Borzekowski & Robinson, 1999).

DIETARY BEHAVIORS

The main foods related to higher childhood BMI are fast foods, sodas, and snack foods (P. M. Anderson & Butcher, 2006). Children's eating behaviors associated with childhood obesity are total energy intake, intake of specific food types (e.g., protective effect of fruit and vegetables), eating or sucking rates (Birch, 1998; Birch & Fisher, 1998), and eating in the absence of hunger (Faith, Scanlon, Birch, Francis, & Sherry, 2004). Only one third of children are meeting dietary recommendations for fruit, vegetables, whole grains, meat, and dairy; even fewer are meeting the requirements for sugar and fat (P. M. Anderson & Butcher, 2006; Birch, 1998).

In the first 5 years of life, children learn a great deal about food and eating; likes and dislikes, when to eat, and how much to eat (Birch, 1998). The development of children's food acceptance patterns stems from a variety of influences, including genetic predispositions, early experiences, and the environment.

Etiology of Eating Behaviors

There are several important factors involved in development of eating habits. Genetic and demographic factors, parent factors, feeding practices (breast-feeding, food restriction, parent control, and modeling), social and physical environment factors, and TV viewing all affect eating behaviors.

Genetic Factors

Humans are predisposed to prefer sweet and fatty tastes from birth and salty tastes from about 4 months old and to reject sour and bitter tastes. These preferences are believed to provide survival advantages. Sweet and fatty foods are high in caloric value, helping people prepare for food shortages; bitter foods may signal toxins. The strong preferences for sweet, fatty, and salty foods helps explain why intake of such foods is so high and why reducing their consumption is so hard (Birch, 1998). *Neophobia* is the predisposition to fear new things. It is important for children to reduce their neophobia toward food through early introduction to many foods and repeated experience with these foods both in the transition to an omnivorous diet from milk and during breast-feeding through the mother's diet. Children may not immediately accept new tastes, and parents should persist, up to 10 times, when introducing a new food (Ziegler, Hanson, Ponza, Novak, & Hendricks, 2006).

Children respond more positively to foods that result in satiety and prefer energy-dense foods (Birch, 1998), but they are able to regulate their energy intake. For example, following a high-energy meal, young children will naturally tend to reduce their intake in subsequent meals. It is important for parents to encourage this natural tendency and to allow children to learn to regulate their own intake and respond to satiety and hunger cues (Birch, 1998). (For a more in-depth discussion of biological and genetic factors, see chap. 1, this volume.)

Demographic Factors

Parent education and ethnicity and child age and gender are related to dietary patterns (Patrick & Nicklas, 2005). Boys tend to eat more fast food (Bowman, Gortmaker, Ebbeling, Pereira, & Ludwig, 2004), and girls prefer and consume more fruits and vegetables (Cooke & Wardle, 2005; Jaramillo et al., 2006; Rasmussen et al., 2006). Low socioeconomic status is associated with greater intake of sugar and fat and lower intake of fruits and vegetables among children (Rasmussen et al., 2006). This pattern may be influenced by the availability and low price of fatty and sweet foods and the higher prices of fruits and vegetables (P. M. Anderson & Butcher, 2006; Drewnowski, 2004). African American households with children, however, have reported higher availability of fruits and vegetables in the home than White households (Ard et al., 2007). Eating patterns appear to become less healthy over Grades 3 to 8 and from childhood (10 years old) to young adulthood (19–28 years old; Demory-Luce et al., 2004; Lytle, Seifert, Greenstein, & McGovern, 2000).

Parent Factors

Parents control access to food, introduction of foods, and education about food to young children, so parental attitudes, knowledge, and beliefs about eating and their child's weight are likely to be important influences. A review suggested that mothers who do not know their children's intake of sweets have children who are 4 times more likely to be overweight as young adults (Faith, Scanlon, et al., 2004). Mothers' education is related to positive feeding behaviors and higher intake of fruit (Cooke et al., 2004). There are gender differences in parental attitudes and feeding practices; for example, mothers are more concerned about their child's weight and restrict certain foods, especially for daughters (Blissett, Meyer, & Haycraft, 2006; Faith, Scanlon et al., 2004). Increases in maternal working habits may partially explain increased obesity because mothers spend less time preparing nutritious meals and more meals are eaten out of the home (P. M. Anderson & Butcher, 2006).

Parent and child weights are strongly related, which is likely due to both genetics and similar eating patterns in a common environment. Eating environments in families with obese parents differ from those in families in which neither parent is obese (Birch & Fisher, 1998). Overweight parents who consume a higher fat diet are also making this diet more available to their children and developing their preference for these types of food (Birch, 1998; Birch & Fisher, 1998). Overweight parents who have problems controlling their own food intake and are concerned about their child's weight status may adopt ineffective, overcontrolling feeding strategies (Birch & Davison, 2001). Interventions to improve children's dietary behaviors have been less successful in children with obese parents (Eliakim, Friedland, Kowen, Wolach, & Nemet, 2004).

Breast-Feeding

Although breast-feeding rates have remained relatively stable while obesity rates have increased (P. M. Anderson & Butcher, 2006), studies show that children who were breast-fed are less likely to be overweight in adolescence (Tulldahl, Pettersson, Andersson, & Hulthen, 1999). There are plausible mechanisms whereby breast-feeding may lead to better eating practices among children (Birch, 1998). For example, flavors from the mother's diet are present in breast milk and may make transition to new foods easier. During breast-feeding, satiety is decided by the child without reference to a fixed amount as in bottle feeding, providing practice for responding to this internal cue. The American Academy of Pediatrics (2005) has recommended breast-feeding to prevent childhood obesity.

Food Restriction and Parental Control

Restricting children's access to snack foods increases the propensity to eat more unhealthy foods when given open access to such foods, even in the absence of hunger (Birch, 1998; Faith, Scanlon, et al., 2004). Conversely, monitoring and positive reinforcement are related to increased healthy food intake and lower BMI (Arredondo et al., 2006; Faith, Berkowitz, et al., 2004). Parental control may make a child less responsive to their internal hunger and satiety cues and more focused on less accessible palatable foods (Birch, 1998). Focusing a child's attention on portion size, rewards, or cleaning the plate may also undermine his or her ability to respond to internal signals (Faith, Scanlon, et al., 2004). Food rewards, for example, result in higher consumption of that food (Birch & Fisher, 1998). Persistent but positive attempts to introduce new healthy foods are more effective than coercive attempts at dietary control (Brown & Ogden, 2004). There is evidence that interventions to improve young children's diets should also target parents' behaviors (Golan & Crow, 2004; see also chaps. 3 and 9, this volume).

Modeling

For young children, eating is usually a social experience in which adults, siblings, and peers can influence child eating through modeling. That children learn to eat chili-flavored foods, a flavor aversive to many humans, is evidence of the importance of family modeling as performed, for example, in Latino families (Birch & Fisher, 1998). Children are more likely to put something in their mouths following the example of their mother rather than a stranger (Birch & Fisher, 1998). Parental modeling is related to fat intake and fruit and vegetable consumption among children (Tibbs et al., 2001). Modeling by other children, especially older children, can be powerful and suggests that child care environments may be an important location for modeling of healthy eating if such foods are made readily available (Birch & Fisher, 1998).

Meal Time Structure

It is estimated that only about half of 9-year-olds in the United States eat a family dinner every day (Gillman et al., 2000). Eating a family meal together, an opportunity to model behavior, has been related to higher levels of vegetable consumption (Campbell, Crawford, & Ball, 2006; Cooke et al., 2004), lower intake of fried foods and soft drinks (Gillman et al., 2000), and lower BMIs (Taveras et al., 2005). Interventions can increase family meal participation (Johnson, Birkett, Evens, & Pickering, 2006).

Social and Physical Environment Context

Children's eating patterns are influenced by characteristics of physical and social environments. A review by Patrick and Nicklas (2005) concluded that children are more likely to eat foods that are easily accessible and that they tend to eat more when larger portions are provided. The availability of healthy foods in the home, child-care setting, school, and local neighborhood are viewed as an essential precursor to a healthy diet (Cawley, 2006; Lindsay et al., 2006). Location of eating may influence intake; for example, fat and soda consumption are higher outside the home (Ziegler, Briefel, Ponza, Novak, & Hendricks, 2006).

In the United States, children grow up in a culture in which fast food is easily available, and enormous soft drink containers are a status symbol (Birch, 1998). Children learn to associate foods with positive and negative social contexts. Repeatedly presenting a food in a positive context, such as celebrations and holiday meals, results in increased liking for those often unhealthy foods (Birch, 1998).

Television Viewing

While watching television children frequently snack, are exposed to extensive advertising for high-fat and high-sugar products, eat fewer fruit and vegetables, eat more salty snacks and soda, and learn to recognize and request brands at an early age (Birch & Fisher, 1998; Cawley, 2006). Compounding these problems, parents who allow unlimited access to television may have fewer concerns about nutrition (Campbell et al., 2006). Media literacy campaigns can improve parents' understanding of the influence of advertising and increase their oversight of children's television viewing (Hindin, Contento, & Gussow, 2004).

Measurement of Dietary Intake

Both parent report and objective methods of assessing young children's eating patterns are available, and some measures can evaluate the feeding context. Observational measures can capture feeding dynamics accurately, but small samples of behavior may not reflect long-term patterns (Faith, Scanlon, et al., 2004).

Multiple 24-hour food recall interviews of caregivers and children are a reliable measurement method (Hodges, 2003). Modified 24-hour recalls of parents, with observation of lunch and dinner and interviews with the primary food preparer for unobserved foods, have been used with young children (Zive, Berry, Sallis, Frank, & Nader, 2002). Diet records can be kept by caregivers over several days to assess usual dietary patterns, and breast-feeding diaries are common (Casiday, Wright, Panter-Brick, & Parkinson, 2004). Food frequency questionnaires can be completed by older children and adolescents or by parents (Campbell et al., 2006; Rockett, Wolf, & Colditz, 1995). All of these methods have well-known limitations.

A variety of self-reported measures examine diet-related variables such as parent beliefs, attitudes, and practices (C. B. Anderson, Hughes, Fisher, & Nicklas, 2005; Birch et al., 2001); eating and feeding styles (Carnell & Wardle, 2007; Golan & Weizman, 1998; Patrick, Nicklas, Hughes, & Morales, 2005;

Wardle, Carnell, & Cooke, 2005; Wardle, Guthrie, Sanderson, & Rapoport, 2001; Wardle, Sanderson, Guthrie, Rapoport, & Plomin, 2002); parental control (Ogden, Reynolds, & Smith, 2006); preferences for foods, food preparation habits, and barriers to eating at home (Cullen et al., 2004; De Bourdeaudhuij et al., 2005); and the family environment (Campbell et al., 2006). Some surveys have been examined for use in minority populations (C. B. Anderson et al., 2005; Rockett et al., 1995; Tibbs et al., 2001). Interviews have been used to assess mother–child feeding patterns (Faith et al., 2003).

Some studies have used observational measures of children's dietary intake and behaviors. The Free Access Procedure measures total energy of the food consumed in an unsupervised 10-minute period (Faith, Scanlon, et al., 2004). Bob and Tom's Method of Assessing Nutrition (BATMAN; Faith, Scanlon, et al., 2004) evaluates child eating behavior and concurrent parental behavior. Grocery receipts have also been used to assess the family food environment (DeWalt et al., 1990).

CONCLUSIONS

The present chapter has made clear the challenge of improving physical activity, sedentary behaviors, and eating patterns among young children. Opportunities for physical activity at school and in the community are decreasing. Technological options for enjoyable sedentary behaviors are increasing. Nutrient-deficient foods that children are biologically programmed to prefer are highly available and are extensively promoted. For almost all the obesity-related behaviors, developmental trends create additional challenges. Physical activity decreases, television viewing and other sedentary behaviors increase during the preteen years, and the healthfulness of dietary patterns deteriorates. Children with low socioeconomic status and minority ethnic and racial backgrounds watch more television and have less healthful diets.

The literature summarized in this chapter identifies opportunities and strategies for intervention that can be further developed. Parental involvement in and facilitation of their children's physical activity can include taking them to places where they can be active and enrolling them in programs or classes. Removing televisions from bedrooms and setting limits on screen time can help parents reduce their children's sedentary behavior. To improve children's dietary behaviors, parents can breast-feed newborns, persistently and positively introduce healthy foods, avoid coercion and using food as rewards, and provide healthful food environments in the home. Recommendations from authoritative groups and based on the present review are summarized in Exhibit 2.1.

The energy gap believed to cause excess weight gain in children is only 110 kilocalories to 165 kilocalories per day (Wang, Gortmaker, Sobol, & Kuntz, 2006). Thus, modest but sustained changes in physical activity, sedentary behavior, and eating habits should be effective in preventing childhood

EXHIBIT 2.1
Preventing Obesity and Promoting Healthful Behaviors in Young Children: Guidelines for Parents and Health Care Practitioners

Recommendations for Physical Activity
- Children should obtain 1 hour of moderate to vigorous physical activity daily (Gidding et al., 2006; Strong et al., 2005).
- Encourage play and participation in activities at home, in school, child-care settings, and throughout the community as opportunities for physical activity (American Academy of Pediatrics, 2003).
- Parents can set good examples for children by being physically active (Koplan et al., 2005).

Recommendations for Television Viewing
- Limit television to 2 hours of high-quality programming each day (American Academy of Pediatrics, 2001; Koplan et al., 2005).
- Keep children under age 2 from watching any television (American Academy of Pediatrics, 2001).
- Refrain from placing television sets in children's bedrooms (American Academy of Pediatrics, 2001).

Recommendations for Dietary Behaviors
- Breast-feed exclusively for the first 4 to 6 months of life (Koplan et al., 2005).
- Provide healthful foods and beverages in the home. Consider nutrient quality and energy density of those foods (Koplan et al., 2005). Have a variety of nutritious, low-energy-dense foods available, such as fruits and vegetables. Limit access to high-calorie and low-nutrient-density foods at home.
- Promote healthful eating behaviors in the home, including having family meals, limiting snacking, and serving controlled portions (Koplan et al., 2005).
- Parents can be good role models for children by eating healthfully (Koplan et al., 2005).
- Expose children to initially disliked foods up to 10 times to break down resistance and encourage healthy food preferences.
- Avoid using food as a reward.

obesity. Although intervention in early childhood is needed, on the basis of the increased prevalence of obesity in this age group, limited tracking of behaviors from childhood to adulthood suggests that interventions should continue during adolescence and may need to continue throughout life. Schools, community organizations, the health care system, corporations, and families need to play an active and informed role in promoting healthful patterns of physical activity, sedentary behaviors, and eating. This involves developing a nonobesogenic environment for children where there are opportunities for daily physical activity, eating nutritious foods with reasonable portion sizes, and alternatives to sedentary pursuits (Koplan et al., 2005).

REFERENCES

American Academy of Pediatrics. (2001). Children, adolescents, and television. *Pediatrics, 107*, 423–426.

American Academy of Pediatrics. (2003). Prevention of pediatric overweight and obesity. *Pediatrics, 112,* 424–430.

American Academy of Pediatrics. (2005). Breastfeeding and the use of human milk. *Pediatrics, 115,* 496–506.

Andersen, R. E., Crespo, C. J., Bartlett, S. J., Cheskin, L. J., & Pratt, M. (1998). Relationship of physical activity and television watching with body weight and level of fatness among children: Results from the Third National Health and Nutrition Examination Survey. *JAMA, 279,* 938–942.

Anderson, C. B., Hughes, S. O., Fisher, J. O., & Nicklas, T. A. (2005). Cross-cultural equivalence of feeding beliefs and practices: The psychometric properties of the child feeding questionnaire among Blacks and Hispanics. *Preventive Medicine, 41*(2), 521–531.

Anderson, P. M., & Butcher, K. E. (2006). Childhood obesity: Trends and potential causes. *The Future of Children, 16*(1), 19–45.

Ard, J. D., Fitzpatrick, S., Desmond, R. A., Sutton, B. S., Pisu, M., Allison, D. B., & Baskin, M. L. (2007). The impact of cost on the availability of fruits and vegetables in the homes of schoolchildren in Birmingham, Alabama. *American Journal of Public Health, 97,* 367–372.

Arredondo, E. M., Elder, J. P., Ayala, G. X., Campbell, N., Baquero, B., & Duerksen, S. (2006). Is parenting style related to children's healthy eating and physical activity in Latino families? *Health Education Research, 21,* 862–871.

Baranowski, T., & Simons-Morton, B. G. (1991). Dietary and physical activity assessment in school-aged children: Measurement issues. *Journal of School Health, 61,* 196–197.

Biddle, S. J. H., Gorely, T., Marshall, S. J., Murdey, I., & Cameron, N. (2004). Physical activity and sedentary behaviors in youth: Issues and controversies. *Journal of the Royal Society for the Promotion of Health, 124,* 29–33.

Birch, L. L. (1998). Development of food acceptance patterns in the first years of life. *Proceedings of the Nutrition Society, 57*(4), 617–624.

Birch, L. L., & Davison, K. K. (2001). Family environmental factors influencing the developing behavioral controls of food intake and childhood overweight. *Pediatric Clinics of North America, 48*(4), 893–907.

Birch, L. L., & Fisher, J. O. (1998). Development of eating behaviors among children and adolescents. *Pediatrics, 101*(3 Pt 2), 539–549.

Birch, L. L., Fisher, J. O., Grimm-Thomas, K., Markey, C. N., Sawyer, R., & Johnson, S. L. (2001). Confirmatory factor analysis of the Child Feeding Questionnaire: A measure of parental attitudes, beliefs and practices about child feeding and obesity proneness. *Appetite, 36*(3), 201–210.

Blissett, J., Meyer, C., & Haycraft, E. (2006). Maternal and paternal controlling feeding practices with male and female children. *Appetite, 47*(2), 212–219.

Borzekowski, D. L. G., & Robinson, T. N. (1999). Viewing the viewers: Ten video cases of children's television viewing behaviors. *Journal of Broadcasting & Electronic Media, 43,* 506–528.

Bowman, S. A., Gortmaker, S. L., Ebbeling, C. B., Pereira, M. A., & Ludwig, D. S. (2004). Effects of fast-food consumption on energy intake and diet quality among children in a national household survey. *Pediatrics, 113,* 112–118.

Brodersen, N. H., Steptoe, A., Williamson, S., & Wardle, J. (2005). Sociodemographic, developmental, environmental, and psychological correlates of physical activity and sedentary behavior at age 11 to 12. *Annals of Behavioral Medicine, 29*(1), 2–11.

Brown, R., & Ogden, J. (2004). Children's eating attitudes and behaviour: A study of the modelling and control theories of parental influence. *Health Education Research, 19*(3), 261–271.

Burdette, H. L., & Whitaker, R. C. (2005). A national study of neighborhood safety, outdoor play, television viewing, and obesity in preschool children. *Pediatrics, 116*(3), 657–662.

Campbell, K. J., Crawford, D. A., & Ball, K. (2006). Family food environment and dietary behaviors likely to promote fatness in 5–6 year-old children. *International Journal of Obesity, 30*(8), 1272–1280.

Carnell, S., & Wardle, J. (2007). Measuring behavioural susceptibility to obesity: Validation of the child eating behaviour questionnaire. *Appetite, 48*(1), 104–113.

Casiday, R. E., Wright, C. M., Panter-Brick, C., & Parkinson, K. N. (2004). Do early infant feeding patterns relate to breast-feeding continuation and weight gain? Data from a longitudinal cohort study. *European Journal of Clinical Nutrition, 58*(9), 1290–1296.

Caspersen, C. J., Powell, K. E., & Christenson, G. M. (1985). Physical activity, exercise, and physical fitness. *Public Health Reports, 100,* 125–131.

Cawley, J. (2006). Markets and childhood obesity policy. *The Future of Children, 16*(1), 69–88.

Certain, L. K., & Kahn, R. S. (2002). Prevalence, correlates, and trajectory of television viewing among infants and toddlers. *Pediatrics, 109,* 634–642.

Cooke, L. J., & Wardle, J. (2005). Age and gender differences in children's food preferences. *The British Journal of Nutrition, 93,* 741–746.

Cooke, L. J., Wardle, J., Gibson, E. L., Sapochnik, M., Sheiham, A., & Lawson, M. (2004). Demographic, familial and trait predictors of fruit and vegetable consumption by pre-school children. *Public Health Nutrition, 7*(2), 295–302.

Coon, K. A., Goldberg, J., Rogers, B. L., & Tucker, K. L. (2001). Relationships between use of television during meals and children's food consumption patterns. *Pediatrics, 107,* E7.

Cooper, P. J., Whelan, E., Woolgar, M., Morrell, J., & Murray, L. (2004). Association between childhood feeding problems and maternal eating disorder: Role of the family environment. *British Journal of Psychiatry, 184,* 210–215.

Cullen, K. W., Klesges, L. M., Sherwood, N. E., Baranowski, T., Beech, B., Pratt, C., et al. (2004). Measurement characteristics of diet-related psychosocial questionnaires among African-American parents and their 8- to 10-year-old daughters: Results from the Girls' Health Enrichment Multi-Site Studies. *Preventive Medicine, 38*(Suppl.), S34–S42.

De Bourdeaudhuij, I., Klepp, K. I., Due, P., Rodrigo, C. P., de Almeida, M., Wind, M., et al. (2005). Reliability and validity of a questionnaire to measure personal, social and environmental correlates of fruit and vegetable intake in 10–11-year-old children in five European countries. *Public Health Nutrition, 8*(2), 189–200.

Dellinger, A. M., & Staunton, C. E. (2002, August 16). Barriers to children walking and biking to school—United States, 1999. *Morbidity and Mortality Weekly Report 51*(32), 701–704.

Demory-Luce, D., Morales, M., Nicklas, T., Baranowski, T., Zakeri, I., & Berenson, G. (2004). Changes in food group consumption patterns from childhood to young adulthood: The Bogalusa Heart Study. *Journal of the American Dietetic Association, 104*(11), 1684–1691.

DeWalt, K. M., D'Angelo, S., McFadden, M., Danner, F. W., Noland, M., & Kotchen, J. M. (1990). The use of itemized register tapes for analysis of household food acquisition patterns prompted by children. *Journal of the American Dietetic Association, 90*(4), 559–562.

Dora, C. A. (1999). A different route to health: Implications of transport policies. *British Medical Journal, 318*, 1686–1689.

Drewnowski, A. (2004). Obesity and the food environment: Dietary energy density and diet costs. *American Journal of Preventive Medicine, 27*(3 Suppl.), 154–162.

Eliakim, A., Friedland, O., Kowen, G., Wolach, B., & Nemet, D. (2004). Parental obesity and higher pre-intervention BMI reduce the likelihood of a multidisciplinary childhood obesity program to succeed—A clinical observation. *Journal of Pediatric Endocrinology & Metabolism, 17*(8), 1055–1061.

Faith, M. S., Berkowitz, R. I., Stallings, V. A., Kerns, J., Storey, M., & Stunkard, A. J. (2004). Parental feeding attitudes and styles and child body mass index: Prospective analysis of a gene–environment interaction. *Pediatrics, 114*(4), e429–e436.

Faith, M. S., Heshka, S., Keller, K. L., Sherry, B., Matz, P. E., Pietrobelli, A., et al. (2003). Maternal–child feeding patterns and child body weight: Findings from a population-based sample. *Archives of Pediatrics and Adolescent Medicine, 157*(9), 926–932.

Faith, M. S., Scanlon, K. S., Birch, L. L., Francis, L. A., & Sherry, B. (2004). Parent–child feeding strategies and their relationships to child eating and weight status. *Obesity Research, 12*(11), 1711–1722.

Gidding, S. S., Dennison, B. A., Birch, L. L., Daniels, S. R., Gillman, M. W., Lichtenstein, A. H., et al. (2006). Dietary recommendations for children and adolescents: A guide for practitioners. *Pediatrics, 117*, 544–559.

Gillman, M. W., Rifas-Shiman, S. L., Frazier, A. L., Rockett, H. R., Camargo, C. A., Jr., Field, A. E., et al. (2000). Family dinner and diet quality among older children and adolescents. *Archives of Family Medicine, 9*(3), 235–240.

Golan, M., & Crow, S. (2004). Targeting parents exclusively in the treatment of childhood obesity: Long-term results. *Obesity Research, 12*(2), 357–361.

Golan, M., & Weizman, A. (1998). Reliability and validity of the Family Eating and Activity Habits Questionnaire. *European Journal of Clinical Nutrition, 52*(10), 771–777.

Gordon-Larsen, P., Nelson, M. C., & Popkin, B. M. (2004). Longitudinal physical activity and sedentary behavior trends: Adolescence to adulthood. *American Journal of Preventive Medicine, 27,* 277–283.

Gortmaker, S. L., Peterson, K., Wiecha, J., Sobol, A. M., Dixit, S., Fox, M. K., et al. (1999). Reducing obesity via a school-based interdisciplinary intervention among youth: Planet Health. *Archives of Pediatrics and Adolescent Medicine, 153*(4), 409–418.

Gustafson, S. L., & Rhodes, R. E. (2006). Parental correlates of physical activity in children and early adolescents. *Sports Medicine, 36*(1), 79–97.

Harper, M. G. (2006). Childhood obesity: Strategies for prevention. *Family and Community Health, 29*(4), 288–298.

Hindin, T. J., Contento, I. R., & Gussow, J. D. (2004). A media literacy nutrition education curriculum for head start parents about the effects of television advertising on their children's food requests. *Journal of the American Dietetic Association, 104*(2), 192–198.

Hodges, E. A. (2003). A primer on early childhood obesity and parental influence. *Pediatric Nursing, 29*(1), 13–16.

Ingram, D. K. (2000). Age-related decline in physical activity: Generalization to nonhumans. *Medicine and Science in Sports and Exercise, 32,* 1623–1629.

Jaramillo, S. J., Yang, S. J., Hughes, S. O., Fisher, J. O., Morales, M., & Nicklas, T. A. (2006). Interactive computerized fruit and vegetable preference measure for African-American and Hispanic preschoolers. *Journal of Nutrition Education and Behavior, 38*(6), 352–359.

Johnson, D. B., Birkett, D., Evens, C., & Pickering, S. (2006). Promoting family meals in WIC: Lessons learned from a statewide initiative. *Journal of Nutrition Education and Behavior, 38*(3), 177–182.

Kann, L., Kinchen, S. A., Williams, B. I., Ross, J. G., Lowry, R., Grunbaum, J. A., et al. (2000, June 9). Youth risk behavior surveillance—United States, 1999. *Morbidity and Mortality Weekly Report. CDC Surveillance Summaries, 49*(5), 1–32.

Koplan, J. P., Liverman, C. T., & Kraak, V. I. (Eds.). (2005). *Preventing childhood obesity.* Washington, DC: National Academies Press.

Lindsay, A. C., Sussner, K. M., Kim, J., & Gortmaker, S. L. (2006). The role of parents in preventing childhood obesity. *The Future of Children, 16,* 169–186.

Lytle, L. A., Seifert, S., Greenstein, J., & McGovern, P. (2000). How do children's eating patterns and food choices change over time? Results from a cohort study. *American Journal of Health Promotion, 14,* 222–228.

Marshall, S. J., Biddle, S. J. H., Gorely, T., Cameron, N., & Murdey, I. (2004). Relationships between media use, body fatness and physical activity in children and youth: Meta-analysis. *International Journal of Obesity, 28,* 1238–1246.

Marshall, S. J., Biddle, S. J. H., Sallis, J. F., McKenzie, T. L., & Conway, T. L. (2002). Clustering of sedentary behaviors and physical activity among youth: A cross-national study. *Pediatric Exercise Science, 14*, 401–417.

McMurray, R. G., Harrell, J. S., Bangdiwala, S. I., & Hu, J. (2003). Tracking of physical activity and aerobic power from childhood through adolescence. *Medicine and Science in Sports and Exercise, 35*, 1914–1922.

Ogden, J., Reynolds, R., & Smith, A. (2006). Expanding the concept of parental control: A role for overt and covert control in children's snacking behaviour? *Appetite, 47*(1), 100–106.

O'Loughlin, J., Gray-Donald, K., Paradis, G., & Meshefedjian, G. (2000). One- and two-year predictors of excess weight gain among elementary school children in multiethnic, low-income, inner-city neighborhoods. *American Journal of Epidemiology, 152*, 739–746.

Patrick, H., & Nicklas, T. A. (2005). A review of family and social determinants of children's eating patterns and diet quality. *Journal of the American College of Nutrition, 24*(2), 83–92.

Patrick, H., Nicklas, T. A., Hughes, S. O., & Morales, M. (2005). The benefits of authoritative feeding style: Caregiver feeding styles and children's food consumption patterns. *Appetite, 44*(2), 243–249.

Pfeiffer, K. A., McIver, K. L., Dowda, M., Almeida, M. J., & Pate, R. (2006). Validation and calibration of the Actical accelerometer in preschool children. *Medicine and Science in Sports and Exercise, 38*, 152–157.

Prentice, A. M., & Jebb, S. A. (1995). Obesity in Britain: Gluttony or sloth? *British Medical Journal, 311*, 437–439.

Puyau, M. R., Adolph, A. L., Vohra, F. A., & Butte, N. F. (2002). Validation and calibration of physical activity monitors in children. *Obesity Research, 10*, 150–157.

Rasmussen, M., Krolner, R., Klepp, K. I., Lytle, L. L., Brug, J., Bere, E., & Due, P. (2006). Determinants of fruit and vegetable consumption among children and adolescents: A review of the literature. Part I: Quantitative studies. *International Journal of Behavioral Nutrition and Physical Activity, 3*, 22.

Roberts, D. F., Foehr, U. G., & Rideout, V. J. (2005). *Generation M: Media in the lives of 8–18 year olds*. Menlo Park, CA: Henry J. Kaiser Family Foundation.

Roberts, D. F., Foehr, U. G., Rideout, V. J., & Brodie, M. (1999). *Kids and media at the new millennium: A comprehensive national analysis of children's media use*. Menlo Park, CA: Henry J. Kaiser Family Foundation.

Robinson, T. N. (1999). Reducing children's television viewing to prevent obesity: A randomized controlled trial. *Journal of the American Medical Association, 282*, 1561–1567.

Rockett, H. R., Wolf, A. M., & Colditz, G. A. (1995). Development and reproducibility of a food frequency questionnaire to assess diets of older children and adolescents. *Journal of the American Dietetic Association, 95*(3), 336–340.

Rosenberg, D. E., Sallis, J. F., Conway, T. L., Cain, K. L., & McKenzie, T. L. (2006). Active transportation to school over 2 years in relation to weight status and physical activity. *Obesity (Silver Spring, Md.), 14*(10), 1771–1776.

Rowe, D. A., Mahar, M. T., Raedeke, T. D., & Lore, J. (2004). Measuring physical activity in children with pedometers: Reliability, reactivity, and replacement of missing data. *Pediatric Exercise Science, 16,* 343–354.

Saelens, B. E., Sallis, J. F., Nader, P. R., Broyles, S. L., Berry, C. C., & Taras, H. L. (2002). Home environmental influences on children's television watching from early to middle childhood. *Journal of Developmental and Behavioral Pediatrics, 23,* 127–132.

Salbe, A. D., Weyer, C., Lindsay, R. S., Ravussin, E., & Tataranni, P. A. (2002). Assessing risk factors for obesity between childhood and adolescence: I. Birth weight, childhood adiposity, parental obesity, insulin, and leptin. *Pediatrics, 110*(2 Pt 1), 299–306.

Sallis, J. F., & Glanz, K. (2006). The role of built environments in physical activity, eating, and obesity in childhood. *The Future of Children, 16,* 89–108.

Sallis, J. F., & Nader, P. R. (1988). Family determinants of health behavior. In D. S. Gochman (Ed.), *Health behavior: Emerging research perspectives* (pp. 107–124). New York: Plenum Press.

Sallis, J. F., Prochaska, J. J., & Taylor, W. C. (2000). A review of correlates of physical activity of children and adolescents. *Medicine and Science in Sports and Exercise, 32*(5), 963–975.

Sallis, J. F., & Saelens, B. E. (2000). Assessment of physical activity by self-report: Status, limitations, and future directions. *Research Quarterly for Exercise and Sport, 71,* S1–S14.

Schmitz, K. H., Lytle, L. A., Phillips, G. A., Murray, D. M., Birnbaum, A. S., & Kubik, M. Y. (2002). Psychosocial correlates of physical activity and sedentary leisure habits in young adolescents: The Teens Eating for Energy and Nutrition at School study. *Preventive Medicine, 34*(2), 266–278.

Strong, W. B., Malina, R. M., Blimkie, C. J., Daniels, S. R., Dishman, R. K., Gutin, B., et al. (2005). Evidence based physical activity for school-age youth. *Journal of Pediatrics, 146*(6), 732–737.

Tammelin, T., Laitinen, J., & Nayha, S. (2004). Change in the level of physical activity from adolescence into adulthood and obesity at the age of 31 years. *International Journal of Obesity and Related Metabolic Disorders, 28*(6), 775–782.

Taveras, E. M., Rifas-Shiman, S. L., Berkey, C. S., Rockett, H. R., Field, A. E., Frazier, A. L., et al. (2005). Family dinner and adolescent overweight. *Obesity Research, 13*(5), 900–906.

Telama, R., Yang, X., Hirvensalo, M., & Raitakari, O. (2006). Participation in organized youth sport as a predictor of adult physical activity: A 21-year longitudinal study. *Pediatric Exercise Science, 17,* 76–88.

Thakkar, R. R., Garrison, M. M., & Christakis, D. A. (2006). A systematic review for the effects of television viewing by infants and preschoolers. *Pediatrics, 118*(5), 2025–2031.

Tibbs, T., Haire-Joshu, D., Schechtman, K. B., Brownson, R. C., Nanney, M. S., Houston, C., et al. (2001). The relationship between parental modeling, eating patterns, and dietary intake among African-American parents. *Journal of the American Dietetic Association, 101*(5), 535–541.

Trudeau, F., Laurencelle, L., & Shephard, R. J. (2004). Tracking of physical activity from childhood to adulthood. *Medicine and Science in Sports and Exercise, 36*, 1937–1943.

Tudor-Locke, C., & Meyers, A. M. (2001). Challenges and opportunities for measuring physical activity in sedentary adults. *Sports Medicine 31*, 91–100.

Tulldahl, J., Pettersson, K., Andersson, S. W., & Hulthen, L. (1999). Mode of infant feeding and achieved growth in adolescence: Early feeding patterns in relation to growth and body composition in adolescence. *Obesity Research, 7*(5), 431–437.

U.S. Department of Health and Human Services. (1996). *Physical activity and health: A report of the Surgeon General.* Atlanta, GA: U.S. Department of Health and Human Services, Centers for Disease Control and Prevention, National Center for Chronic Disease Prevention and Health Promotion.

van Mechelen, W., Twisk, J. W. R., Post, G. B., Snel, J., & Kemper, H. C. G. (2000). Physical activity of young people: The Amsterdam Longitudinal Growth and Health Study. *Medicine and Science in Sports and Exercise, 32*, 1610–1616.

Wang, Y. C., Gortmaker, S. L., Sobol, A. M., & Kuntz, K. M. (2006). Estimating the energy gap among US children: A counterfactual approach. *Pediatrics, 118*, 1721–1733.

Wardle, J., Carnell, S., & Cooke, L. (2005). Parental control over feeding and children's fruit and vegetable intake: How are they related? *Journal of the American Dietetic Association, 105*(2), 227–232.

Wardle, J., Guthrie, C. A., Sanderson, S., & Rapoport, L. (2001). Development of the Children's Eating Behaviour Questionnaire. *Journal of Child Psychology and Psychiatry, 42*(7), 963–970.

Wardle, J., Sanderson, S., Guthrie, C. A., Rapoport, L., & Plomin, R. (2002). Parental feeding style and the inter-generational transmission of obesity risk. *Obesity Research, 10*, 453–462.

Welk, G. J., Corbin, C. B., & Dale, D. (2000). Measurement issues in the assessment of physical activity in children. *Research Quarterly for Exercise and Sport, 71*, 59–73.

Wrotniak, B. H., Epstein, L. H., Paluch, R. A., & Roemmich, J. N. (2004). Parent weight change as a predictor of child weight change in family-based behavioral obesity treatment. *Archives of Pediatrics and Adolescent Medicine, 158*(4), 342–347.

Yang, X., Telama, R., Viikari, J., & Raitakari, O. T. (2006). Risk of obesity in relation to physical activity tracking from youth to adulthood. *Medicine and Science in Sports and Exercise, 38*, 919–925.

Ziegler, P., Briefel, R., Ponza, M., Novak, T., & Hendricks, K. (2006). Nutrient intakes and food patterns of toddlers' lunches and snacks: Influence of location. *Journal of the American Dietetic Association, 106*(1 Suppl. 1), S124–S134.

Ziegler, P., Hanson, C., Ponza, M., Novak, T., & Hendricks, K. (2006). Feeding Infants and Toddlers Study: Meal and snack intakes of Hispanic and non-Hispanic infants and toddlers. *Journal of the American Dietetic Association, 106*(1 Suppl. 1), S107–S123.

Zive, M. M., Berry, C. C., Sallis, J. F., Frank, G. C., & Nader, P. R. (2002). Tracking dietary intake in White and Mexican-American children from age 4 to 12 years. *Journal of the American Dietetic Association, 102*(5), 683–689.

3

SOCIAL AND INTERPERSONAL INFLUENCES ON OBESITY IN YOUTH: FAMILY, PEERS, SOCIETY

ALISON E. FIELD AND NICOLE R. KITOS

Childhood and adolescent obesity have a variety of causes. Among them are genetics; earlier weight status; and family, peer, and societal influences. The objective of this chapter is to delineate the effects of family, peer, and societal influences on the physiological and behavioral choices made by preadolescents and adolescents that may increase their risk of becoming overweight or obese. We review literature on modifiable determinants of obesity and weight gain. Although associations established in clinical trials have been shown to be less prone to confounding and selection bias than observational studies, clinical trials do not easily lend themselves to the examination of family, peer, and societal influences. We place greater weight on longitudinal studies among the observational studies because temporal order of associations can be established.

FAMILIAL INFLUENCES

Parents influence their children's weight through both genes and behaviors. One challenge of studying familial influences is disentangling the role of genes from the role of environmental factors. Moreover, it is challenging to separate determinants of normal and healthy weight gain from those related to excessive weight gain because children and adolescents are expected to grow and gain weight during much of childhood and adolescence. This may be one of the reasons that few behavioral factors have been consistently identified in observational studies as predictors of excessive weight gain or obesity during childhood and adolescence.

Infancy and Early Childhood

Many developmental changes occur during the first 18 years of life. In early childhood, parents have an enormous influence on what their child eats and, consequently, on the child's risk of gaining an excessive amount of weight. However, as children age and spend more time away from home at school, in day care, and in after school programs, parental influence begins to wane.

Children of overweight mothers have been found to be more likely than their leaner peers to become overweight (Dubois & Girard, 2006). This association likely reflects both genetic and behavioral influences. Whitaker (2004) studied low-income children and observed that when mothers were obese in early pregnancy their children were more than twice as likely to be obese at 2 to 4 years of age. In addition, some studies have found that children born to women who were formerly (i.e., prepregnancy) overweight were more likely to be overweight also (Burdette, Whitaker, Hall, & Daniels, 2006).

As described in chapter 2 of this volume, overweight and obese mothers appear to be less likely than their leaner peers to breast-feed their children (Oddy, Landsborough, Kendell, Henderson, & Downie, 2006). This behavioral choice may further increase the infant's risk of becoming overweight. Independent of the mother's weight, several studies have observed that the longer an infant is exclusively breast-fed (or receives breast milk exclusively), the lower the infant's risk is of becoming overweight later in childhood or adolescence (Gillman et al., 2001; Mayer-Davis et al., 2006). However, the association has not been observed in several other studies. Some inconsistency in the findings may have resulted from varying sample size, length of follow-up, and definitions of breast-feeding exposures (i.e., any breast-feeding, exclusively breast-feeding and not supplementing with formula or solids, and duration of breast-feeding).

Feeding practices of parents other than breast-feeding also influence the weight status and weight gain of their infants and young children. Unfortunately, the number of longitudinal studies that have assessed the directionality of a child's weight status and the feeding practices of their parents is limited. Burdette et al. (2006) observed that among 313 preschool children, those whose mothers were overweight before pregnancy had large gains in body fat from age 3 to age 5. Children of mothers with high concerns about their infant overeating or becoming overweight gained significantly more body fat over 2 years than did their peers whose mothers were not as concerned. It is unclear how mothers' concerns translated into actual feeding behaviors, but restriction of certain foods or types of foods may have been one behavior involved. Fisher and Birch (1999) found that higher levels of maternal restriction to food access were associated with greater snack food intake among their 3- to 5-year-old daughters. Moreover, higher maternal food restriction was associated with the mother's own dietary restriction as well as with high levels of body fat among their children. Furthermore, Faith et al. (2004) found that parental restriction predicted body mass index (BMI) increases in children over a 2-year period (from ages 5 to 7). These results suggest that although some of the maternal restriction may be well intentioned (i.e., to prevent excessive weight gain among children with high body fat), restriction may backfire and be associated with greater intake of restricted foods when the child is given access to them. However, Spruijt-Metz, Li, Cohen, Birch, and Goran (2006) found that although concern for the child's weight was positively related to fat mass in a cross-sectional study of 74 White children, concern for weight was inversely related to change in fat mass over a 2- to-3-year follow-up. In a review of studies about parental restrictive feeding style, Faith and Kerns (2005) found that in most studies, child characteristics, such as being overweight, were related to restrictive feeding attitudes and styles of their parents. Taken together, the results suggest that mothers of overweight children are more likely to be concerned about their child's weight and may attempt to restrict the child's food intake. More prospective research is needed to better understand whether maternal restriction is beneficial or detrimental.

Maternal weight concerns and restrictions may influence more than a child's weight status; they may also influence his or her self-esteem and feelings about his or her weight. Research suggests that children as young as 5 years may be negatively influenced by their mother's concern about their weight (Davison, Markey, & Birch, 2000). In the National Growth and Health Study, Schreiber et al. (1996) observed that approximately 40% of Black and White girls who were 9 or 10 years old were trying to lose weight. High BMI and having a mother tell her daughter she was too fat were associated with chronic dieting among the girls. Unfortunately, given the cross-sectional design of the study, it is unclear whether the girls were truly overweight or whether the daughters' weight loss efforts were effective. In a smaller longitudinal study, Francis and Birch (2005) followed and assessed 173 mothers and their daughters at 5, 7, 9, and 11 years of age. They found that mothers preoccupied with their own weight and eating reported higher levels of restricting their daughters' intake and encouraging weight loss in their daughters. Moreover, maternal encouragement of weight loss was positively related to daughters' restrained eating behavior. Although pediatric obesity is a tremendous public health problem, and therefore overeating should be discouraged, restrained eating may promote rather than prevent weight gain. Several longitudinal studies have observed that paradoxically, independent of baseline BMI, dieting is associated with gaining more weight (Davison, Markey, & Birch, 2003); thus, familial factors that promote dieting or restraint may in turn promote greater weight gain.

Preadolescence and Adolescence

The period of preadolescence and adolescence may be particularly important in the prevention of overweight and obesity. The prevalence of adolescent overweight has increased nearly threefold since the late 1980s (Ogden, Carroll, & Flegal, 2008), and weight status during preadolescence and adolescence is a good predictor of adult weight status (Field et al., 2003; Whitaker, 2004). As children become preadolescents and then adolescents, they become more independent and make more of their own choices. Through this period of development, parents have increasingly less control over what their children eat because youths in this age range may be purchasing more food outside of the home, including fast food, sugar-sweetened beverages, and other convenience foods with high caloric content and otherwise questionable nutritional value that may increase the likelihood of excessive weight gain (Berkey et al., 2000). Children in this age group also may decide whether to participate in sports and when and where they want to eat and drink. In addition, they may become more conscious of their weight and as a result adopt behaviors to change their weight or shape. Unlike young children who may want to adopt the behaviors that will please their parents, some adolescents may be more interested in adopting behaviors that their peers will approve of and have less interest in complying with their parents' suggestions. Although parental influences are still important at this age, particularly for preadolescents and adolescents living at home, social pressures, the perceived beliefs and behavior of their friends, media images, and marketing influence behavior at least as much as do parents (Paxton, Schutz, Wertheim, & Muir, 1999).

Eating Behavior

Because parents are more likely than their children to buy and prepare food, they play a key role in promoting healthy or unhealthy dietary patterns by modeling eating patterns and providing access to nutritious foods at home. Many parents inadvertently send conflicting messages about nutrition. In a study of 902 adolescents and their parents or caregivers, Hanson, Neumark-Sztainer, Eisenberg, Story, and Wall (2005) found that 90% of parents and caregivers reported that fruits and vegetables were available at home, but many of the parent and caregivers were not consuming the recommended number of servings of fruits and vegetables. In addition, soft drinks were available in more than half of the homes. Thus, the parents were only partially modeling healthy dietary practices. For the girls in the study, parental intake was a significant predictor of dairy, fruit, and vegetable intake. In contrast, parental reports of fruit and vegetable intake were unrelated to the boys' intakes. More research is needed to understand the gender difference in the effect of parental modeling of healthy dietary practices.

Although parental modeling of eating fruits and vegetables was not assessed, in a study of 3,957 adolescents in Minnesota, Neumark-Sztainer, Wall, Perry, and Story (2003) found that when there was low availability of fruits and vegetables in the home, intake patterns were low regardless of how much the adolescents liked or disliked the taste of fruits and vegetables. However, if availability was high, even adolescents who did not like the taste consumed more fruits and vegetables than their peers in homes with low availability. In a follow-up study, Arcan et al. (2007) observed that parental intake while the participants were adolescents significantly predicted intake of fruits, vegetables, and dairy foods 5 years later. Taken together, the results suggest that availability of fruits and vegetables is necessary, but further research is needed to determine the relationship of parental modeling of dietary practices and the subsequent dietary practices of their children. Unfortunately, many economically disadvantaged communities have few large supermarkets (Chung & Myers, 1999). In such cases, fruits and vegetables may be unavailable or too expensive for parents and caregivers to purchase in sufficient quantities.

Parents can also influence their children's eating patterns by having the family eat meals together. A variety of benefits have been associated with eating meals with family, such as prevention of excessive weight gain (Neumark-Sztainer, Wall, Story, & Fulkerson, 2004) and less adolescent use of tobacco, alcohol, and marijuana (Eisenberg, Olson, Neumark-Sztainer, Story, & Bearinger, 2004). In a cross-sectional analysis of 7,784 girls and 6,647 boys aged 9 to 14 years in the Growing Up Today Study (GUTS), a prospective cohort study, Gillman et al. (2000) observed that preadolescents ate dinner more frequently with their family than did adolescents. Overall, 17% of participants rarely ate dinner with their family, 40% ate with them on most days, and 43% ate with family members daily. Independent of age and gender, children who frequently ate dinner with their family were significantly more likely to eat at least five servings of fruits and vegetables per day and were significantly less likely to drink soda or eat any fried foods away from home. Among 4,746 adolescents in Project EAT, Neumark-Sztainer et al. (2003) found that frequency of family meals was positively associated with intake of fruits and vegetables and inversely associated with soft drink consumption. Males, middle-school students, adolescents whose mothers did not work, and adolescents with higher socioeconomic status (SES), were all more likely to consume family meals. The association between SES and eating family meals is noteworthy given that high SES is inversely related to obesity in Whites and Hispanics (Gordon-Larsen, Adair, & Popkin, 2003; Wang & Zhang, 2006; Yang, Lynch, Schulenberg, Roux, & Raghunathan, 2008). The relationship between family meals and high SES suggests that it is possible that family meals are one mechanism through which high-SES individuals decrease their risk of becoming overweight or obese. Conversely, it is possible that eating family meals together might appear to be associated with healthy eating patterns because it is a proxy for high SES. The limitation of cross-sectional studies is that one cannot determine directionality of associations or explore mechanisms.

The longitudinal data on eating family meals and subsequent weight change are limited and inconclusive. In the GUTS cohort, Taveras et al. (2005) observed that although at baseline the more frequently a child ate dinner with his or her family the less likely he or she was to be overweight, the frequency of eating family dinners did not predict whether the child became overweight during the subsequent year. One possible explanation for the lack of longitudinal association could be that children who are highly active, which would be protective against the development of obesity, may play on sports teams that practice or have games at times that interfere with eating dinner with their family. Mixing these children in with children who do not eat dinner with their family for less healthy reasons would dilute any associations of a protective effect of family dinner. Another possible explanation is that not all family dinners are healthy or have appropriate portion sizes. Obesity is known to cluster in families because of a combination of genetic and environmental influences; thus, it is possible that family dinner in families with overweight or obese parents may be characterized by excessive calories and therefore do not protect against excessive weight gain.

Physical Activity

Although a more thorough discussion of physical and sedentary behavior is contained in chapter 2 of this volume, we review in this section parental influences on activity. Parents should encourage their children to be physically active for a variety of reasons. Although activity is an important component of weight management, it is probably best for parents to promote activity for reasons other than weight control so as not to focus their children too much on weight, which could lead to disordered eating (Keery, Eisenberg, Boutelle, Neumark-Sztainer, & Story, 2006). There are several ways that parents may influence their children's activity levels: modeling the behavior (i.e., being active themselves), providing logistical support (e.g., driving the child to a playing field), and encouraging their child to be active (Trost et al., 2003). Unfortunately, few prospective studies have evaluated the effects of parental influence on activity levels. Several cross-sectional studies of preschool children have observed an association between the activity level of children and that of their parents (Sallis, Prochaska, & Taylor, 2000). However, other studies have failed to find a cross-sectional association between the mother's physical activity level and her child's activity (Sallis, 1993). Several larger studies have evaluated these associations among adolescents. In one study of

900 multiethnic adolescent girls and boys, there was a modest but significant association between the physical activity attitudes and behaviors of adolescents and their parents. Moreover, parental encouragement (as reported by the parent) was positively related to physical activity among girls of all racial–ethnic groups and among White boys and Black boys (McGuire, Hannan, Neumark-Sztainer, Cossrow, & Story, 2002). A stronger association between activity levels of adolescents and those of their parents was observed in a study of 12-year-old students in France. Wagner et al. (2004) found that among 3,000 girls and boys whose parents were both active, 50% were more likely than their peers with less active parents to participate in structured physical activity outside of school. Taken together, the results support an important role parents have in promoting activity among their children.

Given that fewer than 50% of adults in the United States regularly engage in physical activity (Centers for Disease Control and Prevention, 2007), it is possible that the influence of parental activity on offspring is being underestimated because few studies have sufficient numbers of active parents. In addition, data are lacking on whether the activity level and beliefs about activity among mothers and fathers are equally important factors in the health of male and female offspring. However, it does appear that it may be difficult for parents to influence their preadolescent and adolescent daughters to become more active. Fulkerson et al. (2004) assessed 295 preadolescent girls and their mothers and observed that the overweight girls engaged in less activity than nonoverweight girls despite reporting that their friends and guardians thought they should exercise more. Overweight and nonoverweight girls had similar time and logistical support to be active, but compared with their leaner peers, overweight girls more often reported liking activity less, not being good at it, and preferring to do other things. Thus, to promote activity parents may need to do more than offer support. Parents should work with their child to find an activity that he or she enjoys as well as an environment in which the child feels confident about engaging in activity. This may be particularly important among Black adolescent girls, who have been found to engage in less physical activity than their peers of other racial–ethnic groups. Kimm et al. (2002) found that in the National Growth and Health Study, the decline in activity levels was significantly greater among the 1,152 Black girls than the 1,135 White girls in the study. Moreover, the declines in activity were strongly predictive of weight gain.

Sedentary Behavior

Just as parents may help to promote activity through their beliefs, behaviors, and support, they may also inadvertently promote unhealthy lifestyle choices that increase the risk of their child becoming overweight or obese. At least 67% of preadolescents and adolescents live in a home with three or more televisions, and approximately 40% of children (Dennison, Erb, & Jenkins, 2002) and 68% of preadolescents and adolescents have a television in their bedroom (Robert, Foehr, & Rideout, 2005). Some studies have observed that having a television in the bedroom is associated with being overweight among children and preadolescents (Adachi-Mejia et al., 2007). Boys of all ethnic–racial groups, both male and female Black children, and children of lower SES are the most likely to have a television in the bedroom (Barr-Anderson, van den Berg, Neumark-Sztainer & Story, 2008).

The number and placement of televisions in the house is not the only way that parents unintentionally promote being sedentary. Parents who watch a considerable amount of television appear to set fewer limits on their children's access to television. In one study of 173 White girls and their parents, Davison, Francis, and Birch (2005) found that girls whose parents watched a substantial amount of television watched significantly more television than their peers. Given that most Americans spend more time watching television than engaging in physical activity (Snoek, Strien, Janssens, & Engels, 2006), it is possible that modeling of some parental behaviors is doing more to promote than to prevent obesity among children and adolescents.

Weight Concerns and Weight Control Behaviors

Parents should be aware of their own weight-related attitudes and weight control behaviors as well as their attitudes toward their child's weight to avoid unintentional promotion of body dissatisfaction and weight concerns among their children. In GUTS, Field et al. (2005) found that children's perception that their weight was important to their father was associated with becoming very concerned about their weight regardless of their actual BMI. Moreover, both Field et al. (2005) and Keery et al. (2006) observed that preadolescents' and adolescents' perceptions of their mother's weight control behaviors and weight concerns were associated with the young person's own weight concerns and weight control behaviors. In addition, Field et al. (2003) found that independent of a child's or adolescent's BMI, those who diet gain more weight than their peers. These results suggest that offspring of parents with weight concerns may be at greater risk for weight gain by modeling their behaviors on the perception of the parents' behaviors and beliefs.

PEER INFLUENCES

Although peers influence children at all ages, peer influence is greater during preadolescence and adolescence than early childhood. During preadolescence and adolescence, acceptance by peers is highly valued, and to gain this acceptance, adolescents may adopt the perceived beliefs and behaviors practiced by members of their peer group (Paxton et al., 1999).

The desire to be attractive to peers can influence decisions about engaging in healthy as well as unhealthy behaviors. Among preadolescent and adolescent girls, greater importance is placed on body weight and shape among heterosexuals than lesbians (S. B. Austin et al., 2004). As girls enter puberty, they may adopt unhealthy weight control behaviors such as skipping breakfast or using diet pills or laxatives to control their weight (Field, Camargo, Taylor, Berkey, & Colditz, 1999). Moreover, becoming attracted to boys might cause postpubertal girls who have developed androgen-related changes (e.g., body odor, pubic hair) to become less inclined to participate in activities that they believe may make them physically unattractive (Sinton & Birch, 2006). This avoidance could make them especially vulnerable to gaining excessive amounts of weight because their energy expenditure would be decreasing while the hormonal changes of puberty are beginning, causing increases in overall fat mass.

Peer influences on lifestyle behaviors can be negative (Field et al., 1999), but some studies have explored whether peer-based interaction and social pressure can be used to positively affect health and risk behavior (Reisberg, 2000). Because individual values may change in relation to peer-group norms and values (Paxton et al., 1999), peers may play an important role in determining diet and activity patterns of children and adolescents. Unfortunately, only a few studies have assessed peer influences on diet and activity patterns that might influence the risk of obesity (Lau, Quadrel, & Hartman, 1990).

Several interventions have used some sort of peer role models to promote a healthy diet. In the Teens Eating for Energy and Nutrition at School intervention (Birnbaum, Lytle, Story, Perry, & Murray, 2002), which had a school environment interventions arm, a classroom plus school environment interventions arm, and a peer leaders plus a classroom and school environment interventions arm, it was found that children in the peer leaders plus classroom and school environment interventions arm made the largest positive changes in dietary intake. These results suggest that interventions to promote healthy dietary patterns would be wise to involve peers as role models and promoters of the intervention.

Social norms may be an important and understudied determinant of lifestyle related to obesity prevention. A growing body of literature suggests that social norms influence dieting and unhealthy weight control behaviors of teens (Paxton et al., 1999; Sinton & Birch, 2006). The role of peer influence in the decline in physical activity as girls progress through preadolescence and adolescence is less studied. However, as girls progress through childhood to preadolescence and adolescence, they tend to become more aware of their appearance and may become less inclined to participate in activities that could affect their hairstyles, make-up, or nails (Sinton & Birch, 2006). These concerns have not been studied in qualitative or quantitative studies but have been reported to the authors of this chapter by physical education teachers, so it is unclear how common these concerns are and what impact they have on the decline in physical activity among girls. Not all peer influences are necessarily negative, however. Friends may also promote healthy behaviors. Among 354 girls who were 8 to 11 years of age, those whose friends and family supported exercise were more likely than their peers to engage in physical activity (Ievers-Landis et al., 2003). These results suggest that to successfully promote activity and prevent obesity among female youth, it may be prudent to make efforts to change peer norms to support and value being active and eating a healthy diet. However, much more research is needed to better understand the association of peer norms and influences on diet and activity patterns of preadolescent and adolescent boys.

SOCIETAL INFLUENCES

Major influences on children, besides those of family and peers, are the school environment and media. Schools provide opportunities for children to both purchase and consume food, and they are also in a position to influence eating behaviors and activity levels through classroom and sports programs. Outside of school, children spend a considerable amount of time watching television (Robert et al., 2005), which exposes them to advertising for often unhealthy food products. This section discusses these elements and the mechanisms by which they may increase the risk of obesity among children and adolescents.

School Environment

Children and adolescents spend a large part of their day in school; thus, the school environment may play an extremely important role in promoting or preventing obesity. However, many of the school-based obesity prevention interventions have either been unsuccessful or their initial success has not been maintained over time (Stice, Shaw, & Marti, 2006). One potential reason for their lack of long-term success is that many of the food options made available to students are calorie dense or otherwise not extremely nutritious. During the past decade, many schools have allowed vending machines or contracts with soft drink companies and fast food vendors to generate additional revenue in an era of tight funding. A study by the U.S. Government Accountability Office (Bellis, 2005) estimated that 83% of elementary schools, 97% of middle schools, and 99% of high schools have vending machines, school stores, and snack bars where young people can purchase foods of low nutritional value. In addition, approximately 30% of elementary schools, 65% of middle schools, and 75% of high schools have signed "pouring rights" contracts that give companies the rights to sell sugar-sweetened beverages, such as soda, as well as to advertise their products in the school. Approximately 41% of middle schools and 57% of high schools with soft drink contracts receive incentives if certain sales goals are met (Wechsler, Brener, Kuester, & Miller, 2001). Although these contracts were thought to have the ability to generate considerable income because they frequently involve receiving a percentage of the sales revenue, some question the actual financial benefit to schools. Through contracts with soft drink companies, schools raised $3 to $30 per student per year (Bellis, 2005). Recently, however, despite the lure of additional funds, an increasing number of school districts are becoming concerned about the widespread problem of obesity among youth, and some large districts have declined to sign pouring rights contracts and have moved to eliminate sales of soft drinks in the schools (Fried & Nestle, 2002). A growing number of states are now banning or limiting vending machines in schools or regulating the foods and beverages that are available in schools (Vallianatos, 2002). In 2006, the Alliance for a Healthier Generation established new guidelines for the beverage industry that will limit beverage portion size and access to children and adolescents (http://www.healthiergeneration.org/). The following year, the American Beverage Association (2007) reported shipments of full-calorie soda to schools had decreased by 45%, and water shipments increased by 23%. Unfortunately, only one third of contracts between beverage companies and school districts were found to be in compliance with the new guidelines.

Although efforts have been made to improve the federally funded lunch programs in schools, those improvements are unlikely to have a meaningful impact on the weight status of youth if schools continue to offer fast food, sugar-sweetened beverages, and calorie-dense snack foods. According to the 2006 School Health Policies and Programs Study, approximately 12% of elementary schools, 19% of middle schools, and 24% of high schools in the United States offer Pizza Hut, Taco Bell, or other fast food brands in their cafeterias (O'Toole, Anderson, Miller, & Gurthrie, 2007). Fast food vendors potentially offer high-calorie food options. Like soft drink vendors, they may be allowed to advertise in the schools and thus may influence the food and beverage choices of the students when they are outside of school in addition to influencing their eating patterns during the school day. Moreover, children whose schools are connected to Channel One (a commercial public-affairs program designed for adolescents that includes 10 minutes of news and 2 minutes of public service announcements or paid advertising and is shown in 350,000 classrooms throughout the United States) may be exposed to additional advertisements for food products of questionable nutritional value (Story & French, 2004). One study found that 70% of the 45 food commercials shown on Channel One were for fast food, soft drinks, and snack foods (E. W. Austin, Chen, Pinkleton, & Quintero-Johnson, 2006).

Other societal influences on obesity in children within the school environment include school policies regarding vending machine access during the school day and whether students can leave the campus during lunchtime. There are fast food restaurants and stores with snack foods and other less than nutritious food options near many schools, so the influence of an open campus policy is nontrivial. Neumark-Sztainer, French, Hannan, Story, and Fulkerson (2005) evaluated the impact of school policies among a randomly selected sample of 1,088 high school students from 20 high schools in Minnesota and found that students in high schools with open campus lunch policies were significantly more likely than their peers at schools with closed campus policies to eat at fast food restaurants or a convenience store located near schools. This suggests that more attention to proximity and accessibility is needed to limit consumption of nonnutritious food. Neumark-Sztainer et al. additionally observed that students attending schools that turned off soda machines during lunchtime bought significantly fewer soft drinks than their peers in schools that did not limit access. The fact that fast food vendors, sugar-sweetened beverages, and snack foods are allowed in schools and fast food restaurants are located near schools may help to explain the obesity epidemic among youth in the United States.

Another alarming trend seen in schools is that physical education classes and after school programs are being scaled back. In 2000, the School Health Policies and Programs Study found only 6% of middle and high schools reported providing daily physical activity for students throughout the school year. By the sixth grade, mandatory physical education classes begin to steadily decline (Wechsler et al., 2001). Moreover, according to the Youth Risk Behavior Survey, mandatory physical education attendance for high school males fell from 46% in 1991 to 31% in 2003, and high school female attendance decreased 11%, from 37% in 1991 to 26% in 2003 (Lowry et al., 2004; see also chap. 2, this volume). Thus, one of the important contributors to the growing obesity epidemic among children and adolescents may be school environment. Changes within the current school systems need to take place to help prevent excessive weight gain and the development of obesity. Changes include minimizing fast food, snack food, and soda availability on and off campus; replacing food and beverage choices of questionable nutrient value with more nutritious options; and increasing required physical activity both during and after school hours to encourage energy balance.

Media Use

Recent estimates suggest that children and adolescents watch approximately 3 hours per day of television (Robert, Foehr, Rideout, & Brodie, 1999), which exceeds the American Academy of Pediatrics recommendation of less than 2 hours per day (Committee on Public Education, 2001). This high level of media consumption means that preadolescents and adolescents are potentially exposed to 40,000 television advertisements per year (Robert et al., 2005). During television programs specifically aimed at children, it has been estimated that there are an average of 10.65 food advertisements per hour and that 36% of food advertisements on television are for candy, sweets, and soft drinks and 46.5% for convenience foods (Harrison & Marske, 2005). Therefore, the average 6- to 18-year-old child who watches 3 hours per day of television would be exposed to 11,000 food advertisements per year, many of which would be for foods or beverages that may promote weight gain.

Time spent watching television is a robust predictor of weight gain and obesity (Berkey et al., 2000; see also chap. 2, this volume). One reason for the association may be the advertisements that encourage viewers to consume calorie-dense low-nutrient foods and beverages, such as snack foods and soda. A national survey of approximately 2,000 children and adolescents found that 65% reported that the television was on during mealtimes in their house (Robert et al., 1999). A study of 10-year-old French Canadian children by Marquis, Filion, and Dagenais (2005) observed that approximately 18% of the girls and 25% of the boys reported that they ate while watching television 7 days a week and additionally found that the boys and girls who watched the most television made the fewest healthy food choices. In a smaller American study, 36% of dinners and 67% of snacks eaten during the week were consumed in front of the television (Matheson, Killen, Wang, Varady, & Robinson, 2004). Moreover, Snoek et al. (2006) observed that among 10,087 male and female adolescents, number of hours spent watching television was positively related to snacking. The cross-sectional associations did not, however, reveal a clear pattern between eating while watching television and BMI. In a prospective analysis of changes in television programming and changes in foods commonly advertised on television among 9,263 preadolescents and adolescents in GUTS, S. L. Gortmaker, H. S. H. Lee, G. C. Sorensen, W. C. Willett, and G. A Colditz (personal communication, June 23, 2005) observed that for each 1-hour increase in television viewing over the 1-year follow-up period, children's daily energy intake increased by approximately 50 calories, and those who increased their viewing time by 2 hours increased their intake by 100 calories per day. Thus, it appears that one mechanism through which television viewing promotes weight gain and obesity is by promoting increased caloric intake.

CONCLUSION

Consuming more calories than one expends results in weight gain; therefore, prevention interventions should focus on energy balance rather than on specific dietary factors. Interventions should include goals to improve parent diet and activity patterns so that parents may act as appropriate role models for their children. School policies can have a large impact on development of overweight and obesity in children by eliminating high-calorie snacks, soda, and fast food in addition to adopting closed-campus policies to limit access to foods with questionable nutrient value. Schools should also offer more opportunities for students to be physically active during and after school. Future research should focus on better understanding what factors motivate youth to make lasting lifestyle changes, such as becoming more physically active, that are maintained after an intervention has ended. In addition, more research is needed to understand how to promote a healthy interest in physical and mental health without promoting excessive concerns with weight and shape. Two studies (S. B. Austin et al., 2004, 2007) have suggested that obesity prevention programs that do not discuss weight per se were effective at preventing the development of obesity among girls and decreased the risk of using unhealthy weight control behaviors. The next step is to investigate whether such programs are effective across a range of ages, racial–ethnic groups, and gender and whether the effects persist over time.

REFERENCES

Adachi-Mejia, A., Longacre, M., Gibson, J., Beach, M., Titus-Ernstoff, L., & Dalton, M. (2007). Children with a TV in their bedroom at higher risk for being overweight. *International Journal of Obesity, 31,* 644–651.

American Beverage Association. (2007). *School beverage guidelines progress report 2006–2007.* Retrieved April 24, 2008, from http://www.ameribev.org/industry-issues/school-beverage-guidelines/download.aspx?id=157

Arcan C., Neumark-Sztainer D., Hannan P., van den Berg P., Story M., & Larson N. (2007). Parental eating behaviours, home food environment and adolescent intakes of fruits, vegetables and dairy foods: Longitudinal findings from Project EAT. *Public Health Nutrition, 10,* 1257–1265.

Austin, E. W., Chen, Y., Pinkleton, B., & Quintero Johnson, J. (2006). Benefits and costs of Channel One in a middle school setting and the role of media-literacy training. *Pediatrics, 117,* 423–433.

Austin, S. B., Kim, J., Weicha, J., Troped, P. J., Feldman, H. A., & Peterson, K. E. (2007). School-based overweight and preventive intervention lowers incidence of disordered weight-control behaviors in early adolescent girls. *Archives of Pediatrics and Adolescent Medicine, 161,* 865–869.

Austin, S. B., Ziyadeh, N., Kahn, J., Camargo, C. A., Jr., Colditz, G. A., & Field, A. (2004). Sexual orientation, weight concerns, and eating-disordered behaviors in adolescent girls and boys. *Journal of the American Academy of Child and Adolescent Psychiatry, 43,* 1115–1123.

Barr-Anderson, D. J., van den Berg, P., Neumark-Sztainer, D., & Story, M. (2008). Characteristics associated with older adolescents who have a television in their bedrooms. *Pediatrics, 121,* 718–724.

Bellis, D. B. (2005). *School meal programs: Competitive foods are widely available and generate substantial revenues for schools.* Retrieved November 2, 2006, from http://www.gao.gov/new.items/d05563.pdf

Berkey, C., Rockett, H., Field, A., Gillman, M., Frazier, A., & Camargo, C. A., Jr. (2000). Activity, dietary intake, and weight changes in a longitudinal study of preadolescent and adolescent boys and girls. *Pediatrics, 105*(4), E56.

Birnbaum, A., Lytle, L., Story, M., Perry, C., & Murray, D. (2002). Are differences in exposure to a multicomponent school-based intervention associated with varying dietary outcomes in adolescents? *Health Education and Behavior, 29*, 427–443.

Burdette, H. L., Whitaker, R. C., Hall, W. C., & Daniels, S. R. (2006). Maternal infant-feeding style and children's adiposity at 5 years of age. *Archives of Pediatrics & Adolescent Medicine, 160*, 513–520.

Centers for Disease Control and Prevention. (2007, November 23). Prevalence of regular physical activity among adults—U.S., 2001 and 2005. *Morbidity and Mortality Weekly Report, 56*, 1209–1212.

Chung, C., & Myers, S. (1999). Do the poor pay more for food? An analysis of grocery store availability and food price disparities. *Journal of Consumer Affairs, 32*, 276–296.

Committee on Public Education. (2001). American Academy of Pediatrics: Children, adolescents, and television. *Pediatrics, 107*, 423–426.

Davison, K. K., Francis, L. A., & Birch, L. L. (2005). Links between parents' and girls' television viewing behaviors: A longitudinal examination. *Journal of Pediatrics, 147*, 436–442.

Davison, K. K., Markey, C. N., & Birch, L. L. (2000). Etiology of body dissatisfaction and weight concerns among 5-year-old girls. *Appetite, 35*, 143–151.

Davison, K. K., Markey, C. N., & Birch, L. L. (2003). A longitudinal examination of patterns in girls' weight concerns and body dissatisfaction from ages 5 to 9 years. *International Journal of Eating Disorders, 33*, 320–332.

Dennison, B. A., Erb, T. A., & Jenkins, P. L. (2002). Television viewing and television in bedroom associated with overweight risk among low-income preschool children. *Pediatrics, 109*, 1028–1035.

Dubois, L., & Girard, M. (2006). Early determinants of overweight at 4.5 years in a population-based longitudinal study. *International Journal of Obesity* (London), 30, 610–617.

Eisenberg, M., Olson, R., Neumark-Sztainer, D., Story, M., & Bearinger, L. (2004). Correlations between family meals and psychosocial well-being among adolescents. *Archives of Pediatrics & Adolescent Medicine, 158*, 792–796.

Faith, M., Berkowitz, R., Stallings, V., Kerns, J., Storey, M., & Stunkard, A. (2004). Parental feeding attitudes and styles and child body mass index: Prospective analysis of a gene–environment interaction. *Pediatrics, 114*, 429–436.

Faith, M., & Kerns, J. (2005). Infant and child feeding practices and childhood overweight: The role of restriction. *Maternal and Child Nutrition, 1*, 164–168.

Field, A., Austin, S. B., Striegel-Moore, R., Taylor, C., Camargo, C. A., Jr., & Laird, N. (2005). Weight concerns and weight control behaviors of adolescents and their mothers. *Archives of Pediatrics & Adolescent Medicine, 159*, 1121–1126.

Field, A., Austin, S. B., Taylor, C., Malspeis, S., Rosner, B., Rockett, H., et al. (2003). Relation between dieting and weight change among preadolescents and adolescents. *Pediatrics, 112*, 900–906.

Field, A., Camargo, C. A., Jr., Taylor, C., Berkey, C., & Colditz, G. A. (1999). Relation of peer and media influences to the development of purging behaviors among preadolescent and adolescent girls. *Archives of Pediatrics & Adolescent Medicine, 153*, 1184–1189.

Fisher, J., & Birch, L. (1999). Restricting access to foods and children's eating. *Appetite, 32*, 405–419.

Francis, L. A., & Birch, L. L. (2005). Maternal influences on daughters' restrained eating behavior. *Health Psychology, 24*, 548–554.

Fried, E., & Nestle, M. (2002). The growing political movement against soft drinks in schools. *JAMA, 288*, 2176–2181.

Fulkerson, J., French, S., Story, M., Hannan, P. J., Neumark-Sztainer, D., & Himes, J. (2004). Weight-bearing physical activity among girls and mothers: Relationships to girls' weight status. *Obesity Research, 12*, 258–266.

Gillman, M., Rifas-Shiman, S., Camargo, C. A., Jr., Berkey, C., Frazier, A., & Rockett, H. (2001). Risk of overweight among adolescents who were breastfed as infants. *JAMA, 285*, 2461–2467.

Gillman, M. W., Rifas-Shiman, S. L., Frazier, A. L., Rockett, H. R., Camargo, C. A., Jr., Field, A. E., et al. (2000). Family dinner and diet quality among older children and adolescents. *Archives of Family Medicine, 9*, 235–240.

Gordon-Larsen, P., Adair, L., & Popkin, B. (2003). The relationship of ethnicity, socioeconomic factors, and overweight in US adolescents. *Obesity Research, 11*, 121–129.

Hanson, N., Neumark-Sztainer, D., Eisenberg, M., Story, M., & Wall, M. (2005). Associations between parental report of the home food environment and adolescent intakes of fruits, vegetables and dairy foods. *Public Health and Nutrition, 8*, 77–85.

Harrison, K., & Marske, A. (2005). Nutritional content of foods advertised during the television programs children watch most. *American Journal of Public Health, 95*, 1568–1574.

Ievers-Landis, C. Burant, C., Drotar, D., Morgan, L., Trapl, E., & Kwoh, C. (2003). Social support, knowledge, and self-efficacy as correlates of osteoporosis preventive behaviors among preadolescent females. *Journal of Pediatric Psychology, 28*, 335–345.

Keery, H., Eisenberg, M., Boutelle, K., Neumark-Sztainer, D., & Story, M. (2006). Relationships between maternal and adolescent weight-related behaviors and concerns: The role of perception. *Journal of Psychosomatic Research, 61*, 105–111.

Kimm, S. Y., Glynn, N. W., Kriska, A. M., Barton, B. A., Kronsberg, S. S., Daniels, S. R., et al. (2002). Decline in physical activity in Black girls and White girls during adolescence. *New England Journal of Medicine, 347*, 709–715.

Lau, R., Quadrel, M., & Hartman, K. (1990). Development and change of young adults' preventive health beliefs and behavior: Influence from parents and peers. *Journal of Health and Social Behavior, 31*, 240–259.

Lowry, R., Brener, N., Lee, S., Epping, J., Fulton, J., & Eaton, D. (2004, September 17). Participation in high school physical education—United States 1991–2003. *Morbidity & Mortality Weekly Report, 53*, 844–847.

Marquis, M., Filion, Y., & Dagenais, F. (2005). Does eating while watching television influence children's food related behaviors? *Canadian Journal of Dietetic Practice and Research, 66*, 12–18.

Matheson, D., Killen, J., Wang, Y., Varady, A., & Robinson, T. (2004). Children's food consumption during television viewing. *American Journal of Clinical Nutrition, 79*, 1088–1094.

Mayer-Davis, E., Rifas-Shiman, S., Zhou, L., Hu, F., Colditz, G. A., & Gillman, M. (2006). Breast-feeding and risk for childhood obesity. *Diabetes Care, 29*, 2231–2237.

McGuire, M., Hannan, P., Neumark-Sztainer, D., Cossrow, N., & Story, M. (2002). Parental correlates of physical activity in a racially/ethnically diverse adolescent sample. *Journal of Adolescent Health, 30*, 253–261.

Neumark-Sztainer, D., French, S., Hannan, P., Story, M., & Fulkerson, J. (2005). School lunch and snacking patterns among high school students: Associations with school food environment and policies. *International Journal of Behavioral Nutrition and Physical Activity, 2*, 14–20.

Neumark-Sztainer, D., Wall, M., Perry, C., & Story, M. (2003). Correlates of fruit and vegetable intake among adolescents. Findings from Project EAT. *Preventive Medicine, 37*, 198–208.

Neumark-Sztainer, D., Wall, M., Story, M., & Fulkerson, J. (2004). Are family meal patterns associated with disordered eating behaviors among adolescents? *Journal of Adolescent Health, 35*, 350–359.

Oddy, W., Landsborough, L., Kendell, G., Henderson, S., & Downie, J. (2006). The association of maternal overweight and obesity with breastfeeding duration. *Journal of Pediatrics, 149*, 185–191.

Ogden, C. L., Carroll, M. D., & Flegal, K. M. (2006). High body mass index for age among U.S. children and adolescents, 2003–2006. *JAMA, 299*, 2401–2405.

O'Toole, T. P., Anderson, S., Miller, C., & Gurthrie, J. (2007). Nutrition services and foods and beverages available at school: Results from the School Health Policies and Programs Study 2006. *Journal of School Health, 77*, 500–521.

Paxton, S., Schutz, H., Wertheim, E., & Muir, S. (1999). Friendship clique and peer influences on body image concerns, dietary restraint, extreme weight-loss behaviors, and binge eating in adolescent girls. *Journal of Abnormal Psychology, 108*, 255–266.

Reisberg, L. (2000). Colleges use peer pressure to encourage healthy behavior. *Chronicle of Higher Education, 46*, A60–A61.

Robert, D., Foehr, U., & Rideout, V. (2005). *Generation M: Media in the lives of 8–18 year olds*. Menlo Park, CA: Kaiser Family Foundation.

Robert, D., Foehr, U., Rideout, V., & Brodie, M. (1999). *Kids & media @ the new millennium*. Menlo Park, CA: Kaiser Family Foundation.

Sallis, J. (1993) Epidemiology of physical activity and fitness in children and adolescents. *Critical Review of Food Science Nutrition, 33*, 403–408.

Sallis, J., Prochaska, J., & Taylor, W. (2000). A review of correlates of physical activity of children and adolescents. *Medical Science in Sport and Exercise, 32*, 963–975.

Schreiber, G., Robins, M., Striegel-Moore, R., Obarzanek, E., Morrison, J. & Wright, D. (1996). Weight modification efforts reported by Black and White preadolescent girls: National Heart, Lung, and Blood Institute Growth and Health Study. *Pediatrics, 98,* 63–70.

Sinton, M., & Birch, L. (2006). Individual and sociocultural influences on pre-adolescent girls' appearance schemas and body dissatisfaction. *Journal of Youth and Adolescence, 35,* 165–175.

Snoek, H., Strien, T., Janssens, J., & Engels, R. (2006). The effect of television viewing on adolescents' snacking: Individual differences explained by external, restrained and emotional eating. *Journal of Adolescent Health, 39,* 448–451.

Spruijt-Metz, D., Li, C., Cohen, E., Birch, L., & Goran, M. (2006). Longitudinal influence of mother's child-feeding practices on adiposity in children. *Journal of Pediatrics, 148,* 314–320.

Stice, E., Shaw, H., & Marti, N. (2006). A meta-analytic review of obesity prevention programs for children and adolescents: The skinny on interventions that work. *Psychological Bulletin, 132,* 667–691.

Story, M., & French, S. (2004). Food advertising and marketing directed at children and adolescents in the US. *International Journal of Behavioral Nutrition and Physical Activity, 1,* 3–20.

Taveras, E. M., Rifas-Shiman, S. L., Berkey, C. S., Rockett, H. R., Field, A. E., Frazier, A. L., et al. (2005). Family dinner and adolescent overweight. *Obesity Research, 13,* 900–906.

Trost, S., Sallis, J., Pate, R., Freedson, P., Taylor, W., & Dowda, M. (2003). Evaluating a model of parental influence on youth physical activity. *American Journal of Preventive Medicine, 25,* 277–282.

Vallianatos, M. (2002). *Healthy school food policies: A checklist.* Retrieved January 5, 2007, from http://departments.oxy.edu/uepi/cfj/publications/healthy_school_food_policies_05.pdf

Wagner, A., Klein-Platat, C., Arveiler, D., Haan, M., Schlienger, J., & Simon, C. (2004). Parent–child physical activity relationships in 12-year-old French students do not depend on family socioeconomic status. *Diabetes Metabolism, 30,* 359–366.

Wang, Y., & Zhang, Q. (2006). Are American children and adolescents of low socioeconomic status at increased risk of obesity? Changes in the association between overweight and family income between 1971 and 2002. *American Journal of Clinical Nutrition, 84,* 707–716.

Wechsler, H., Brener, N., Kuester, S., & Miller, C. (2001). Food service and foods and beverages available at school: Results from the School Health Policies and Programs Study 2000. *Journal of School Health, 71,* 313–324.

Whitaker, R. (2004). Predicting preschooler obesity at birth: The role of maternal obesity in early pregnancy. *Pediatrics, 114,* 29–36.

Yang, S., Lynch, J., Schulenberg, J., Roux, A. V., & Raghunathan, T. (2008). Emergence of socioeconomic inequalities in smoking and overweight and obesity in early adulthood: The national longitudinal study of adolescent health. *American Journal of Public Health, 98,* 468–477.

II

PSYCHOSOCIAL, INTERPERSONAL, AND INTRAPERSONAL EFFECTS OF OBESITY

4

PSYCHOSOCIAL CONSEQUENCES OF OBESITY AND WEIGHT BIAS: IMPLICATIONS FOR INTERVENTIONS

JESS HAINES AND DIANNE NEUMARK-SZTAINER

Obesity is associated with adverse physical and psychological consequences. Although the physical consequences are a direct result of obesity, the psychological consequences are primarily a result of weight bias. Interventions are needed that aim to prevent adolescent and childhood obesity as well as decrease the various forms of weight-related stigmatization that occur in our society. To aid in the development of such interventions, a clear understanding of the associations among obesity, weight-related stigmatization, and adverse psychosocial consequences is also needed.

Our research team has focused on trying to better understand the experience of being overweight in a thin-oriented society. Much of our work has sought to increase our understanding of the psychosocial consequences of obesity and weight bias to guide the development of interventions aimed at preventing obesity and other weight-related disorders among children and adolescents. For example, we have explored the frequency and impact of weight-related teasing in children and adolescents to determine the magnitude of the problem, whether it is worthy of addressing within interventions, and how best to address weight-teasing to decrease its occurrence. We have used quantitative, qualitative, and intervention research methodologies to explore weight-related stigmatization, psychosocial concerns, and health-compromising behaviors among overweight youth. Quantitative surveys of large population-based samples have been useful in examining associations between obesity and its psychosocial consequences (Neumark-Sztainer et al., 1997; Neumark-Sztainer, Story, Hannan, Perry, & Irving, 2002). In-depth interviews and focus groups with smaller samples of children and adolescents have provided additional information about their experiences dealing with weight-based stigmatization (Haines, Neumark-Sztainer, & Thiel, 2007; Neumark-Sztainer, Story, & Faibisch, 1998; Neumark-Sztainer, Story, Faibisch, Ohlson, & Adamiak, 1999). Our intervention research with children and adolescents has informed us about issues such as body image concerns and weight teasing, areas that we are continuously trying to address more effectively through work with youth as well as with their teachers, coaches, youth group leaders, health care providers, and parents (Haines, Neumark-Sztainer, Perry, Hannan, & Levine, 2006; Neumark-Sztainer, 2005; Neumark-Sztainer, Sherwood, Coller, & Hannan, 2000; Neumark-Sztainer, Story, Hannan, & Rex, 2003).

In this chapter, we examine the psychosocial consequences of obesity and weight bias identified in our own research and in the work of others. We first present some of the key research findings examining the social consequences of being overweight within a society that values thinness. We then examine the implications of being overweight and of being exposed to weight-related stigmatization on psychological well-being and discuss implications for working toward the prevention of obesity, weight bias, and their associated psychosocial consequences.

STIGMATIZATION AND MISTREATMENT BY PEERS

Obesity is negatively stereotyped in Western cultures, and this negative stereotyping appears to begin early in life. Studies have found that children as young as 3 years attribute negative characteristics, such as "lazy," "dirty," "stupid," "ugly," "liar," and "cheat," to overweight children (Brylinsky, 1994; Greenleaf, Chambliss, Rhea, Martin, & Morrow, 2006; Richardson, Goodman, Hastorf, & Dornbusch, 1961; Staffieri, 1967; Turnbull, Heaslip, & McLeod, 2000).

In a series of landmark studies conducted in the early 1960s, 10- and 11-year-old children were shown six drawings of children and were asked to rank them according to how well they liked each child (Richardson et al., 1961). The drawings included a healthy child, an obese child, and four children with various physical disabilities or disfigurements. The children ranked the obese child last on likeability, behind the children with physical impairments including facial disfigurement and use of a wheelchair. In 2001, Latner and Stunkard replicated this study among 458 fifth- and sixth-grade students and found that stigmatization of obesity by children had increased over the 40 years since the original study was completed. In the 2001 study, the obese child was ranked last on likeability and, of great concern, was liked significantly less than in the 1961 study (Latner & Stunkard, 2003).

It is unclear how these hypothetical scenarios reflect the real-life experiences of obese youth. One study has suggested that attitudes may be less negative in real-life situations than in these more abstract situations; Lawson (1980) found no relationship between the stereotypes attached to drawings and same-item judgments of overweight peers among a sample of 84 children in Grades 2 through 6. Thus, the desirable norms relating to body shape did not appear to be used to evaluate their fellow classmates. Similarly, Phillips and Hill (1998) found that overweight preadolescent girls received peer nominations of popularity comparable to those of normal-weight girls. Conversely, as described in the following paragraphs, numerous studies have found that overweight youth are subject to various forms of mistreatment by their peers, including social isolation or marginalization, weight-related teasing, and bullying.

Social Marginalization

Social marginalization has been defined as youth excluding their peers as a result of viewing them as different or undesirable (Robinson, 2006). A study of elementary school students suggests that overweight children are marginalized by their peers; compared with average-weight children of the same age, overweight children in Grades 2 through 5 received lower ratings as potential playmates and were chosen more often as the least-preferred playmates in their class (Strauss, 1985).

This rejection and social marginalization appears to continue into adolescence. In a population-based cohort study of more than 17,000 adolescents, researchers used participants' listings of their five best male and female friends to explore social networks of overweight and normal-weight adolescents (Strauss & Pollack, 2003). Results suggest that overweight adolescents were more socially isolated than their normal-weight peers. Overweight adolescents received significantly fewer friendship nominations and were more likely to receive zero friendship nominations than normal-weight adolescents. In addition, studies examining the association between relational victimization, defined as intentionally using friendship status as a way to inflict harm (e.g., excluding a peer from a social activity) have found significant positive associations between relational victimization and weight status among adolescents (Janssen, Craig, Boyce, & Pickett, 2004; Pearce, Boergers, & Prinstein, 2002), particularly among females, who are more likely than males to engage in this type of victimization (Crick, 1997; Galen & Underwood, 1997).

Our own work has demonstrated that overweight adolescents perceive that they are treated differently because of their weight. We conducted qualitative interviews with overweight adolescent girls to explore their weight-related experiences. Many of the girls described hurtful and inaccurate assumptions that people make on the basis of their size, such as being "unclean" or "smelly" (Neumark-Sztainer et al., 1998). A number of girls also described being socially marginalized because of their weight. For example, one girl described being excluded from a peer group because of her weight:

> At my other school that I used to go to, there were some girls that . . . all they hung around with was thin people. . . . I talked to one other girl that was with them and like we were friends. But they would tell her not to hang around me because it makes her look bad, because she's thin and I was fat. . . . I just told her . . . if she didn't want to talk to me or hang around with me, then that's okay . . . cuz those were her friends more cuz I had just come to that school. So she went with them and I kind of felt bad. (Neumark-Sztainer, 1998)

We also found evidence of social marginalization of overweight adolescents in a large, population-based sample of 7th-, 9th-, and 11th-grade students who completed a statewide survey about adolescent health. Our results suggest that obese girls and boys are significantly less likely to spend time with friends than their average-weight peers (Falkner et al., 2001).

In addition to decreased social interaction with peers, overweight adolescents may also have reduced opportunity for romantic relationships. Research suggests that overweight adolescents, particularly overweight girls, appear to be perceived as less desirable partners for romantic relationships. In a study of 786 high school students, Sobal, Nicolopoulos, and Lee (1995) found that adolescents, in particular boys, expressed low comfort levels in dating overweight peers, and comfort levels were lowest for dating a very overweight individual. Pearce et al. (2002) also examined romantic relationships in an ethnically diverse group of 416 adolescents and found that obese girls were less likely to date than their peers. Obese boys, however, did not report dating less than their peers. Pearce et al. (2002) speculated that this may be because boys are not judged by potential romantic partners according to their weight to the same extent as girls.

Weight-Related Teasing and Bullying

Overweight youth are at greater risk for being involved in more overt forms of aggression, including weight-related teasing and bullying. In a recent study we conducted with 151 fourth- through sixth-grade students, teasing by peers was reported by 45% of overweight children compared with only 15% of average weight children (Haines, 2005). Hayden-Wade et al. (2005) found a similar positive association between teasing and weight among elementary school children. Teasing also disproportionately affects overweight adolescents. In a large, population-based study of middle and high school students, we found that teasing by peers was reported by 63% of overweight adolescent girls compared with 21% of average weight adolescent girls. Among boys, teasing by peers was reported by 58% of overweight boys and 13% of average-weight boys (Neumark-Sztainer, Falkner, et al., 2002).

Griffiths, Wolke, Page, Horwood, and the ALSPAC Study Team (2006), in their prospective study of elementary school children, found that children of higher weight, both boys and girls, were more often victims of bullying. Obese boys were also more likely to be the perpetrators of bullying than their average-weight peers. Janssen et al. (2004) found similar results in their study of adolescents: Overweight and obese adolescents were more likely to be both the victims and the perpetrators of bullying behavior compared with their average-weight peers. Overweight youths' increased likelihood of being a bully–perpetrator may be due to their physical dominance over their peers or in response to being bullied (Griffiths et al., 2006; Janssen et al., 2004).

STIGMATIZATION AND MISTREATMENT WITHIN EDUCATIONAL AND HEALTH CARE SETTINGS

Children and adolescents facing weight-related stigmatization should be able to seek guidance and comfort within educational and health care settings. Because of the important role of educators and health care providers and their ongoing contact with youth, both can have a large effect on overweight youth. However, studies have suggested that some educators and health care providers may have negative attitudes regarding obesity that can interfere with their ability to provide overweight youth with the help that they may need (Neumark-Sztainer & Haines, 2004).

Our research group explored weight-related attitudes among 115 middle school and high school teachers and school health workers (Neumark-Sztainer, Harris, & Story, 1999). Approximately one fifth of the school staff expressed the view that obese persons are more emotional, less tidy, less likely to succeed at work, and have different personalities than nonobese persons. About one quarter of the respondents viewed obese persons as having more family problems than nonobese persons and agreed with the statement, "One of the worst things that could happen to a person would be for him/her to become obese" (Neumark-Sztainer et al., 1999). Strong negative prejudices toward obese individuals have been found among university students enrolled in physical education or exercise science programs (Chambliss, Finley, & Blair, 2004; O'Brien, Hunter, & Banks, 2007). Given that many of these university students will become physical education teachers, this finding has important implications for youth: Antifat biases among physical education staff could be a barrier to enjoyment or involvement in physical activity among overweight and obese children and adolescents. In addition to affecting interactions with overweight students, school staff's own attitudes about weight may also influence the overall school environment by dictating whether the staff will intervene when weight stigmatization by other students occurs.

Similar negative attitudes and stereotypes toward obese individuals have been found among various groups of health professionals, including nurses (Bagley, Conklin, Isherwood, Pechiulis, & Watson, 1989; Maroney & Golub, 1992), dietitians and dietetic students (McArthur & Ross, 1997; Oberrieder, Walker, Monroe, & Adeyanju, 1995), and physicians and medical students (Price, Desmond, Krol, Snyder, & O'Connell, 1987; Wigton & McGaghie, 2001) as well as researchers and other health professionals specializing in obesity treatment and prevention (Schwartz, Chambliss, Brownell, Blair, & Billington, 2003). In a study that examined physicians' attitudes toward obese patients, more than half of the 620 physicians surveyed viewed obese patients as noncompliant, unattractive, and ugly (Foster et al., 2003). There is some evidence that this antifat prejudice may affect the care that health professionals provide. For example, a study that explored physicians' potential treatment of overweight patients using case reports of patients that differed only in weight found that physicians reported that they would feel more negative toward overweight patients and that they would spend less time with them (Hebl & Xu, 2001). Although little is known about how the antifat bias of health care professionals affects youths' health care–seeking behavior, a number of studies have found that obese women are more likely than nonobese women to cancel or delay health care appointments, particularly for preventive services, such as breast and gynecological screening tests (Amy, Aalborg, Lyons, & Keranen, 2006; Fontaine, Faith, Allison, & Cheskin, 1998; Olson, Schumaker, & Yawn, 1994). Barriers for seeking appropriate health care identified by obese women include disrespectful treatment, embarrassment at being weighed or about their weight, negative attitudes of providers, unsolicited advice to lose weight, and medical equipment that is too small (Amy et al., 2006; Olson et al., 1994). Conversely, a study that examined adult patients' reports of the level of care that they received from their physicians found that only overweight men reported that physicians spent less time with them than with average-weight men; overweight women did not report receiving a lower level of care (Hebl, Xu, & Mason, 2003). Further study is needed to assess how negative attitudes within the health professions affect the care provided to adult as well as youth populations.

Given that health care providers and educators have opportunities for providing overweight youth with support and guidance regarding healthy weight management behaviors, strategies to improve the health care and educational experiences of overweight children and adolescents are worthy of exploration. Some suggested changes for those who treat or educate obese children and adolescents include enhanced understanding of the various forms of stigma that overweight youth endure (Schwartz et al., 2003; Teachman, Gapinski, Brownell, Rawlins, & Jeyaram, 2003), familiarity with community resources available to youth, and treating youth with respect and compassion. Suggested changes that are specific to health care professionals include improved knowledge of multidisciplinary treatments and creating more accessible environments for obese youth by providing armless chairs and larger examination gowns (Frank, 1993). On the basis of our own research, in which we found that the majority of overweight youth have experienced weight stigmatization, we would further suggest that health care providers approach an overweight child under the assumption that the child has been the victim of some type of weight mistreatment and is sensitive to comments about his or her weight. Although it may be important to discuss the health benefits of being at a healthy weight, the conversation should take into account the child's sensitivity to weight-related comments and include some positive words about the child's appearance and other personal traits. It may be better to focus on strategies for behavioral change rather than weight change, and the difficulties inherent to both types of changes should be honestly discussed. Finally, time should be taken to discuss weight-related mistreatment experiences and strategies for coping and responding to such incidents. Children and adolescents need to know that regardless of their size, they should not be mistreated by anyone because of their weight.

PSYCHOLOGICAL CONSEQUENCES OF OBESITY AND WEIGHT-RELATED STIGMATIZATION

In light of the pervasive weight-related stigmatization faced by many overweight youth, differences in psychological concerns might be anticipated. In this section we describe associations between obesity and global psychological concerns such as self-esteem and depression. In addition, we review some of the research that has examined associations between weight stigmatization and psychological consequences.

Self-Esteem

Self-esteem is influenced by one's perceptions about how others regard and treat one. The previous discussion clearly indicates that many overweight youth perceive that others make negative assumptions about them and treat them differently because of their weight. Thus, we might expect to find large differences in self-esteem between overweight and nonoverweight youth. Furthermore, we might expect to find stronger associations among adolescents than among children, given that appearance, fitting in with the norm, and social interactions tend to be key issues among this age group. In a review of the literature examining associations between obesity and self-esteem among children and adolescents, French et al. (1995) did find stronger associations among adolescents then among children. However, findings were not consistent across studies. About half of the cross-sectional studies (13 out of 25) showed lower self-esteem in obese children and adolescents than in their nonobese counterparts. No studies reported higher levels of self-esteem in obese youth than in nonobese youth. Results from the few prospective studies that were reviewed by French et al. were inconsistent.

Findings from more recent population-based studies are also somewhat inconsistent. A 2004 study that followed a large sample of elementary school children aged 5 to 10 years at baseline for 3 years found that weight was negatively associated with self-esteem at both baseline and follow-up. This relationship was stronger at follow-up, suggesting that risk of low self-esteem is higher for overweight adolescents than for children (Hesketh, Wake, & Waters, 2004). Findings from a second prospective study involving a large sample of youth also suggest that age may moderate the association between overweight and self-esteem (Strauss, 2000). Self-esteem scores were not significantly different among 9- to 10-year-old obese and nonobese children, whereas there were significant differences 4 years later. This study also found that ethnicity may moderate this association: Self-esteem was negatively associated with weight status in Hispanic and Caucasian adolescent girls but not in African American girls (Strauss, 2000). Still another study found that self-esteem is lower in overweight adolescents but only if the influence of body image is not controlled for (Pesa, Syre, & Jones, 2000). Thus, findings from observational research suggest that obesity tends to be associated with lower self-esteem, particularly in adolescents, but associations tend to be modest and inconsistent across studies. Additional research that explores associations between various domains of self-esteem (e.g., athletic, social, appearance) and weight status may be needed to help uncover possible differences in self-esteem among overweight and nonoverweight youth.

Psychological Consequences of Weight-Related Stigmatization

Two studies by our research team demonstrate the potential for weight teasing to strongly affect the psychological well-being of adolescents (Eisenberg, Neumark-Sztainer, Haines, & Wall, 2006; Eisenberg, Neumark-Sztainer, & Story, 2003). Cross-sectional analyses of a large sample of adolescents found that being teased about body weight by family members or peers was consistently associated with poorer scores in self-esteem, depressive symptoms, and higher percentages of youth reporting suicide ideation and suicide attempts. These associations held for both boys and girls, across racial and ethnic groups and weight groups. Body mass index was not significantly associated with most outcome measures after teasing was entered into multivariate models, indicating that the experience of being teased about weight, rather than actual body weight, appears to be the relevant factor for self-esteem, depressive symptoms, and suicidal ideation and attempts (Eisenberg et al., 2003). Longitudinal analyses that examined these associations 5 years later found that teasing at baseline predicted lower self-esteem and higher depressive symptoms at follow-up, suggesting that weight teasing during adolescence can have a lasting effect on the emotional health of youth (Eisenberg et al., 2006).

IMPLICATIONS FOR INTERVENTIONS

The high prevalence of weight-related stigmatization and its strong associations with adverse psychological consequences point to a strong need for interventions aimed at (a) decreasing weight stigmatization by others and (b) providing support for overweight individuals facing weight stigmatization.

Decreasing Weight-Related Stigmatization

Because few interventions designed to reduce weight-related stigmatization among youth have been developed and evaluated (Irving, 2000; McVey & Tweed, 2005; Piran, 1999; Smolak, Levine, & Schermer, 1998), our research group conducted interviews and focus groups with elementary school children and their teachers and parents to gain their insight about how best to address weight-based stigmatization in a school-based intervention. Teachers and parents recommended that the school implement more explicit rules regarding teasing as a way to reduce weight stigmatization. Teachers also suggested promoting size acceptance among the students. Students suggested educating students on the impact teasing can have on peers. One student stated,

> Like put ourselves in their shoes. . . . think about how it would feel to be teased each and every day. . . . I think you should tell them that it would really hurt if you were teased everyday for the rest of the year. Something like that. (Haines et al., 2007, p. 16)

Students also discussed strategies for dealing with teasing. Teaching skills to defend themselves or others from teasing were discussed as ways to help students deal with teasing when it occurred (Haines et al., 2007).

On the basis of the results of this qualitative research, our research group developed Very Important Kids (V.I.K.), a school-based intervention that was designed to prevent weight stigmatization and promote healthy weight-related behaviors among all fourth- through sixth-grade students regardless of weight status. The program included four components: (a) an extracurricular after school program, (b) a theater production, (c) school outreach, and (d) family outreach. The interactive after school sessions ran for 1 day a week for 10 weeks and used role-plays and small group discussions to enhance children's empathy for those who are teased and to develop their skills to intervene in weight-teasing situations. The after school sessions also included activities to promote a healthy body image and healthy weight-related behaviors among the children. The children also participated in a theater program that involved working with a local theater company, Illusion Theater, to develop a play based on their own experiences with teasing. School-level strategies used to change social norms regarding teasing and weight included (a) an educational workshop for school staff on the impact of weight-stigmatization and strategies to reduce teasing at school; (b) a school-wide, no-teasing campaign developed by the students; and (c) a school-wide reading of a fictional book about teasing (Lovell, 2001) followed by a discussion led by the classroom teachers. The V.I.K. intervention also had a family component that included postcards, family nights, and the promotion of key V.I.K. messages at parent–teacher nights.

The effectiveness of the V.I.K. intervention was evaluated in a pilot study that used a pre–post quasi-experimental design with one school assigned to each condition: intervention and assessment-only control. The V.I.K. intervention was found to be effective in reducing teasing; the prevalence of teasing in the control school increased from 21.1% to 29.8% over the 8-month study period, whereas in the intervention condition, school levels of teasing decreased from 30.2% to 20.6% (Haines et al., 2006). There was also a significant increase in self-efficacy to affect weight-teasing norms and a decrease in perceived peer weight-related norms (i.e., teasing and dieting behaviors) in the intervention school relative to the control school. Although research using a larger sample of schools is needed to confirm these results, these findings provide promising evidence that interventions that incorporate individual, home, and school-level strategies focused on changing social norms regarding weight and weight-based teasing may be effective in reducing weight-related stigmatization among youth.

Another potential method for decreasing weight stigmatization and ensuing discriminatory practices is to alter the negative manner in which youth view obesity. Attribution theory suggests that youths' attitudes toward an overweight peer would be more favorable if they view the problem as beyond the peer's control (Weiner, Perry, & Magnusson, 1988). Consequently, changing youths' beliefs about the controllability of obesity has been explored as a way to reduce negative stereotyping of obesity. Interventions using this approach have been brief and involve presenting youth with information about the controllability of obesity using written vignettes, audiotapes, videos, or a 10-minute oral presentation (Anesbury & Tiggemann, 2000; Bell & Morgan, 2000; DeJong, 1993; Sigelman, 1991). In general, these interventions have been able to alter children's beliefs about the controllability of obesity, but their impact on the children's attitudes and negative stereotyping of obesity has been minimal. Longer and more intensive interventions may be needed to alter youths' attitudes toward their obese peers.

Providing Support for Overweight Individuals

Family members of overweight youth as well as educators, health care providers, and peers can provide support in coping with weight-related stigmatization to decrease its potential impact on psychosocial well-being. Support from these key individuals is also needed to help overweight youth make healthy lifestyle choices that will prevent excessive weight gain (e.g., getting regular physical activity, reducing television viewing).

Two population-based studies (Fulkerson, Strauss, Neumark-Sztainer, Story, & Boutelle, 2007; Mellin, Neumark-Sztainer, Story, Ireland, & Resnick, 2002), found that overweight adolescents who had supportive families were more resilient and had better psychosocial outcomes than overweight adolescents whose families were less supportive. Overweight children reared in supportive families, in which family members refrain from making negative comments about the child's appearance and weight, will feel better about themselves and be less likely to suffer the psychosocial consequences associated with being overweight. At the same time, families of overweight children need to provide opportunities and gentle encouragement for healthy eating and physical activity. The balance between these messages may present challenges for parents. An important approach that should be explored is the creation of home-based interventions that aim to help parents walk this fine line to promote their children's health. The research findings from our own team and other studies have led to the development of four cornerstones for parents who want to help their children have a healthy body image and a healthy body weight and form the basis for a parenting book (Neumark-Sztainer, 2005). The four cornerstones are (a) model healthy behaviors for your children, (b) provide an environment that makes it easy for your children to make healthy choices, (c) focus less on weight and more on behavior and overall health, and (d) provide a supportive environment with lots of talking and even more listening (Neumark-Sztainer, 2005, p. 120). More attention needs to be directed toward the parents of children and adolescents to help them help their children. Parents live in the same world as their children and are exposed to the same weight-related pressures. Parents may be concerned about the physical and psychological well-being of their children, particularly if they are overweight, and need tools for helping and not hindering their children's efforts to adopt healthful behaviors, feel good about themselves, and live productive and fulfilling lives.

As discussed previously, some health care providers and educators hold negative attitudes regarding obesity that can interfere with their ability to act in a supportive manner toward overweight patients and students. However, the majority of health care providers and educators do not hold negative attitudes and are interested in learning how they can be more supportive. At conferences and meetings, clinicians often ask researchers how best to work with the overweight children and adolescents that they see in their practices, and conference sessions on this topic tend to be popular and well-attended. In a survey of school staff, our research group found that the majority of school-based health care providers and teachers were interested in attending a staff training on the prevention of weight-related disturbances (Neumark-Sztainer, Harris et al., 1999). Material on how to prevent weight stigmatization and how to promote the psychosocial well-being of overweight youth could clearly be incorporated into such sessions. Suggested activities include self-examination of their own weight-related attitudes and experiences growing up, dissemination of accurate facts about the harmful consequences of weight teasing among youth, and identification of ways to discuss and promote healthy weight-related behaviors in a sensitive manner. A tool that we have used in our trainings with school staff to help them explore their weight-related prejudices is the Implicit Association Test, which is a timed word-classification task designed to uncover implicit weight prejudices (Schwartz et al., 2003).

New Moves, a school-based program for overweight girls or girls at risk for becoming overweight as a result of low levels of physical activity, is built on the philosophy that overweight youth require a supportive and accepting environment to adopt healthy weight-related behaviors. New Moves aims to (a) bring about positive change in physical activity and eating behaviors to improve weight status and overall health, (b) help girls function in a thin-oriented society and feel good about themselves, and (c) help girls avoid unhealthy weight control behaviors. Initial findings demonstrated that the program was well-received by adolescent girls, their parents, and the school staff. However, initial findings also indicated a need for a more intensive, multicomponent intervention and a more comprehensive evaluation to detect a change in behavioral and physical outcomes (Neumark-Sztainer et al., 2003).

New Moves has been revised and now includes an intensive intervention phase in which girls participate in an all-female physical education class with sessions on nutrition, physical activity, and body image and a maintenance phase that includes weekly meetings over lunch. The girls also participate in individual counseling sessions with a New Moves coach throughout both phases of the study. During these sessions, the New Moves coaches establish a nonconfrontational and supportive climate in which the girls feel comfortable talking about their experiences and challenges in trying to change their weight-related behaviors. We are in the process of evaluating the New Moves program in a randomized controlled trial with 12 high schools in Minnesota.

CONCLUSION

Obesity and weight bias have been found to be associated with an array of adverse psychosocial consequences in youth. Additional research is needed to further elucidate these associations. In their recent comprehensive review of weight stigmatization in youth, Puhl and Latner (2007) identified a number of key areas for future research, which we outline in Table 4.1.

TABLE 4.1
Summary of Research Areas to Be Addressed
in Weight Stigma Among Youth

Domain	Research areas
Nature or extent of stigma	Longitudinal studies to examine gender differences in weight stigma
	Prospective work to determine whether antifat attitudes change throughout childhood and reasons for potential changes
	Cross-cultural examinations of vulnerability to weight stigma
	Assessment of ethnicity and endorsement of stigma across gender, age, weight
	Examination of relationship between body weight, stigma, and internalization of stigma among overweight youth
	Examination of the formation of attributions about causality of obesity, how attributions influence biased attitudes, whether modification of attributions improves attitudes in youth
	Identification of origins of weight bias and interpersonal differences that influence perceptions of stigma toward youth
	Assessment of discriminatory practices and unfair treatment toward obese youth
	Experimental work to clarify attitude–behavior consistency in weight bias
	Examination of individual differences in the vulnerability to weight bias and its consequences
	Validation of self-report measures of stigmatizing attitudes using corroborative evidence from friends, parents, or teachers
	Examination of possible evolutionary explanations to account for origin of biased beliefs about obesity

(continues)

TABLE 4.1
Summary of Research Areas to Be Addressed
in Weight Stigma Among Youth   *(Continued)*

Domain	Research areas
Sources of stigma	Identification of prevalence, nature, and severity of stigma by educators
	Multiple assessment measures to investigate differential treatment of obese youth in classrooms and educational admissions procedures
	Examination of the nature and impact of stigma communicated by parents
	Identification of whether weight stigma extends to parents of obese youth
	Identification of other sources of bias toward obese youth (e.g., health care providers, coaches, camp counselors, employers)
Psychosocial consequences of stigma	Examination of whether stigma increases vulnerability to low self-esteem, depression, and body dissatisfaction
	Examination of stigma as a moderator for adverse psychosocial outcomes
	Assessment of the effect of different forms of weight-based victimization on emotional, social, and academic outcomes for obese youth of different ages and ethnicity
	Assessment of whether reductions in weight stigma improve social, emotional, and academic outcomes among obese youth
	Identification of protective factors that buffer obese children from negative consequences of stigma
	Examination of whether different types and sources of weight stigma have a differential impact on psychosocial outcomes
Academic and socioeconomic status outcomes	Identification of whether weight bias is a possible mediator of the relationship between obesity and economic and academic attainment
	Prospective investigation of the relationship between cognitive and academic ability, weight, and socioeconomic status
	Testing methods for reducing weight bias in education settings, with dependent variables that include academic as well as psychological outcomes
Eating behaviors	Investigation of the effects of verbal commentary or teasing on eating behavior using prospective investigations
	Investigation of stigmatizing parental behaviors and their effect on disordered eating
	Experimental research investigating the possible influence of negative commentary on eating behavior or binge eating

TABLE 4.1
Summary of Research Areas to Be Addressed
in Weight Stigma Among Youth   *(Continued)*

Domain	Research areas
Physical health and stigma	Examination of pathways that weight stigma affects physical health
	Identification of how weight stigma affects stress levels in youth
	Examination of how chronic exposure to weight stigma influences cardiovascular health outcomes in youth
	Assessment of whether health outcomes are worse for children who experience stigma at higher levels of obesity
	Identification of whether obese children who internalize stigma are at increased risk for health problems versus those who do not internalize
	Examination of health implications of weight stigma for children of different genders, ages, and ethnic backgrounds
	Examination of whether different types and sources of weight stigma have differential effects on cardiovascular reactivity of children
Stigma reduction	Identification and assessment of strategies to reduce weight-based victimization by peers in school settings
	Integration and testing of stigma-reduction interventions as part of existing school-based diversity curricula
	Assessment of stigma-reduction methods to improve attitudes in educators
	Identification of ways to reduce weight stigma among parents, family members, and other caregivers of obese youth
	Examination of effectiveness of different message frames for stigma reduction efforts (e.g., inducing empathy, education about causes of obesity, awareness of inaccuracy of stereotypes)
	Identification of most effective modes of delivery for stigma reduction messages (e.g., videos, presentations, reading materials, Internet)
	Assessment of effectiveness of Internet-based interventions to reduce bias
	Assessment of the effect of stigma reduction on emotional, social, health, and academic outcomes in youth

Note. Adapted from "Stigma, Obesity, and the Health of the Nation's Children," by R. M. Puhl and J. D. Latner, 2007, *Psychological Bulletin, 133*, p. 573. Copyright 2007 by the American Psychological Association.

Although additional research is needed to further elucidate these associations, interventions aimed at preventing obesity and its psychosocial consequences are needed now. Peers, school staff, health care professionals, and parents all serve as important targets for interventions aimed at decreasing weight stigmatization and increasing support for youth dealing with weight-related issues. In addition, intervention studies, evaluating the impact of obesity prevention and treatment in youth, need to include strong and comprehensive evaluation designs to assess program impact and to ensure that there are no unintentional harmful effects on psychosocial outcomes. It is crucial to develop and widely implement interventions that simultaneously strive to prevent both obesity and weight bias among children and adolescents.

REFERENCES

Amy, N. K., Aalborg, A., Lyons, P., & Keranen, L. (2006). Barriers to routine gynecological cancer screening for White and African-American obese women. *International Journal of Obesity (London)*, 30, 147–155.

Anesbury, T., & Tiggemann, M. (2000). An attempt to reduce negative stereotyping of obesity in children by changing controllability beliefs. *Health Education Research*, 15, 145–152.

Bagley, C., Conklin, D., Isherwood, R., Pechiulis, D., & Watson, L. (1989). Attitudes of nurses toward obesity and obese patients. *Perceptual and Motor Skills*, 68, 954.

Bell, S. K., & Morgan, S. B. (2000). Children's attitudes and behavioral intentions toward a peer presented as obese: Does medical explanation for the obesity make a difference? *Journal of Pediatric Psychology*, 25, 137–145.

Brylinsky, J. A. (1994). The identification of body build stereotypes in young children. *Journal of Research in Personality*, 28, 170–181.

Chambliss, H. O., Finley, C. E., & Blair, S. N. (2004). Attitudes toward obese individuals among exercise science students. *Medicine and Science in Sports and Exercise*, 36, 468–474.

Crick, N. R. (1997). Engagement in gender normative versus nonnormative forms of aggression: Links to social-psychological adjustment. *Developmental Psychology*, 33, 610–617.

DeJong, W. (1993). Obesity as a characterological stigma: The issue of responsibility and judgments of task performance. *Psychological Reports*, 73, 963–970.

Eisenberg, M. E., Neumark-Sztainer, D., Haines, J., & Wall, M. (2006). Weight-teasing and emotional well-being in adolescents: Longitudinal findings from Project EAT. *Journal of Adolescent Health*, 38, 675–683.

Eisenberg, M. E., Neumark-Sztainer, D., & Story, M. (2003). Associations of weight-based teasing and emotional well-being among adolescents. *Archives of Pediatrics and Adolescent Medicine*, 157, 733–738.

Falkner, N. H., Neumark-Sztainer, D., Story, M., Jeffery, R. W., Beuhring, T., & Resnick, M. D. (2001). Social, educational and psychological correlates of weight status in adolescents. *Obesity Research, 9*, 32–42.

Fontaine, K. R., Faith, M. S., Allison, D. B., & Cheskin, L. J. (1998). Body weight and health care among women in the general population. *Archives of Family Medicine, 7*, 381–384.

Foster, G. D., Wadden, T. A., Makris, A. P., Davidson, D., Sanderson, R. S., Allison, D. B., & Kessler, A. (2003). Primary care physicians' attitudes about obesity and its treatment. *Obesity Research, 11*, 1168–1177.

Frank, A. (1993). Futility and avoidance—medical professionals in the treatment of obesity. *JAMA, 269*, 2132–2133.

French, S. A., Story, M., & Perry, C. L. (1995). Self-esteem and obesity in children and adolescents: A literature review. *Obesity Research, 3*, 479–490.

Fulkerson, J. A., Strauss, J., Neumark-Sztainer, D., Story, M., & Boutelle, K. N. (2007). Correlates of psychosocial well-being among overweight adolescents: The role of the family. *Journal of Consulting and Clinical Psychology, 75*, 181–186.

Galen, B. R., & Underwood, M. K. (1997). A developmental investigation of social aggression among children. *Developmental Psychology, 33*, 589–600.

Greenleaf, C., Chambliss, H., Rhea, D. J., Martin, S. B., & Morrow, J. R., Jr. (2006). Weight stereotypes and behavioral intentions toward thin and fat peers among White and Hispanic adolescents. *Journal of Adolescent Health, 39*, 546–552.

Griffiths, L. J., Wolke, D., Page, A. S., Horwood, J. P., and the ALSPAC Study Team. (2006). Obesity and bullying: Different effects for boys and girls. *Archives of Disease in Childhood, 91*, 121–125.

Haines, J. (2005). *V.I.K. (Very Important Kids): Pilot program to impact weight-related teasing, dieting, internalization of media messages, and body satisfaction among children.* Unpublished doctoral dissertation, University of Minnesota, Minneapolis.

Haines, J., Neumark-Sztainer, D., Perry, C. L., Hannan, P. J., & Levine, M. P. (2006). V.I.K. (Very Important Kids): A school-based program designed to reduce teasing and unhealthy weight-control behaviors. *Health Education Research, 21*, 884–895.

Haines, J., Neumark-Sztainer, D., & Thiel, L. (2007). Addressing weight-related issues in an elementary school: What do students, parents, and school staff recommend? *Eating Disorders, 15*, 5–21.

Hayden-Wade, H. A., Stein, R. I., Ghaderi, A., Saelens, B. E., Zabinski, M. F., & Wilfley, D. E. (2005). Prevalence, characteristics, and correlates of teasing experiences among overweight children vs. non-overweight peers. *Obesity Research, 13*, 1381–1392.

Hebl, M. R., & Xu, J. (2001). Weighing the care: Physicians' reactions to the size of a patient. *International Journal of Obesity and Related Metabolic Disorders, 25*, 1246–1252.

Hebl, M. R., Xu, J., & Mason, M. F. (2003). Weighing the care: Patients' perceptions of physician care as a function of gender and weight. *International Journal of Obesity and Related Metabolic Disorders, 27*, 269–275.

Hesketh, K., Wake, M., & Waters, E. (2004). Body mass index and parent-reported self-esteem in elementary school children: Evidence for a causal relationship. *International Journal of Obesity and Related Metabolic Disorders, 28*, 1233–1237.

Irving, L. M. (2000). Promoting size acceptance in elementary school children: The EDAP Puppet Program. *Eating Disorders, 8*, 221–232.

Janssen, I., Craig, W. M., Boyce, W. F., & Pickett, W. (2004). Associations between overweight and obesity with bullying behaviors in school-aged children. *Pediatrics, 113*, 1187–1194.

Latner, J. D., & Stunkard, A. J. (2003). Getting worse: The stigmatization of obese children. *Obesity Research, 11*, 452–456.

Lawson, M. C. (1980). Development of body build stereotypes, peer ratings, and self-esteem in Australian children. *Journal of Psychology, 104*, 111–118.

Lovell, P. (2001). *Stand tall, Molly Lou Melon*. New York: Putnam.

Maroney, D., & Golub, S. (1992). Nurses' attitudes toward obese persons and certain ethnic groups. *Perceptual and Motor Skills, 75*, 387–391.

McArthur, L., & Ross, J. (1997). Attitudes of registered dietitians toward personal overweight and overweight clients. *Journal of the American Dietetic Association, 97*, 63–66.

McVey, G., & Tweed, S. (2005, April). *Healthy Schools–Healthy Kids: Findings from an RCT of a comprehensive eating disorder prevention program in middle school*. Paper presented at the Academy for Eating Disorders International Conference on Eating Disorders, Montreal, Quebec, Canada.

Mellin, A. E., Neumark-Sztainer, D., Story, M., Ireland, M., & Resnick, M. D. (2002). Unhealthy behaviors and psychosocial difficulties among overweight youth: The potential impact of familial factors. *Journal of Adolescent Health, 31*, 145–153.

Neumark-Sztainer, D. (1998). Qualitative interviews with overweight adolescent girls [Unpublished data]. University of Minnesota, Minneapolis.

Neumark-Sztainer, D. (2005). *"I'm, like, SO fat!": Helping your teen make healthy choices about eating and exercise in a weight-obsessed world*. New York: Guilford Press.

Neumark-Sztainer, D., Falkner, N., Story, M., Perry, C., Hannan, P. J., & Mulert, S. (2002). Weight-teasing among adolescents: Correlations with weight status and disordered eating behaviors. *International Journal of Obesity and Related Metabolic Disorders, 26*, 123–131.

Neumark-Sztainer, D., & Haines, J. (2004). Psychosocial and behavioral consequences of obesity. In J. Thompson (Ed.), *Handbook of eating disorders and obesity* (pp. 349–371). New York: Wiley.

Neumark-Sztainer, D., Harris, T., & Story, M. (1999). Beliefs and attitudes about obesity among teachers and school health care providers working with adolescents. *Journal of Nutrition Education, 31*, 3–9.

Neumark-Sztainer, D., Sherwood, N. E., Coller, T., & Hannan, P. J. (2000). Primary prevention of disordered eating among pre-adolescent girls: Feasibility and short-term impact of a community based intervention. *Journal of the American Dietetic Association, 100,* 1466–1473.

Neumark-Sztainer, D., Story, M., & Faibisch, L. (1998). Perceived stigmatization among overweight African American and Caucasian adolescent girls. *Journal of Adolescent Health, 23,* 264–270.

Neumark-Sztainer, D., Story, M., Faibisch, L., Ohlson, J., & Adamiak, M. (1999). Issues of self-image among overweight African American and Caucasian adolescent girls: A qualitative study. *Journal of Nutrition Education, 31,* 311–320.

Neumark-Sztainer, D., Story, M., French, S., Hannan, P., Resnick, M., & Blum, R. W. (1997). Psychosocial concerns and health compromising behaviors among overweight and non-overweight adolescents. *Obesity Research, 5,* 237–249.

Neumark-Sztainer, D., Story, M., Hannan, P. J., Perry, C. L., & Irving, L. M. (2002). Weight-related concerns and behaviors among overweight and non-overweight adolescents: Implications for preventing weight-related disorders. *Archives of Pediatrics and Adolescent Medicine, 156,* 171–178.

Neumark-Sztainer, D., Story, M., Hannan, P. J., & Rex, J. (2003). New Moves: A school-based obesity prevention program for adolescent girls. *Preventive Medicine, 37,* 41–51.

Oberrieder, H., Walker, R., Monroe, D., & Adeyanju, M. (1995). Attitude of dietetics students and registered dietitians toward obesity. *Journal of the American Dietetic Association, 95,* 914–916.

O'Brien, K. S., Hunter, J. A., & Banks, M. (2007). Implicit anti-fat bias in physical educators: Physical attributes, ideology and socialization. *International Journal of Obesity (London), 31,* 308–314.

Olson, C. L., Schumaker, H. D., & Yawn, B. P. (1994). Overweight women delay medical care. *Archives of Family Medicine, 3,* 888–892.

Pearce, M. J., Boergers, J., & Prinstein, M. J. (2002). Adolescent obesity, overt and relational peer victimization, and romantic relationships. *Obesity Research, 10,* 386–393.

Pesa, J. A., Syre, T. R., & Jones, E. (2000). Psychosocial differences associated with body weight among female adolescents: The importance of body image. *Journal of Adolescent Health, 26,* 330–337.

Phillips, R. G., & Hill, A. J. (1998). Fat, plain, but not friendless: Self-esteem and peer acceptance of obese pre-adolescent girls. *International Journal of Obesity, 22,* 287–293.

Piran, N. (1999). Eating disorders: A trial of prevention in a high-risk school setting. *Journal of Primary Prevention, 20,* 75–90.

Price, J., Desmond, S., Krol, R., Snyder, F., & O'Connell, J. (1987). Family practice physicians' beliefs, attitudes, and practices regarding obesity. *American Journal of Preventive Medicine, 3,* 339–345.

Puhl, R. M., & Latner, J. D. (2007). Stigma, obesity, and the health of the nation's children. *Psychological Bulletin, 133,* 557–580.

Richardson, S. A., Goodman, N., Hastorf, A. H., & Dornbusch, S. M. (1961). Cultural uniformity in reaction to physical disabilities. *American Sociological Review, 26,* 241–247.

Robinson, S. (2006). Victimization of obese adolescents. *Journal of School Nursing, 22,* 201–206.

Schwartz, M. B., Chambliss, H. O., Brownell, K. D., Blair, S. N., & Billington, C. (2003). Weight bias among health professionals specializing in obesity. *Obesity Research, 11,* 1033–1039.

Sigelman, C. K. (1991). The effect of causal information on peer perceptions of children with physical problems. *Journal of Applied Developmental Psychology, 12,* 237–253.

Smolak, L., Levine, M. P., & Schermer, F. (1998). A controlled evaluation of an elementary school primary prevention program for eating problems. *Journal of Psychosomatic Research, 44,* 339–353.

Sobal, J., Nicolopoulos, V., & Lee, J. (1995). Attitudes about overweight and dating among secondary students. *International Journal of Obesity, 19,* 376–381.

Staffieri, J. R. (1967). A study of social stereotype in children. *Journal of Perspectives in Social Psychology, 7,* 101–107.

Strauss, C. C. (1985). Personal and interpersonal characteristics associated with childhood obesity. *Journal of Pediatric Psychology, 10,* 337–343.

Strauss, R. S. (2000). Childhood obesity and self-esteem. *Pediatrics, 105,* e15.

Strauss, R. S., & Pollack, H. A. (2003). Social marginalization of overweight children. *Archives of Pediatrics and Adolescent Medicine, 157,* 746–752.

Teachman, B. A., Gapinski, K. D., Brownell, K. D., Rawlins, M., & Jeyaram, S. (2003). Demonstrations of implicit anti-fat bias: The impact of providing causal information and evoking empathy. *Health Psychology, 22,* 68–78.

Turnbull, J. D., Heaslip, S., & McLeod, H. A. (2000). Pre-school children's attitudes to fat and normal male and female stimulus figures. *International Journal of Obesity and Related Metabolic Disorders, 24,* 1705–1706.

Weiner, B., Perry, R., & Magnusson, J. (1988). An attributional analysis of reactions to stigmas. *Journal of Personality and Social Psychology, 55,* 738–748.

Wigton, R. S., & McGaghie, W. C. (2001). The effect of obesity on medical students' approach to patients with abdominal pain. *Journal of General Internal Medicine, 16,* 262–265.

5

BODY IMAGE IN PEDIATRIC OBESITY

SYLVIA HERBOZO AND J. KEVIN THOMPSON

As obesity has rapidly increased in the past 3 decades, greater attention has been given to its prevalence and potential negative consequences, especially among youth. The adverse effects of obesity on physical health are well documented and often emphasized in recent movements to reduce the high levels of obesity. It has become evident that there are also significant psychosocial consequences that are equally important to highlight, and these factors (e.g., teasing, stigmatization) may have an immediate impact on the individual's functioning. Specifically, one outcome of being overweight or obese, which appears to be related strongly to psychosocial issues, is dissatisfaction with physical appearance. The phrase *body image* has been used to characterize the subjective evaluation of one's appearance (J. K. Thompson, Heinberg, Altabe, & Tantleff-Dunn, 1999). In this chapter, we explore the issue of body image in pediatric obesity.

BODY IMAGE

Children and adolescents are not immune to the weight and shape concerns often expressed by adults. Weight and shape concerns, especially in the form of body dissatisfaction, have been reported during childhood and adolescence (Ricciardelli & McCabe, 2001; Smolak & Levine, 2001). Research suggests that overweight and obese youth are more likely than nonoverweight youngsters to experience such appearance concerns. A recent large population-based study of middle and high school students by Crow, Eisenberg, Story, and Neumark-Sztainer (2006) indicated that both overweight boys (25.2%) and girls (46.5%) had higher levels of body dissatisfaction than did nonoverweight boys (8.6%) and girls (24.8%). Vander Wal and Thelen (2000) found significant differences in concerns about being or becoming overweight as well as body dissatisfaction among children of elementary school age, with overweight children expressing greater weight concerns and body dissatisfaction than average weight children.

The strong association between body image concerns and adiposity is also evident in studies focusing exclusively on girls (Burrows & Cooper, 2002; Striegel-Moore, Schreiber, Crawford, Obarzanek, & Rodin 2000). In a study of high school adolescent girls, J. K. Thompson et al. (2007) found that overweight and obese girls had greater body dissatisfaction than did average weight girls. Using the Eating Disorder Examination for Children (CH-EDE) with girls aged 11 to 12, Burrows and Cooper (2002) reported greater weight and shape concerns in overweight girls than in normal-weight girls. Similar findings based on the CH-EDE have been reported for children as young as 6 (Tanofsky-Kraff et al., 2004).

These elevated rates of body dissatisfaction, particularly among overweight youth, warrant attention. Longitudinal studies (e.g., Holsen, Kraft, & Roysamb, 2001; Stice, 2001; Stice & Bearman, 2001) indicate that low body satisfaction predicts poor psychological functioning and disordered eating behaviors during adolescence. For instance, Stice and Bearman (2001) found low body satisfaction predicted depressive symptoms in adolescent girls. In a study of adolescent girls and boys, Neumark-Sztainer et al. (2006) reported that body dissatisfaction was associated with unhealthy weight control behaviors and binge eating as well as fewer health-promoting behaviors, including physical activity and fruit and vegetable intake. There was also little evidence that body dissatisfaction served as a motivator for engaging in healthy weight management behaviors.

TEASING

As do overweight adults, overweight youth also face weight stigmatization and discrimination that are likely to elicit or contribute to weight and shape concerns. Weight-based teasing is particularly common among children and adolescents and more prevalent for girls and boys with higher body mass indexes (BMIs; Neumark-Sztainer & Haines, 2004; see chap. 4, this volume). Research on weight-based teasing increasingly suggests that this type of interaction can be harmful and have serious consequences for the physical and mental well-being of young people (J. K. Thompson et al., 2007).

Weight-based teasing has been strongly associated with body image problems, disordered eating behaviors, and poor psychological functioning in earlier studies with adults (e.g., Fabian & Thompson, 1989; Stormer & Thompson, 1996; J. K. Thompson & Psaltis, 1988) as well as in more recent studies with adolescents (e.g., Haines, Neumark-Sztainer, Eisenberg, & Hannan, 2006; Neumark-Sztainer, Falkner, et al., 2002). Fabian and Thompson (1989) reported that teasing frequency was significantly related to body satisfaction, eating disturbance, and depression in adolescent girls. More recently, Eisenberg, Neumark-Sztainer, and Story (2003) found that weight-based teasing during adolescence was associated with low body satisfaction, low self-esteem, high depressive symptoms, and suicide ideation and attempts (for further discussion, see chap. 4, this volume).

A covariance structure modeling study by J. K. Thompson, Coovert, and Stormer (1999) indicated that the effect of appearance-related teasing on body image and eating disturbance was mediated by appearance-based comparisons. Body image was also identified as a mediational link between appearance-related teasing and eating disturbance. These findings coincide with those of other covariance structure modeling studies on adolescent girls (e.g., J. K. Thompson, Coovert, Richards, Johnson, & Cattarin, 1995; van den Berg, Wertheim, Thompson, & Paxton, 2002) that suggest appearance-based teasing may lead to the development of body image and eating disturbance.

The potentially long-lasting effects of childhood teasing on body image in adulthood have also been demonstrated. In a sample of college females and males, Gleason, Alexander, and Somers (2000) examined the effects of three types of childhood teasing (competency, weight, and appearance) on self-esteem and body image. They found that more frequent teasing significantly predicted lower self-esteem and poorer body image for both females and males. It is interesting that for females only, teasing about both appearance and competence predicted problems with self-esteem. As did studies with obese samples, Grilo, Wilfley, Brownell, and Rodin (1994) found that greater frequency of weight and size teasing was associated with more negative appearance evaluation and body dissatisfaction in adult obese women. Wardle, Waller, and Fox (2002) also examined teasing in obese women and reported that earlier age of obesity onset was associated with body dissatisfaction and teasing during childhood for both the early onset group (overweight by age 16 per self-report) and the entire sample. (For a review on additional psychological effects of weight-based teasing, see chap. 4, this volume.)

UNHEALTHY WEIGHT CONTROL BEHAVIORS

Given their higher rates of body dissatisfaction, obese children and adolescents may be at risk for using unhealthy weight control methods to quickly attain a more socially acceptable body shape. Dieting and restricting behaviors (e.g., fasting, skipping meals) as well as extreme weight control behaviors (e.g., diet pills, self-induced vomiting, laxatives) have been associated with weight status in adolescent girls and boys (Boutelle, Neumark-Sztainer, Story, & Resnick, 2002; Eisenberg, Neumark-Sztainer, Story, & Perry, 2005; Mellin, Neumark-Sztainer, Story, Ireland, & Resnick, 2002; Neumark-Sztainer et al., 1997; Neumark-Sztainer, Story, Hannan, Perry, & Irving, 2002). In a comparison study of adolescents varying in weight status, Boutelle et al. (2002) found the highest percentages of dieting and extreme weight loss strategies among obese adolescents, which were followed by overweight adolescents and then nonoverweight adolescents. For instance, obese girls and boys reported more dieting (54.5% and 31.3%) and self-induced vomiting (7.6% and 2.9%) than did nonoverweight girls and boys (35.9% and 8.6%, 3.4% and 1.5%, respectively). Eisenberg et al. (2005) also found that adolescent girls with higher BMIs engaged in more unhealthy weight control behaviors than those with lower BMIs. Other studies comparing overweight and average weight children have also shown higher rates of dieting among overweight children (e.g., Crow et al., 2006; Vander Wal & Thelen, 2000).

On the basis of a series of population-based studies with adolescents, Neumark-Sztainer and colleagues have reported that overweight adolescents who have experienced weight-based teasing are more likely to engage in disordered eating behaviors consisting of unhealthy weight control methods (e.g., fasting, self-induced vomiting, laxatives, smoking more cigarettes) and binge eating compared with overweight adolescents who were not teased (Neumark-Sztainer & Haines, 2004). For instance, Neumark-Sztainer, Falkner, et al. (2002) found that approximately 80% of overweight girls and 61.5% of overweight boys were teased frequently about their weight and engaged in unhealthy weight control behaviors. The associations between weight-based teasing and disordered eating behaviors remained statistically significant after adjusting for BMI and sociodemographic characteristics. There is also longitudinal evidence that illustrates the harmful effects of weight-based teasing. Haines, Neumark-Sztainer, Eisenberg, and Hannan (2006) reported that weight-based teasing predicted disordered eating behaviors, including unhealthy weight control methods, frequent dieting, and binge eating at 5-year follow-up with distinct patterns across gender.

As would be expected because of the different body ideals for females and males, dieting behaviors are more common among overweight and obese girls than among boys with the same weight status during preadolescence and adolescence (Boutelle et al., 2002; Crow et al., 2006; Mellin et al., 2002). In fact, the rates of dieting for girls are usually close to double the rates for boys. Neumark-Sztainer et al. (1999) found that 49.3% of overweight girls and 21.5% of overweight boys were dieting while in 7th, 9th, and 11th grades. Similarly, a much higher percentage of obese adolescent girls (52.1%) were dieting than obese boys (31.3%). Mellin et al. (2002) reported that overweight adolescent girls reported higher rates of extreme dieting (10.6%) and skipping breakfast (55%) than overweight adolescent boys (4.2% and 42%, respectively). As with overweight adolescent girls, overweight girls of elementary school age are more likely to diet than overweight boys of similar ages (Vander Wal & Thelen, 2000). The same patterns have been found for more problematic weight loss behaviors, such as self-induced vomiting and laxatives (Boutelle et al., 2002; Field et al., 1999; Neumark-Sztainer et al., 1999).

RISK FACTOR MODELS OF BODY IMAGE
AND EATING DISTURBANCE

Various potential risk factors have been proposed for the onset of body image and eating disturbance. In a recent meta-analysis, Stice (2002) examined the literature on potential risk factors and maintenance factors for eating pathology. All of the longitudinal and experimental studies identified in this analysis dealt with bulimic symptoms, binge eating, or eating disorder composites. The results of Stice's meta-analysis indicated that body dissatisfaction, negative affect, perfectionism, and impulsivity are risk factors for eating pathology. With regard to body image, elevated body mass is considered to be a risk factor for body dissatisfaction. It was also found that perceived sociocultural pressure to be thin and thin-ideal internalization are causal risk factors for both body dissatisfaction and eating pathology. Negative affect is viewed as a causal risk factor for body dissatisfaction and caloric intake.

Only a few sociocultural models have been developed to explain how identified risk factors promote eating and body image disturbance. The dual pathway model of bulimic pathology (Stice, Nemeroff, & Shaw, 1996) and tripartite influence model of body image and eating disturbance (J. K. Thompson, Heinberg, et al., 1999) have received empirical support. Stice (1994) proposed the dual pathway model of bulimia pathology in which body mass, internalization of the thin ideal, perceived pressure to be thin, body dissatisfaction, dietary restraint, and negative affect interact to predict bulimic symptoms. Stice et al. (1996) tested the dual pathway model of bulimia nervosa in a sample of female undergraduate students using structural equation modeling and found that the model accounted for 71% of the variance in bulimic symptoms. In addition, the dual pathway model was examined by Stice et al. in female high school and college students who were classified as either bulimic, subclinical bulimic, or control participants. The findings provided additional evidence for the dual pathway model and demonstrated that it applies to diagnostic levels of bulimia. Using latent variable modeling, Stice, Shaw, and Nemeroff (1998) tested the dual pathway model in a longitudinal study with high school adolescent girls. The results indicated that as hypothesized by the model, dietary restraint and negative affect mediated the effects of body mass, perceived pressure, ideal body internalization, and body satisfaction on future bulimic symptoms. Dietary restraint and negative affect were shown to directly predict bulimic symptoms.

The tripartite influence model (Thompson et al., 1999) argues that peer, parental, and media influences lead to body image and eating problems through the social processes of appearance comparisons and thin-ideal internalization. It is proposed that the three sources of influence result in appearance comparisons and thin-ideal internalization, which in turn contribute to the onset of body dissatisfaction. The subsequent body dissatisfaction is hypothesized to promote restriction and bulimic symptoms. This integration of sociocultural factors with individuals' psychological factors has been identified as one of the unique contributions of this model (Stice, 2001). Initial work on the tripartite model was conducted by van den Berg et al. (2002) with a sample of adults. More recently, the model has received support in two samples of adolescent girls (Keery, van den Berg, & Thompson, 2004; Shroff & Thompson, 2006) and a sample of Japanese college students (Yamamiya, Shroff, & Thompson, 2008).

One limitation of this area is that the studies often have not specifically evaluated the role of weight status as a predictor in the models tested. At times, BMI may be tested as a variable, but seldom are groups formed to determine whether models fit better or worse for overweight, obese, or normal-weight participants. In addition, few risk models have tested males or individuals of diverse ethnicities.

ASSESSMENT AND TREATMENT OF BODY IMAGE DISTURBANCE

A great deal of work has focused on the creation and evaluation of assessment strategies, prevention programs, and treatments for body image disturbance in adolescence (e.g., Stice, 2002; J. K. Thompson & Smolak, 2001; see also Yanover & Thompson, 2009); however, the prevention and treatment programs have largely focused on issues of body image related to eating disturbances and not on the particular issues that overweight and obese adolescent youth encounter. In this section, we detail some of the specific measurement strategies and prevention and treatment options useful for understanding or altering body image concerns.

As noted throughout this volume, several specific assessment strategies have been developed for the measurement of some component of body image disturbance in youth (see also Yanover & Thompson, 2009). These include such measures as the Eating Disorder Inventory–Body Dissatisfaction subscale, the Multidimensional Body Self-Relations Questionnaire: Appearance Evaluation subscale, and various figural rating scales. Table 5.1 lists the most common scales plus some of the more recently developed scales. When assessing body image in overweight or obese youngsters, it is important to take a broad conceptual approach, including measures that tap into the weight dimension as well as other aspects of body image, such as muscularity concerns and dissatisfaction (Cafri & Thompson, 2007).

Prevention and treatment strategies have only recently begun to deal with the particular issues faced by overweight and obese youngsters. In contrast (see Levine & Harrison, 2004; Levine & Smolak, 2009), there has been a wealth of work in the area of evaluation of prevention programs for children and adolescents at risk for eating disorders. These programs, such as the dissonance induction program developed by Stice and colleagues (e.g., Stice & Hoffman, 2004), generally focus on strategies to increase body size acceptance by challenging societal pressures for thinness. Clearly, these types of approaches are not appropriate for objectively overweight or obese youth.

Few recent programs have emerged that address the body image issues confronted in pediatric obesity. Neumark-Sztainer and colleagues (see chap. 4, this volume) have developed a program called New Moves that not only has ways to help girls function in a society focused on thinness but also deals with positive change in physical activity and eating behaviors to improve weight status and overall health and to help girls avoid unhealthy weight control behaviors. In addition, Neumark-Sztainer and colleagues have developed Very Important Kids (V.I.K.), a multilevel ecological program designed to prevent teasing (Haines, Neumark-Sztainer, Eisenberg, & Hannan, 2006; Haines, Neumark-Sztainer, Perry, et al., 2006). This program has been found to reduce teasing at a targeted school compared with a matched comparison school (Haines, Neumark-Sztainer, Eisenberg, & Hannan, 2006; Haines, Neumark-Sztainer, Perry, et al., 2006). V.I.K. also increased students' self-efficacy in regard to changing weight-teasing norms and reduced negative peer norms and behavior about weight (for a more detailed review of V.I.K., see chap. 4, this volume). It is clear that more work needs to be done at the school, individual, and family levels to reduce body dissatisfaction in overweight and obese children and adolescents.

CONCLUSION AND DIRECTIONS FOR FUTURE RESEARCH

Recent studies have clearly illustrated the negative psychosocial and behavioral consequences of obesity in youth. Children and adolescents with higher BMIs, especially girls, are more likely to experience weight and shape concerns and weight-related stigmatization, placing them at greater risk for dieting and unhealthy weight control behaviors, in addition to other health-compromising behaviors. These findings highlight the need for obesity interventions to screen for disordered eating behaviors and other

TABLE 5.1

Frequently Used Body Image Measures

Type and name of instrument	Author(s)	Description	Reliability	Standardization sample
		Figural ratings		
None given	Collins (1991)	7 male child and 7 female child figure drawings ranging from thin to obese	TR (3 days): self = .71; ideal/self = .59; ideal/ other child = .38	1,118 preadolescent children, mean age = 7.97
Kid's Eating Disorder Survey	Childress, Brewerton, Hodges, and Jarrell (1993)	8 male and 8 female figure drawings	TR (4 months): .83 for entire survey; not given for figures only	3,129 children, Grades 5–8
Body Rating Scale	Sherman, Iacono, and Donnelly (1995)	2 scales; 9 female figures representing preadolescent (11) and adolescent (17) females	Interrater	108 females, age 11, and 102 females, age 17
Contour Drawing Rating Scale	M. A. Thompson and Gray (1995)	9 male and 9 female figures	TR (2–14 weeks): current = .77–.84; ideal = .65–.78	1,056 females, ages 11–14 (Wertheim, Paxton, & Tilgner, 2004)
Body Image Assessment– Children	Veron-Guidry and Williamson (1996)	2 scales; 9 silhouettes of male and females, children and preadolescents	TR (immediate): current = .94, ideal = .93; (1 week): current = .79, current/ ideal = .67	22 males and females ages 8–10 100 males and females, ages 8–10
Body Image Scale	Sands, Tricker, Sherman, Armatas, and Maschette (1997)	7 side profiles of prepubescent boys and girls	TR (3 months): current = .56; (6 months): current = .40	26 females and 35 males, ages 10–12
Body Mass Index Silhouette Matching Test	Peterson, Ellenberg, and Crossan (2003)	27-item interval scale with 4 gender-specific figures to anchor	TR: males current = .79, females current = .85; males ideal = .83, females ideal = .82	75 females and 140 males, Grades 9–12

Subjective and attitudinal measures

Measure	Citation	Description	Reliability	Sample
Eating Disorder Inventory (EDI, EDI-2, and EDI-3) Body Dissatisfaction Scale	Garner, Olmstead, and Polivy (1984); Garner (1991); Garner (2004)	9-item subscale assesses feeling about satisfaction with body size; items are 6-point, forced choice; reading level is 5th grade	IC: Adolescents (11–18) Females: .91 Males: .86 Children (8–10) Females: .84 Males: .72	196 males and 414 females, ages 11–18 (Shore & Porter, 1990) 95 males and 109 females, ages 8–10 (Wood, Becker, & Thompson, 1996)
Body Shape Questionnaire (BSQ)	Cooper, Taylor, Cooper, and Fairburn (1987)	34-item self-report questionnaire about the phenomenal experience of "feeling fat"; scored on a 6-point Likert scale from never (1) to always (6)	No data	81 eating disordered patients age 18 and under (Bunnell, Cooper, Hertz, & Shenker, 1992)
Multidimensional Body Self-Relations Questionnaire (MBSRQ) Appearance Evaluation subscale	Cash (2008)	Global measure of satisfaction with your looks	IC = .76 TR (4–5 weeks): .89	393 Grade 9 females, mean age = 14.5 (Banasiak, Wertheim, Koerner, & Voudouris, 2000)
Eating Disorders Inventory for Children (EDI-C). Body Dissatisfaction Scale	1. Garner (1991) 2. Thurfjell, Edlund, Arinell, Hägglöf, and Engström (2003; Swedish translation)	Same 9-item subscale as EDI. Wording was rephrased for Grades 1–2 reading level	1. No data 2. IC: ED group = .91, Control group = .92	1. None 2. 211 girls and 9 boys diagnosed with ED, ages 13–17; 2,073 girls, Grades 7–12
Body Image Questionnaire	Huddy, Nieman, and Johnson (1993)	20 items on a 3-point Likert scale from agree (1) to disagree (3)	TR (6 weeks): .97	69 boys, 43 girls, ages 12–14 (Duncan, Woodfield, O'Neill, & Al-Nakeeb, 2002)
Body Satisfaction Scale	Siegel, Yancey, Aneshensel, and Schuler (1999)	Participants rate satisfaction with four aspects of pubertal development using response scale ranging from 1 (very dissatisfied) to 4 (very satisfied)	IC: .73 to .80	469 males and 407 females, ages 12 to 17

(continues)

TABLE 5.1

Frequently Used Body Image Measures *(Continued)*

Type and name of instrument	Author(s)	Description	Reliability	Standardization sample
Body Esteem Scale for Adolescents and Adults	Mendelson, Mendelson, and White (2001)	3-factor scale assessing weight, appearance, and attribution	IC: weight = .94; appearance = .92; attribution = .81	763 females and 571 males, ages 12–25
Body Uneasiness Test (BUT)	Cuzzolaro, Vetrone, Marano, and Garfinkel (2006)	34 items assessing body shape or weight dissatisfaction, avoidance, compulsive control behaviors, feelings of detachment and another 37 items assessing concern about specific body parts or functions	IC = .79–.90 for BUT-A; .69–.90 for BUT-B TR (1 week) = BUT-A .71–.91 (nonclinical); .80–.94 (clinical): BUT-B .78–.94 (nonclinical); .68–.92 (clinical)	IC: 491 females and 40 males (clinical); 2,017 females and 1,257 males (nonclinical), ages 13–80 TR: subset from initial sample of 32 females and 6 males (clinical); 56 females and 24 males (nonclinical)
Muscularity measures				
Drive for Muscularity— Body Image subscale	1. McCreary and Sasse (2000) 2. Cafri, van den Berg, and Thompson (2006)	7-item subscale assessing satisfaction with appearance related to a muscular physique	1. IC = .84 (whole scale) 2. IC = .90	1. 101 girls and 96 boys, ages 16–24 2. 269 boys ages 13–18
Muscle Appearance Satisfaction Scale	Mayville, Williamson, White, Netmeyer, and Drab (2002)	5-subscale measure assessing symptoms of muscle dysmorphia	Adolescents (13–18) all ICs > .70	269 boys ages 13–18 (Cafri, van den Berg, & Thompson, 2006)

Note. TR = test–retest; IC = internal consistency.

health-compromising behaviors, provide education on healthy eating and physical activity, and focus on discussing body and self-acceptance issues. It is imperative that interventions not place too much emphasis on dieting behaviors in the context of weight management, which may unintentionally elicit behaviors that lead to unhealthy eating behaviors. Interventions should also be culturally sensitive as they promote healthy eating in minority groups with higher rates of obesity.

Furthermore, the higher rates of disordered eating behaviors among overweight and obese youth compared with average-weight youth indicate that eating problems can co-occur (see chap. 6, this volume). It is also evident that individuals may transition from one eating problem to another, which is likely due to the shared risk factors among weight-related disorders. Given the findings that obesity and eating disorders are not mutually exclusive, researchers in this area have argued for collaboration between the two fields to address these weight-related disorders (Neumark-Sztainer, 2003; Neumark-Sztainer, Levin, & Paxton, 2006). Clinicians should attempt to reduce the potential stigmatizing nature of obesity in prevention and intervention work with youth. No evidence indicates that any type of stigmatizing experience, teasing, or commentary regarding weight has any positive influence on motivation to reduce weight or to engage in effective weight-reduction strategies. No evidence indicates that enhancing body image dissatisfaction has any positive effects on weight loss strategies or outcomes. Puhl and Latner (2007) recently conducted a comprehensive review of the issue of weight stigmatization in youth, and their article is essential reading for anyone conducting research or working clinically in the area of pediatric obesity (for a review of Puhl and Latner's work, see chap. 4, this volume). As concluded by Puhl and Latner, there are many different avenues for future research in the area of weight stigmatization and its negative effects in pediatric obesity.

REFERENCES

Banasiak, S. J., Wertheim, E. H., Koerner, J., & Voudouris, N. J. (2001). Test–retest reliability and internal consistency of a variety of measures of dietary restraint and body concerns in a sample of adolescent girls. *International Journal of Eating Disorders, 29*, 85–89.

Boutelle, K., Neumark-Sztainer, D., Story, M., & Resnick, M. (2002). Weight control behavior among obese, overweight, and nonoverweight adolescents. *Journal of Pediatric Psychology, 27*, 531–540.

Bunnell, D., Cooper, P., Hertz, S., & Schenker, I. (1992). Body shape concerns among adolescents. *International Journal of Eating Disorders, 11*, 79–83.

Burrows, A., & Cooper, M. (2002). Possible risk factors in the development of eating disorders in overweight adolescent girls. *International Journal of Obesity, 26*, 1268–1273.

Cafri, G., & Thompson, J. K. (2007). Measurement of the muscular ideal. In J. K. Thompson & G. Cafri (Eds.), *The muscular ideal: Psychological, social and medical perspectives* (pp. 107–120). Washington, DC: American Psychological Association.

Cafri, G., van den Berg, P., & Thompson, J. K. (2006). Pursuit of muscularity in adolescent boys: Relations among biopsychosocial variables and clinical outcomes. *Journal of Clinical Child and Adolescent Psychology, 35*, 283–291.

Cash, T. F. (2008). *The users' manuals for the Multidimensional Body–Self Relations Questionnaire, Situational Inventory.* Available at http://www.body-image.com

Childress, A. C., Brewerton, T. D., Hodges, E. L., & Jarrell, M. P. (1993). The Kids' Eating Disorders Survey (KEDS): A study of middle school students. *Journal of the American Academy of Child and Adolescent Psychiatry, 32*, 843–850.

Collins, M. E. (1991). Body figure perceptions and preferences among preadolescent children. *International Journal of Eating Disorders, 10*, 199–208.

Cooper, P. J., Taylor, M. J., Cooper, Z., & Fairburn, C. G. (1987). The development and validation of the Body Shape Questionnaire. *International Journal of Eating Disorders, 6*, 485–494.

Crow, S., Eisenberg, M. E., Story, M., & Neumark-Sztainer, D. (2006). Psychosocial and behavioral correlates of dieting among overweight and nonoverweight adolescents. *Journal of Adolescent Health, 38*, 569–574.

Cuzzolaro, M., Vetrone, G., Marano, G., & Garfinkel, P. E. (2006). The Body Uneasiness Test (BUT): Development and validation of a new body image assessment scale. *Eating and Weight Disorders, 11*, 1–13.

Duncan, M. J., Woodfield, L. A., O'Neill, S. J., & Al-Nakeeb, Y. (2002). Test–retest stability of body image scores in a sample of 12- to 14-yr.-olds. *Perceptual and Motor Skills, 95*, 1007–1012.

Eisenberg, M. E., Neumark-Sztainer, D., & Story, M. (2003). Associations of weight-based teasing and emotional well-being among adolescents. *Archives of Pediatrics & Adolescent Medicine, 137*, 733–738.

Eisenberg, M. E., Neumark-Sztainer, D., Story, M., & Perry, C. (2005). The role of social norms and friends' influences on unhealthy weight-control behaviors among adolescent girls. *Social Science and Medicine, 60*, 1165–1173.

Fabian, L. J., & Thompson, J. K. (1989). Body image and eating disturbance in young females. *International Journal of Eating Disorders, 8*, 63–74.

Field, A. E., Camargo, C. A., Jr., Taylor, C. B., Berkey, C. S., Frazier, A. L., Gillman, M. W., & Colditz, G. A. (1999). Overweight, weight concerns, and bulimic behaviors among girls and boys. *Journal of the American Academy of Child and Adolescent Psychiatry, 38*, 754–760.

Garner, D. (1991). *Manual for the Eating Disorder Inventory–2 (EDI-2).* Odessa, FL: Psychological Assessment Resources.

Garner, D. (2004). *Manual for the Eating Disorder Inventory–3 (EDI-3).* Odessa, FL: Psychological Assessment Resources.

Garner, D. M., Olmstead, M. P., & Polivy, J. (1983). Development and validation of a multidimensional eating disorder inventory for anorexia nervosa and bulimia. *International Journal of Eating Disorders, 2*(2) 15–34.

Gleason, J. H., Alexander, A. M., & Somers, C. L. (2000). Later adolescents' reactions to three types of childhood teasing: Relations with self-esteem and body image. *Social Behavior and Personality, 28,* 471–480.

Grilo, C. M., Wilfley, D. E., Brownell, K. D., & Rodin, J. (1994). Teasing, body image, and self-esteem in a clinical sample of obese women. *Addictive Behavior, 19,* 443–450.

Haines, J., Neumark-Sztainer, D., Eisenberg, M. E., & Hannan, P. J. (2006). Weight teasing and disordered eating behaviors in adolescents: Longitudinal findings from Project EAT (Eating Among Teens). *Pediatrics, 117,* 209–215.

Haines, J., Neumark-Sztainer, D., Perry, C. L., Hannan, P. J., & Levine, M. P. (2006). V.I.K. (Very Important Kids): A school-based program designed to reduce teasing and unhealthy weight-control behaviors. *Health Education Research, 21,* 884–895.

Holsen, I., Kraft, P., & Roysamb, E. (2001). The relationship between body image and depressed mood in adolescence: A 5-year longitudinal panel study. *Journal of Health Psychology, 6,* 613–627.

Huddy, D. C., Nieman, D. C., & Johnson, R. L. (1993). Relationship between body image and percent body fat among college male varsity athletes and non-athletes. *Perceptual and Motor Skills, 77,* 851–857.

Keery, H., van den Berg, P., & Thompson, J. K. (2004). An evaluation of the tripartite influence model of body dissatisfaction and eating disturbance with adolescent girls. *Body Image, 1,* 237–251.

Levine, M. P., & Smolak, L. (2009). Recent developments and promising directions in the prevention of negative body image and disordered eating in children and adolescents. In L. Smolak & J. K. Thompson (Eds.), *Body image, eating disorders, and obesity in youth* (2nd ed., pp. 215–240). Washington, DC: American Psychological Association.

Levine, M. P., & Harrison, K. (2004). Media's role in the perpetuation and prevention of negative body image and disordered eating. In J. K. Thompson (Ed.), *Handbook of eating disorders and obesity* (pp. 695–717). Hoboken, NJ: Wiley.

Mayville, S. B., Williamson, D. A., White, M. A., Netmeyer, R., & Drab, D. L. (2002). Development of the Muscle Appearance Satisfaction Scale: A self-report measure for the assessment of muscle dysmorphia symptoms. *Assessment, 9,* 351–360.

McCreary, D. R., & Sasse, D. K. (2000). An exploration of the drive for muscularity in adolescent boys and girls. *Journal of American College Health, 48,* 297–304.

Mellin, A. E., Neumark-Sztainer, D., Story, M., Ireland, M., & Resnick, M. (2002). Unhealthy behaviors and psychosocial difficulties among overweight adolescents: The potential impact of familial factors. *Journal of Adolescent Health, 31,* 145–153.

Mendelson, B. K., Mendelson, M. J., & White, D. R. (2001). Body-Esteem Scale for adolescents and adults. *Journal of Personality Assessment, 76,* 90–106.

Neumark-Sztainer, D. (2003). Obesity and eating disorders prevention: An integrated approach? *Adolescent Medicine: State of the Art Reviews, 14,* 159–173.

Neumark-Sztainer, D., Falkner, N., Story, M., Perry, C., Hannan, P. J., & Mulert, S. (2002). Weight-teasing among adolescents: Correlations with weight status and disordered eating behaviors. *International Journal of Obesity and Related Metabolic Disorders, 26,* 123–131.

Neumark-Sztainer, D., & Haines, J. (2004). Psychosocial and behavioral consequences of obesity. In J. K. Thompson (Ed.), *Handbook of eating disorders and obesity* (pp. 349–371). Hoboken, NJ: Wiley.

Neumark-Sztainer, D., Levin, M. P., & Paxton, S. (2006). Prevention of body dissatisfaction and disordered eating: What next? *Eating Disorders, 14,* 265–285.

Neumark-Sztainer, D., Story, M., Falkner, N. H., Beuhring, T., & Resnick, M. D. (1999). Sociodemographic and personal characteristics of adolescents engaged in weight loss and weight/muscle gain behaviors: Who is doing what? *Prevention Medicine, 28,* 40–50.

Neumark-Sztainer, D., Story, M., French, S., Hannan, P., Resnick, M., & Blum, R. W. (1997). Psychosocial concerns and health-compromising behaviors among overweight and nonoverweight adolescents. *Obesity Research, 5,* 237–249.

Neumark-Sztainer, D., Story, M., Hannan, P. J., Perry, C. L., & Irving, L. M. (2002). Weight-related concerns and behaviors among overweight and nonoverweight adolescents. *Archives of Pediatrics & Adolescent Medicine, 156,* 171–178.

Neumark-Sztainer, D., Wall, M., Guo, J., Story, M., Haines, J., & Eisenberg, M. (2006). Obesity, disordered eating, and eating disorders in a longitudinal study of adolescents: How do dieters fare 5 years later? *Journal of the American Dietetic Association, 106,* 559–568.

Peterson, M., Ellenberg, D., & Crossan, S. (2003). Body-image perceptions: Reliability of a BMI-based silhouette-matching test. *American Journal of Health Behavior, 27,* 355–363.

Puhl, R. M., & Latner, J. D. (2007). Stigma, obesity and the health of the nation's children. *Psychological Bulletin, 133,* 557–580.

Ricciardelli, L. A., & McCabe, M. P. (2001). Children's body image concerns and eating disturbance: A review of the literature. *Clinical Psychology Review, 21,* 325–344.

Sands, R., Tricker, J., Sherman, C., Armatas, C., & Maschette, W. (1997). Disordered eating patterns, body image, self-esteem, and physical activity in preadolescent school children. *International Journal of Eating Disorders, 21,* 159–166.

Sherman, D. K., Iacono, W. G., & Donnelly, J. M. (1995). Development and validation of body rating scales for adolescent females. *International Journal of Eating Disorders, 18,* 327–333.

Shore, R. A., & Porter, J. E. (1990). Normative and reliability data for 11 to 18 year olds on the Eating Disorder Inventory. *International Journal of Eating Disorders, 9,* 201–207.

Shroff, H., & Thompson, J. K. (2006). Peer influences, body-image dissatisfaction, eating dysfunction and self-esteem in adolescent girls. *Journal of Health Psychology, 11,* 533–551.

Siegel, J. M., Yancey, A. K., Aneshensel, C. S., & Schuler, R. (1999). Body image, perceived pubertal timing, and adolescent mental health. *Journal of Adolescent Health, 25,* 255–266.

Smolak, L., & Levine, M. P. (2001). Body image in children. In J. K. Thompson & L. Smolak (Eds.), *Body image, eating disorders, and obesity in youth: Assessment, prevention, and treatment* (pp. 41–66). Washington, DC: American Psychological Association.

Stice, E. (1994). Review of the evidence for a sociocultural model of bulimia nervosa and an exploration of the mechanisms of action. *Clinical Psychology Review, 14*, 633–661.

Stice, E. (2001). Risk factors for eating pathology: Recent advances and future directions. In R. H. Striegel-Moore & L. Smolak (Eds.), *Eating disorders: Innovative directions in research and practice* (pp. 51–74). Washington, DC: American Psychological Association.

Stice, E. (2002) Risk and maintenance factors for eating pathology: A meta-analytic review. *Psychological Bulletin, 128*, 825–848.

Stice, E., & Bearman, S. K. (2001). Body-image and eating disturbances prospectively predict increases in depressive symptoms in adolescent girls: A growth curve analysis. *Developmental Psychology, 37*, 597–607.

Stice, E., & Hoffman, E. (2004) Eating disorder prevention programs. In J. K. Thompson (Ed.), *Handbook of eating disorders and obesity* (pp. 33–57). Hoboken, NJ: Wiley.

Stice, E., Nemeroff, C., & Shaw, H. E. (1996). Test of the dual pathway model of bulimia nervosa: Evidence for dietary restraint and affect regulation mechanisms. *Journal of Social and Clinical Psychology, 15*, 340–363.

Stice, E., Shaw, H., & Nemeroff, C. (1998). Dual pathway model of bulimia nervosa. Longitudinal support for dietary restraint and affect-regulation mechanisms. *Journal of Social and Clinical Psychology, 17*, 129 149.

Stormer, S. M., & Thompson, J. K. (1996). Explanations of body image disturbance. A test of maturational status, negative verbal commentary, social comparison, and sociocultural hypotheses. *International Journal of Eating Disorders, 19*, 193–202.

Striegel-Moore, R. H., Schreiber, G. B., Lo, A., Crawford, P., Obarzanek, E., & Rodin, J. (2000). Eating disorder symptoms in a cohort of 11 to 16 year old Black and White girls: The NIH Growth and Health Study. *International Journal of Eating Disorders, 27*, 49–66.

Tanofsky-Kraff, M., Yanovski, S. Z., Wifley, D. E., Marmarosh, C., Morgan, C. M., & Yanovski, J. A. (2004). Eating-disordered behaviors, body fat, and psychopathology in overweight and normal-weight children. *Journal of Counseling and Clinical Psychology, 72*, 53–61.

Thompson, J. K., Coovert, M. D., Richards, K. J., Johnson, S., & Cattarin, J. (1995). Development of body image, eating disturbance, and general psychological functioning in female adolescents: Covariance structure modeling and longitudinal investigations. *International Journal of Eating Disorders, 18*, 221–236.

Thompson, J. K., Coovert, M. D., & Stormer, S. M. (1999). Body image, social comparison, and eating disturbance: A covariance structure modeling investigation. *International Journal of Eating Disorders, 26*, 43–51.

Thompson, J. K., Heinberg, L., Altabe, M., & Tantleff-Dunn, S. (1999). *Exacting beauty: Theory, assessment, and treatment of body image disturbance*. Washington, DC: American Psychological Association.

Thompson, J. K., & Psaltis, K. (1988). Multiple aspects and correlates of body figure ratings: A replication and extension of Fallon and Rozin (1985). *International Journal of Eating Disorders, 7*, 813–818.

Thompson, J. K., Shroff, H., Herbozo, S., Cafri, G., Rodriguez, J., & Rodriguez, M. (2007). Relations among multiple peer influences, body dissatisfaction, eating disturbance and self-esteem: A comparison of overweight/obese and average weight adolescent girls. *Journal of Pediatric Psychology, 1*, 1–6.

Thompson, J. K., & Smolak, L. (Eds.). (2001). *Body image, eating disorders, and obesity in youth*. Washington, DC: American Psychological Association.

Thompson, M. A., & Gray, J. J. (1995). Development and validation of a new body-image assessment scale. *Journal of Personality Assessment, 64*, 258–269.

Thurfjell, B., Edlund, B., Arinell, H., Hägglöf, B., & Engström, I. (2003). Psychometric properties of Eating Disorder Inventory for Children (EDI-C) in Swedish girls with and without a known eating disorder. *Eating and Weight Disorders, 8*, 296–303.

van den Berg, P., Wertheim, E. H., Thompson, J. K., & Paxton, S. J. (2002). Development of body image, eating disturbance, and general psychological functioning in adolescent females: A replication using covariance structure modeling in an Australian sample. *International Journal of Eating Disorders, 32*, 46–51.

Vander Wal, J. S., & Thelen, M. H. (2000). Eating and body image concerns among obese and average-weight children. *Addictive Behaviors, 25*, 775–778.

Veron-Guidry, S., & Williamson, D. A. (1996). Development of a body image assessment procedure for children and preadolescents. *International Journal of Eating Disorders, 20*, 287–293.

Wardle, J., Waller, J., & Fox, E. (2002). Age of onset and body dissatisfaction in obesity. *Addictive Behaviors, 27*, 561–573.

Wertheim, E. H., Paxton, S. J., & Tilgner, L. (2004). Test–retest reliability and construct reliability of Contour Drawing Rating Scales scores in a sample of early adolescent girls. *Body Image, 1*, 199–205.

Wood, K. C., Becker, J. A., & Thompson, J. K. (1996). Body image dissatisfaction in preadolescent children. *Journal of Applied Developmental Psychology, 17*, 85–100.

Yamamiya, Y., Shroff, H., & Thompson, J. K. (2008). The tripartite influence model of body image and eating disturbance: A replication with a Japanese sample. *International Journal of Eating Disorders, 41*, 88–91.

Yanover, T., & Thompson, J. K. (2009). Assessment of body image in children and adolescents. In L. Smolak & J. K. Thompson (Eds.), *Body image, eating disorders, and obesity in youth* (2nd ed., pp. 177–192). Washington, DC: American Psychological Association.

6

PSYCHOLOGICAL COMORBIDITY AND CHILDHOOD OVERWEIGHT

REBECCA M. RINGHAM, MICHELE D. LEVINE,
AND MARSHA D. MARCUS

There has been substantial interest in the relationship between psychiatric and psychological problems and pediatric obesity. In large part, study of the links between pediatric obesity and psychiatric disorders has followed from the well-described associations between adult weight problems and mood or eating disorders. Given that the prevalence and severity of pediatric obesity are increasing, there has been a corresponding increase in research concerning relationships among mood disorders, eating disorders, and pediatric weight problems.

Although the *Diagnostic and Statistical Manual of Mental Disorders* (4th ed., text revision; *DSM–IV–TR*; American Psychiatric Association [APA], 2000) defines numerous disorders of childhood, the available information on the association of psychiatric disorders specific to childhood obesity is limited, with one exception. Literature detailing a relationship between mental retardation, particularly the Prader-Willi syndrome, and obesity (e.g., Brambilla et al., 1997; Theodoro, Talebizadeh, & Butler, 2006) is substantial. However, consideration of this research is beyond the scope of the present chapter. Thus, in this chapter, we selectively review the literature on the co-occurrence of pediatric obesity and psychiatric disorders or psychological distress with a particular focus on depression and eating disorders. We first review the relationship between obesity and depression in childhood. Next, we consider studies of the relationship between obesity and eating disorders in childhood, particularly binge eating disorder, and we highlight the relationships among depression, binge eating, and weight. Finally, we briefly note the literature pertaining to the relationship between attention-deficit/hyperactivity disorder (ADHD) and childhood obesity and the relationship between quality of life and childhood obesity and present recommendations for addressing lifestyle change in obese children with psychological comorbidities.

It is important to clarify several terms used in the chapter. First, we use the term *children* to refer to youth between the ages of 8 and 18 years. The majority of the literature has evaluated psychiatric symptoms and obesity among children ages 8 years and above, and rates of obesity increase as children age (Ogden et al., 2006). However, a number of studies have examined psychological comorbidities of obesity in children younger than 8 years, and we note any relevant studies of children in this age range. Second, definitions of pediatric obesity as well as terms to describe excess adiposity in children have varied over time. Historically, childhood *obesity* usually was characterized by a percentage over ideal body weight using various reference charts. In 2000, with the publication of pediatric growth charts using body mass index (BMI), *overweight* (the term *obesity* was not used) was defined as at or above the 95th percentile of BMI for age and sex, and *at risk for overweight* was defined as greater than or equal to the 85th percentile and less than the 95th percentile for age and sex (Kuczmarski et al., 2000; Kuczmarski & Flegal, 2000).

Recently, the American Medical Association (AMA; 2007) provided definitions for pediatric overweight and obesity. According to these guidelines, *obesity* in children is defined as greater than or equal to the 95th percentile of BMI for age and sex, or BMI exceeding 30 (whichever is smaller). A child is considered *overweight* if his or her BMI is greater than or equal to the 85th percentile, but less than the 95th percentile, for age and sex. Given that many of the articles reviewed in the following sections were published before the use of BMI percentiles or the AMA guidelines, studies using all of the described definitions are included in the chapter.

DEPRESSION AND CHILDHOOD OBESITY

The well-established relationship between overweight and depression among adults has stimulated research on the relationship between depression and obesity among children. In adults, cross-sectional data show elevated rates of depression among overweight women seeking weight loss and in community samples of overweight individuals when compared with nonoverweight individuals (Carpenter, Hasin, Allison, & Faith; 2000; Istavan, Zavela, & Weidner, 1992). There also is evidence that depression and other negative mood states can precipitate overeating (Davis, Freeman, & Garner, 1988; Lingswiler, Crowther, & Stephens, 1989) and thereby contribute to weight gain. In other investigations, depression has been found to predict the onset of overweight (Hasler et al., 2004) and overweight to predict the onset of depression (Roberts, Deleger, Strawbridge, & Kaplan, 2003). Thus, among adults, depression and depressive symptoms have been implicated as both a cause and consequence of overweight. Alternatively, depression and overweight run in families, and it may be that some individuals have a shared diathesis for both disorders.

Less is known about the relationship between depression and obesity in children. There is a common belief that obese children are unhappy with their weight and experience more psychological distress and depression than do normal-weight children (Wadden & Stunkard, 1987), but it also is possible that depression leads to obesity in some children. However, as reviewed later in this chapter, the relationship between depression and obesity in children depends on the nature of the sample, the degree of obesity of the child, and other factors.

Clinical Versus Community Samples

The majority of studies examining the co-occurrence of depression and obesity in children have assessed depressive symptoms or clinical depression among children seeking weight loss treatment. Generally, children seeking treatment for obesity report higher levels of depressive symptoms than do normal-weight children (Britz et al., 2000; Erermis et al., 2004; Zeller, Roehrig, Modi, Daniels, & Inge, 2006). However, it is unclear whether children seeking treatment for obesity report more symptoms than obese children who do not present for weight loss treatment. Some studies have found statistically significant differences in depressive symptoms between treatment-seeking and non-treatment-seeking obese children (Sheolow, Hassink, Wallace, & DeLancey, 1993; Wallace, Sheslow, & Hassink, 1993), whereas other studies have not (Britz et al., 2000; Erermis et al., 2004). Clearly, not all obese children who seek weight loss treatment are depressed, and several factors may confound examination of depressive symptoms among obese children seeking weight loss treatment.

One factor that may influence the relationship between obesity and depression in clinical samples is that distressed people (or in this case, parents of distressed children) are likelier than those who are not distressed to seek treatment. Compared with population norms, rates of psychiatric disorders are higher among individuals who seek treatment relative to those who do not (Vila et al., 2004). Thus, it may be that obese children appear to have higher rates of depression than do other children because of the high rate of psychiatric disorders among those who seek treatment. Although obese children in clinical samples generally report more depression than do children in non-clinical samples, it is unclear whether they report more depression than children who present for treatment for other medical or psychiatric illnesses. To address this question, Vila et al. (2004) documented psychiatric problems, including depression and depressive symptoms, in 155 children seeking treatment for obesity and compared these rates with those reported by normal weight insulin-dependent diabetic children seen in an outpatient diabetes management clinic. Compared with children with diabetes, overweight children had significantly higher scores on questionnaires assessing behavioral problems and anxiety and had more overall psychological distress. However, rates of depressive symptoms were similar among children seeking either medical or obesity treatment. This study suggests that obese children seeking weight loss treatment may be at increased risk for behavioral problems and anxiety compared with children with a high-burden medical illness, but levels of depression appear to be similar among medically ill and obese children. Nonetheless, additional research is needed to draw definitive conclusions about rates of obesity-related distress in treatment-seeking children.

Although there appear to be elevated levels of depressive symptoms among obese children presenting for weight loss treatment, the relationship between depression and obesity among community samples of children is unclear. Several studies have found that overweight children report more depressive symptoms than do normal weight children (e.g., Erickson, Robinson, Haydel, & Killen, 2000; Swallen, Reither, Haas, & Meier, 2005), but others have not observed elevated rates of depressive symptoms in overweight children (e.g., Lamertz, Jacobi, Yassouridis, Arnold, & Henkel, 2002; Wardle, Williamson, Johnson, & Edwards, 2006). Thus, the association between obesity and depression among children depends on the sample studied. Obese children who present for weight loss treatment appear to be more depressed than obese children who are not seeking weight loss treatment, but the relationship between obesity and depression among obese children in general is equivocal.

Depression and Severity of Obesity

Research on the association between depression and severity of obesity in children has followed from research that has been conducted among adults. In adults, despite differences in the nature of the samples and assessments of depression used, the relationship between depression and overweight is strongest among the most obese individuals (Onyike, Crum, Lee, Lyketsos, & Eaton, 2003; Sullivan et al., 1993). Overweight children who seek weight loss treatment are often heavier than non-treatment-seeking overweight children (Zeller et al., 2006), but as noted earlier, several studies have found similar levels of depression in clinical and nonclinical samples of overweight children. Erermis et al. (2004) examined psychopathology among obese treatment-seeking children, obese children not seeking treatment, and nonobese children and found that higher depression scores were related to higher BMI. In summary, the severity of childhood obesity appears to be associated with increased comorbid psychopathology and psychological distress.

Other Factors Affecting the Relationship Between Depression and Childhood Obesity

A number of studies have evaluated the relationships among demographic variables, mood, and weight in adults and children. For example, Friedman and Brownell (1995) identified sex, socioeconomic status (SES), and ethnicity as potential moderators of the relationship between obesity and depression in adults. As reviewed later in this chapter, although there is less evidence evaluating the role of these factors in relation to obesity in children, they may have an impact on the rates of depression observed in obese children.

The relationship between depression and obesity differs for adult men and women (Istavan et al., 1992), and there is evidence that overweight girls report more depression than do overweight boys (e.g., Falkner et al., 2001). Anderson, Cohen, Naumova, and Must (2006) found that anxiety disorders and depression were associated with obesity in females but not males. However, another longitudinal study (Mustillo et al., 2003) found increased levels of depressive symptoms in chronically overweight boys but not in girls. Still another study (Wardle et al., 2006) failed to find any sex differences in the associations between overweight and depressive symptoms. Thus, the interaction of sex, mood, and weight in children remains unclear.

There is a strong association between obesity and depression among Caucasian adults with higher SES (Ross, 1994). However, studies have failed to find significant differences in the association between depression and overweight in different ethnic groups among children (Wardle et al., 2006), although it is widely known that minority children are at increased risk for obesity (Kimm et al., 2001). However, as Wardle and Cooke (2005) noted, the role of SES and ethnicity on mood and weight in children has not been sufficiently evaluated.

Aberrant eating behaviors and attitudes also may influence the relationship between depression and weight in children. Increased eating and weight concerns are associated with obesity in adults, and numerous studies have suggested that these cognitions are related to mood and may influence the relationship between depression and obesity in children. For example, in Erickson et al.'s (2000) study of third graders, after controlling for the degree of concern about weight, BMI was no longer significantly associated with depressive symptoms in girls. Similarly, Needham and Crosnoe (2005) found that BMI was associated with depressive symptoms among children in a school-based sample, but after controlling for dieting behaviors, this relationship was no longer significant. Finally, a number of studies have documented the relationship among binge eating, depression, and obesity in children, and as discussed later in this chapter, the findings suggest that the relationship between weight and depression may be strongly influenced by the child's eating behaviors. Thus, it appears that as in adults, increased eating and weight concerns are associated with obesity in children.

Teasing also has been implicated as a factor in the association between depression and weight in children. Many overweight children report that they have been teased frequently about their weight (Neumark-Sztainer et al., 2002), and there is a positive relationship between a history of weight-related teasing and depressive symptoms (Eisenberg, Neumark-Sztainer, & Story, 2003; Roth, Coles, & Heimberg, 2002). Eisenberg, Neumark-Sztainer, Haines, and Wall (2006) demonstrated that students who reported being teased about their weight tended to have more depressive symptoms 5 years later than did their peers who were not teased. However, the exact nature of the relationship among teasing, weight, and depression is unclear. It may be that obese children are more likely to be teased about their weight and subsequently to become depressed. Alternatively, children who are teased may become depressed and subsequently gain weight.

In summary, a number of factors may affect the relationship between childhood obesity and depression. Given that findings documenting a differential association between depression and obesity for boys and girls or for children of different ethnicities and SES backgrounds have not been replicated consistently, the precise roles of sex, SES, ethnicity, and other factors in pediatric obesity require elucidation. In contrast, consistent findings suggest that a history of teasing or concerns about weight or eating increase the likelihood of an association between obesity and depression in children.

Longitudinal Relationships Between Depression and Childhood Obesity

Although the cross-sectional studies reviewed in the foregoing have documented relationships between depressive symptoms and obesity in children, it is unclear whether obesity contributes to the subsequent development of depression or vice versa. To consider the direction of the association between obesity and depression, we review evidence suggesting a contribution of depressive symptoms to the development of obesity, followed by evidence documenting the relationship between childhood obesity and the subsequent development of depression.

Some studies have found that children who report depressive symptoms at baseline have larger increases in BMI 1 to 5 years later compared with children who do not report depressive symptoms at baseline (Goodman & Whitaker, 2002; Richardson et al., 2003). Stice, Presnell, Shaw, and Rohde (2005) assessed a number of psychological variables including depressive symptoms and behavioral variables among girls 11 to 15 years old and followed them over 4 years. They reported that depressive symptoms was one of several factors that predicted overweight onset.

In another study, Pine, Goldstein, Wolk, and Weissman (2001) examined the relationship between major depression in childhood and BMI in adulthood. Using a sample that included individuals who were of normal weight or at risk for overweight as children and who had either major depressive disorder or no psychiatric disorder, these investigators found that participants diagnosed with childhood major depression had a twofold increased risk of overweight as adults compared with nondepressed children. Moreover, duration of childhood depression predicted adult BMI.

However, childhood depression is not the only psychological factor implicated in the development of obesity, and there are relationships between a number of childhood psychiatric disorders and adult obesity (Anderson et al., 2006). For example, Pine, Cohen, Brook, and Coplan (1997) found that symptoms of conduct disorders during adolescence, rather than depression, were associated with overweight in early adulthood. Mustillo et al. (2003) examined overweight-related trajectories from childhood to adolescence in Caucasian children 9 to 16 years old from the general population. Chronic overweight in childhood was associated with oppositional defiant disorder in boys and girls and depressive disorders in boys only. Thus, it may be that general childhood psychopathology rather than depression per se contributes to the onset, development, or maintenance of obesity. Furthermore, the mechanisms by which psychiatric disorders lead to obesity are unclear. It may be that children with difficulties in self-regulation in general tend to overeat or that there may be a shared and overlapping diathesis for psychiatric and weight disorders.

Other longitudinal studies have been designed to examine the role of obesity in the development of depression. Herva et al. (2006) completed a longitudinal study of body weight and depression and found that overweight at 14 years of age was associated with depressive symptoms at 31 years of age. Females who were overweight at both 14 and 31 years of age were at greatest risk for depression. However, the authors did not measure depression at baseline, and it is unknown what impact baseline symptoms may have had on depression at 31 years of age. In contrast, Stice and Bearman (2001) found that elevated body mass in adolescent girls did not predict depression 20 months or 4 years later. Similarly, after controlling for baseline depression, Goodman and Whitaker (2002) found no association between overweight and the development of depression 1 year later. Rather, as noted earlier, they found childhood depression to be a risk factor for the development of overweight. Thus, it appears that being obese as a child is not strongly associated with the development of depression.

EATING DISORDERS AND CHILDHOOD OBESITY

Binge eating is defined as the consumption of an unusually large amount of food in a circumscribed period of time coupled with a feeling of loss of control over eating (Fairburn & Wilson, 1993; Spitzer et al., 1992; Stunkard, 1959). Binge eating is included in the diagnostic criteria for bulimia nervosa and binge eating disorder in the *DSM–IV–TR* (APA, 2000), but the two disorders are distinct. *Bulimia nervosa* is characterized by persistent, frequent binge eating; regular and extreme compensatory behaviors (e.g., purging, laxative misuse); and overconcern about body shape and weight (APA, 2000). In contrast, *binge eating disorder* (BED) is characterized by recurrent binge eating without the regular compensatory behaviors that are seen in bulimia nervosa (APA, 2000).

Binge eating is associated with considerable medical and psychiatric morbidity (J. G. Johnson, Spitzer, & Williams, 2001; Newman et al., 1996) and has a robust relationship to overweight in adults (de Zwann et al., 1994; Smith, Marcus, Lewis, Fitzgibbon, & Schreiner, 1998). Adult individuals who binge eat are likelier to be obese than are nonbinge eaters, and individuals with BED are more likely to report a history of childhood overweight than are individuals with other eating disorders (Fairburn et al., 1998). Studies of the relationship between binge eating and obesity in children have followed from the association observed among adults.

However, because children differ in important ways from adults, we first discuss the definition of binge eating in children, followed by a review of the relevant literature on the relationship of binge eating with overweight in children. The variability in reported rates of binge eating in obese children is wide, and the identification and classification of childhood eating disturbances remains challenging (Rosen, 2003). Specifically, it is often difficult to diagnose and categorize eating disorders in general, and this is more difficult in children because of the variability in children's emotional and cognitive development and daily eating behaviors. In light of recent arguments for more flexible, developmentally appropriate criteria for eating disorders in children (Bryant-Waugh, 2006), attention to key behaviors of eating disorders in children is needed (Marcus & Kalarchian, 2003). Thus, some studies have attempted to target a specific aspect of binge eating, namely loss of control, as a marker of aberrant eating in children.

The majority of what is known about the relationship between binge eating and overweight in children comes from studies of children seeking treatment for obesity and studies of school-based samples of children. Despite varying definitions and assessments of binge eating, there is consensus that a subgroup of children report binge eating and loss of control, and that binge eating and loss of control in children, as in adults, are associated with obesity. Furthermore, increasing evidence suggests that binge eating in children is associated with depression and that mood, eating, and weight are interrelated in children as well as in adults.

Binge Eating and Childhood Obesity

Several studies have documented that children seeking treatment for obesity are at increased risk for aberrant eating behaviors (Decaluwe & Braet, 2003; Glasofer et al., 2007; Isnard et al., 2003; Levine, Ringham, Kalarchian, Wisniewski, & Marcus, 2006). These elevated rates of binge eating are consistent with data from adults seeking weight loss treatment that have shown that approximately 30% of adults seeking treatment for overweight at university centers report binge eating (e.g., Marcus, Moulton, & Greeno, 1995). Similarly, studies of community samples of children have found that heavier children report more binge eating and purging behaviors than do normal weight children (Ackard, Neumark-Sztainer, Story, & Perry, 2003; Field et al., 1999; Lamerz et al., 2005; Shisslak et al., 1998). Thus, treatment-seeking and non-treatment-seeking obese children appear to have higher rates of binge eating and purging behaviors than do their normal weight peers.

There also is preliminary evidence that loss of control may be the most salient aspect of aberrant eating in children (Marcus & Kalarchian, 2003), and several studies have documented a positive association between loss of control over eating and obesity. For example, using an interview technique to assess eating behaviors, Tanofsky-Kraff et al. (2004) examined eating disorder pathology in overweight and normal weight children aged 6 to 13 years. Eating episodes involving loss of control over eating were more prevalent in overweight children and were associated with increased adiposity and eating disorder cognitions. Morgan et al. (2002) also evaluated loss of control over eating in overweight children ages 6 to 10 years and found that 33.1% of children reported loss of control over eating and that 5.3% met BED criteria. Children who reported loss of control over eating had significantly higher BMIs than those who did not. Moreover, after controlling for BMI, children with episodes of loss of control reported more anxiety, negative mood, depressive symptoms, body dissatisfaction, and weight and shape concerns than children with no loss of control. Thus, children endorsing loss of control over their eating also have reported significant psychological symptomatology, including symptoms of depression, and are more likely to be obese than children who do not report loss of control over eating.

The relationships among binge eating, depression, and obesity that have been documented in adults also are evident in children. In clinical and community samples, children reporting binge eating have been heavier and are more likely to report eating disorder cognitions, depressive symptoms, and other psychological problems (Decaluwe & Braet, 2003; Isnard et al., 2003; Tanofsky-Kraff et al., 2004). Furthermore, there is evidence that binge eating and obesity are heritable conditions, and there is modest overlap in the genetic risk factors that increase liability to these conditions (Bulik, Sullivan, & Kendler, 2003). However, it is unclear whether children who are depressed binge eat and become obese or if obese children become depressed and binge eat.

Longitudinal Relationships Between Eating Disorders and Childhood Obesity

Studies in adults have shown that binge eating is a risk factor for obesity (McGuire, Wing, Klem, Lang, & Hill, 1999; Stice, Agras, & Hammer, 1999). The converse also appears to be true—that obesity is a risk factor for binge eating in adults (e.g., Fairburn et al., 1998). Evidence from two longitudinal studies of binge eating and obesity in children suggests that the relationship may be reciprocal. Tanofsky-Kraff et al. (2006) examined psychological predictors of body fat gain among children ages 6 to 12 years. At a baseline assessment, participants were weighed; measured using dual-energy X-ray absorptiometry; and completed a number of self-report questionnaires assessing depressive symptoms, dieting, bulimia nervosa, binge eating, and eating attitudes. The children were followed for an average of 4.2 years, and changes in body fat were documented. Binge eating and dieting predicted increases in body fat. Neither depressive symptoms nor disturbed eating attitudes were significant predictors of increases in body fat. In contrast, among a large sample of adolescent girls followed for 5 years, self-reported depressive symptoms, but not binge eating symptoms, predicted overweight onset (Stice et al., 2005).

Thus, the results from the two studies to date that have examined mood, binge eating, and weight in children over a period of time lead to differing conclusions. In one study, binge eating, but not depression, was associated with obesity, whereas in the other study, depressive symptoms, but not binge eating, were associated with obesity. It may be that differences in age and sex in the respective samples explain conflicting findings. Specifically, the adolescent girls in the Stice et al. (2005) study may be more similar to adults than to younger children. Moreover, as mentioned previously, some evidence suggests that sex may affect the relationship between mood and weight gain such that depressive symptoms are more likely to be related to obesity among girls than boys. Finally, differences in the assessment of mood and eating behaviors may have affected results. Tanofsky-Kraff et al. (2006) relied on a self-report questionnaire to document binge behaviors and depressive symptoms, whereas Stice et al. used an interview method to determine depressive symptoms and binge behaviors. Interview measures of loss of control over eating are more stringent than are self-report measures. Thus, differences in the prevalence of binge eating among children in the two studies may be due to the assessment method. Although the specifics conflict, these findings highlight that obesity is related to both binge eating and depression, and it is likely that obesity, mood, and binge eating interact over time.

ATTENTION-DEFICIT/HYPERACTIVITY DISORDER AND CHILDHOOD OBESITY

Several studies have examined childhood obesity and ADHD. Children with ADHD may be at increased risk for obesity as a result of fewer opportunities to engage in structured sport activities, social isolation, or unusual dietary patterns (Curtin, Bandini, Perrin, Tybor, & Must, 2005). Furthermore, impulsive behavior is a symptom of ADHD, conduct disorder, and oppositional defiant disorder. Given the relationship between impulsivity and binge eating (Bulik, Sullivan, Weltzin, and Kaye, 1995; Vitousek & Manke, 1994), the impulsivity among children with externalizing disorders may contribute to overeating, which leads to the development of obesity in children. Animal, genetic, and neuroimaging studies suggest that the dopaminergic system plays a role in both the biology of ADHD and the reward system of food-seeking behavior (Holtkamp et al., 2004). Thus, factors that are believed to contribute to children's ADHD symptoms may also affect the neurobiology of reward, increasing the reinforcing properties of food and resulting in increased food intake.

In general, findings concerning the co-occurrence of ADHD and obesity in children are mixed. Some studies have found that the prevalence of at-risk-for-overweight and overweight in children with ADHD does not appear to be higher than in age-matched reference populations (e.g., Curtin et al., 2005), whereas others have documented an increased risk for overweight in children with ADHD (Holtkamp et al., 2004). Agranat-Meged et al. (2005) examined comorbidity between childhood obesity and ADHD among children hospitalized for severe obesity. Among 26 children, 57.7% had ADHD (compared with 10% of the general population for same school age group). Thus, as highlighted previously, treatment-seeking samples of obese children have displayed higher prevalence rates of psychological comorbidities including ADHD, but the relationship of ADHD to obesity has been less clear among children who do not present for weight loss treatment.

QUALITY OF LIFE AND CHILDHOOD OBESITY

Quality of life in relation to health or disease is defined as the subjective impact of these conditions on physical, mental, and social well-being (Testa & Simonson, 1996), and there are several studies examining the relationship between health-related quality of life and obesity in children. In community studies of obese versus nonobese children, differences in quality of life are few (e.g., Pinhas-Hamiel et al., 2006). However, compared with their normal weight peers, overweight children seeking treatment for weight have reported decreased quality of life in most domains (Pinhas-Hamiel et al., 2006). In fact, some have suggested that the effects of obesity on quality of life in children are comparable to those observed among children with cancer (Schwimmer, Burwinkle, & Varni, 2003).

Quality of life among children is negatively related to degree of obesity, with heavier children experiencing a lower quality of life on some but not all domains. For example, Williams, Wake, Hesketh, Maher, and Waters (2005) found differences across BMI groups for physical and social domains but not for school and emotional domains. Swallen et al. (2005) also found significant differences among BMI groups for general health and functional limitations but not for psychosocial domains including school and social functioning, self-esteem, and depression. Thus, as is the case with regard to the relationship between depression and binge eating and severity of obesity, heavier children appear to be at greater risk for decreased quality of life, particularly in the domains of physical and functional health.

RECOMMENDATIONS FOR LIFESTYLE INTERVENTIONS FOR CHILDHOOD OBESITY

Given that depression, aberrant eating, potentially ADHD, and quality of life are related to pediatric obesity among children who present for weight loss treatment, it is important to examine the potential implications of the associations between psychiatric problems and weight loss in children. In adults, treatment of overweight often leads to a decrease in depression (Dymek, le Grange, Neven, & Alverdy, 2001; Stunkard, Faith & Allison, 2003). However, the mechanism for changes in mood is unclear, and weight loss interventions may have a direct impact on mood or an indirect effect via weight loss.

As in adults, behavioral interventions targeting weight loss in children appear to have a beneficial impact on mood (e.g., Epstein, Paluch, Saelens, Ernst, & Wilfley, 2001). Butryn and Wadden (2005) reviewed the literature on the effects of dieting on eating behavior and psychological status in children. Overall, the authors reported that weight loss programs for overweight children were associated with significant improvements in psychosocial status, including depression. For example, Levine, Ringham, Kalarchian, Wisniewski, and Marcus (2001) evaluated the efficacy of a family-based behavioral intervention for severe pediatric obesity. Children who completed the program reported significant improvements in depression and other psychological factors. These psychosocial improvements were maintained at follow-up despite a tendency to regain weight following the end of treatment. Thus, family-based behavioral weight management interventions appear to have a positive benefit on depression among children, regardless of their impact on longer-term weight loss maintenance.

Although less is known regarding the effects of weight loss treatment on binge eating in children, there has been concern that weight loss programs may influence the development of binge eating and purging behaviors in children. To date, these concerns have not been substantiated. Butryn and Wadden (2005) reviewed the literature on the effects of dieting on eating behaviors in children and concluded that weight loss programs do not increase eating disorder behaviors and attitudes in children and adolescents. Indeed, one study demonstrated that moderately overweight adolescents who successfully restricted dietary intake reported significant decreases in bulimic symptoms compared with weight-matched participants who did not successfully restrict intake (Stice, Martinez, Presnell, & Groesz, 2006).

Thus, the recommendations for lifestyle interventions among obese children with co-occurring psychological disorders are few. For the majority of children, difficulties with mood or binge eating likely are not contraindications for family-based behavioral intervention. If an obese child reports significant depressive symptoms or binge eating behaviors, consideration of targeted interventions addressing mood and problematic eating behaviors may be indicated. Healthy eating and physical activity are recommended for all children and may have particular benefits for children with emotional problems.

Nevertheless, clinicians may want to assess problem eating in children. Modified criteria for BED in children younger than 14 years have been proposed (Marcus & Kalarchian, 2003), and these criteria have received preliminary research support (Shapiro et al., 2007; Tanofsky-Kraff et al., 2007). Specifically, inclusion criteria include (a) recurrent episodes of binge eating characterized by food seeking in the absence of hunger and a sense of lack of control over eating; (b) binge episodes associated with one or more of the following: food seeking in response to negative affect, food seeking as a reward, and sneaking or hiding food; and (c) symptom duration of at least 3 months. Exclusion criteria are that eating is not associated with the regular use of inappropriate compensatory behaviors and does not occur exclusively during the course of anorexia nervosa or bulimia nervosa. However, clinical interviews using these criteria or research interviews such as the Child Eating Disorder Examination (Bryant-Waugh, Cooper, Taylor, & Lask, 1996) may be impractical for most clinicians. Alternatively, self-report questionnaires such as the Child Eating Attitudes Test (Maloney, McGuire, & Daniels, 1988) and the Questionnaire for Eating and Weight Patterns—Adolescent Version (W. G. Johnson, Grieve, Adams, & Sandy, 1999) may be used to screen for binge eating problems in children.

In conclusion, research evidence supports relationships among childhood obesity and several childhood psychological disorders including depression; binge eating; and to some extent, ADHD, although the precise nature of these relationships remains unknown. Psychological comorbidity does not appear to be an obstacle in the treatment of childhood overweight, however, and lifestyle interventions targeting healthy eating and activity are recommended for all children.

REFERENCES

Ackard, D. M., Neumark-Sztainer, D., Story, M., & Perry, C. (2003). Overeating among adolescents: Prevalence and associations with weight-related characteristics and psychological health. *Pediatrics, 111*(1), 67–74.

Agranat-Meged, A. N., Deitcher, C., Goldzweig, G., Leibenson, L., Stein, M., & Galili-Weisstub, E. (2005). Childhood obesity and attention deficit/hyperactivity disorder: A newly described comorbidity in obese hospitalized children. *International Journal of Eating Disorders, 37*, 357–359.

American Medical Association. (2007). *Expert committee recommendations on the assessment, prevention, and treatment of child and adolescent overweight and obesity*. Retrieved July 9, 2007, from http://www.ama-assn.org/ama1/pub/upload/mm/433/ped_obesity_recs.pdf

American Psychiatric Association. (2000). *Diagnostic and statistical manual of mental disorders* (4th ed., text revision). Washington, DC: Author.

Anderson, S. E., Cohen, P., Naumova, E. N., & Must, A. (2006). Association of depression and anxiety disorders with weight change in a prospective community-based study of children followed up into adulthood. *Archives of Pediatric and Adolescent Medicine, 160*, 285–291.

Brambilla, P., Bosio, L., Manzoni, P., Pietrobelli, A., Beccaria, L., & Chiumello, G. (1997). Peculiar body composition in patients with Prader-Labhart-Willi syndrome. *American Journal of Clinical Nutrition, 65*, 1369–1374.

Britz, A., Siegfried, W., Ziegler, A., Lamertz, C., Herpertz-Dahlmann, B. M., Remschmidt, H., et al. (2000). Rates of psychiatric disorders in a clinical study group of adolescents with extreme obesity and in obese adolescents ascertained via a population based study. *International Journal of Obesity and Related Metabolic Disorders, 24*, 1707–1714.

Bryant-Waugh, R. J. (2006). Eating disorders in children and adolescents. In S. Wonderlich, J. E. Mitchell, M. De Zwann, & H. Steiger (Eds.), *Annual review of eating disorders* (pp. 131–144), Abingdon, England: Radcliffe.

Bryant-Waugh, R. J., Cooper, P. J., Taylor, C. L., & Lask, B. D. (1996). The use of the eating disorder examination with children: A pilot study. *International Journal of Eating Disorders, 19*, 391–397.

Bulik, C. M., Sullivan, P. F., & Kendler, K. S. (2003). Genetic and environmental contributions to obesity and binge eating. *International Journal of Eating Disorders*, 33, 293–298.

Bulik, C. M., Sullivan, P. F., Weltzin, T. E., & Kaye, W. H. (1995). Temperament in eating disorders. *International Journal of Eating Disorders*, 17, 251–261.

Butryn, M. L., & Wadden, T. A. (2005). Treatment of overweight in children and adolescents: Does dieting increase the risk of eating disorders? *International Journal of Eating Disorders*, 37(4), 285–293.

Carpenter, K. M., Hasin, D. S., Allison, D. B., & Faith, M. S. (2000). Relationship between obesity and DSM–IV major depressive disorder, suicide ideation, and suicide attempts: Results from a general population study. *American Journal of Public Health*, 90, 251–257.

Curtin, C., Bandini, L. G., Perrin, E. G., Tybor, D. J., & Must, A. (2005). Prevalence of overweight in children and adolescents with attention deficit hyperactivity disorder and autism spectrum disorders: A chart review. *BMC Pediatrics*, 5, 48.

Davis, R., Freeman, R. J., & Garner, D. M. (1988). A naturalistic investigation of eating behavior in bulimia nervosa. *Journal of Consulting and Clinical Psychology*, 56, 273–279.

Decaluwe, V., & Braet, C. (2003). Prevalence of binge-eating disorder in obese children and adolescents seeking weight-loss treatment. *International Journal of Obesity*, 27, 404–409.

de Zwann, M., Mitchell, J. E., Seim, H. C., Specker, S. M., Pyle, R. L., Raymond, N. C., & Crosby, R. B. (1994). Eating related and general psychopathology in obese females with binge eating disorders. *International Journal of Eating Disorders*, 15, 43–52.

Dymek, M., le Grange, D., Neven, K., & Alverdy, J. (2001). Quality of life and psychosocial adjustment in patients after Roux-en-Y gastric bypass: A brief report. *Obesity Surgery*, 11, 32–39.

Eisenberg, M. E., Neumark-Sztainer, D., Haines, J., & Wall, M. (2006). Weight-teasing and emotional well being in adolescents: Longitudinal findings from project EAT. *Journal of Adolescent Health*, 38, 675–683.

Eisenberg, M. E., Neumark-Sztainer, D., & Story, M. (2003). Associations of weight-based teasing and emotional well-being among adolescents. *Archives of Pediatrics & Adolescent Medicine*, 157, 733–738.

Epstein, L. H., Paluch, R. A., Saelens, B. E., Ernst, M. M., & Wilfley, D. E. (2001). Changes in eating disorder symptoms with pediatric obesity treatment. *Journal of Pediatrics*, 139, 58–65.

Erermis, S., Cetin, N., Tamar, M., Bukusoglu, N., Akdeniz, F., & Goksen, D. (2004). Is obesity a risk factor for psychopathology among adolescents? *Pediatrics International*, 46, 296–301.

Erickson, S. J., Robinson, T. N., Haydel, K. F., & Killen, J. D. (2000). Are overweight children unhappy? *Archives of Pediatrics & Adolescent Medicine*, 154, 931–935.

Fairburn, C. G., Doll, H. A., Welch, S. L., Hay, P. J., Davies, B. A., & O'Connor, M. E. (1998). Risk factors for binge eating disorder; A community-based, case-control study. *Archives of General Psychiatry, 55*, 425–432.

Fairburn, C. G., & Wilson, G. T. (1993). Binge eating: Definition and classification. In C. G. Fairburn & G. T. Wilson (Eds.), *Binge eating: Nature, assessment, and treatment* (pp. 3–14). New York: Guilford Press.

Falkner, N. H., Neumark-Sztainer, D., Story, M., Jeffrey, R. W., Beuhring, T., & Resnick, M. D. (2001). Social, educational, and psychological correlates of weight status in adolescents. *Obesity Research, 9*, 32–42.

Field, A. E., Camargo, C. A., Jr., Taylor, C. B., Berkey, C. S., Frazier, A. L., Gillman, M. W., & Colditz, G. A. (1999). Overweight, weight concerns, and bulimic behaviors among girls and boys. *Journal of the American Academy of Child and Adolescent Psychiatry, 38*, 754–760.

Friedman, M. A., & Brownell, K. D. (1995). Psychological correlates of obesity: Moving to the next research generation. *Psychological Bulletin, 117*, 3–20.

Glasofer, D. R., Tanofsky-Kraff, M., Eddy, K. T., Yanovski, S. Z., Theim, K. R., Ghorbani, S., et al. (2007). Binge eating in overweight treatment-seeking adolescents. *Journal of Pediatric Psychology, 32*, 95–105.

Goodman, E., & Whitaker, R. C. (2002). A prospective study of the role of depression in the development and persistence of adolescent obesity. *Pediatrics, 109*(3), 497–504.

Hasler, G., Pine, D. S., Gamma, A., Milos, G., Ajdacic, V., Eich, D., et al. (2004). The associations between psychopathology and being overweight: A 20-year prospective study. *Psychological Medicine, 34*, 1047–1057.

Herva, A., Laitinen, J., Miettunen, J., Veijola, J., Karvonen, J. T., Laksy, K., & Joukamaa, M. (2006). Obesity and depression: Results from the longitudinal Northern Finland 1966 birth cohort study. *International Journal of Obesity (2005), 30*, 520–527.

Holtkamp, K., Konrad, K., Muller, B., Heussen, N., Herpertz, S., Herpertz-Dahlmann, B., & Hebebrand, J. (2004). Overweight and obesity in children with attention-deficit/hyperactivity disorder. *International Journal of Obesity and Related Metabolic Disorders, 28*, 685–689.

Isnard, P., Michel, G., Frelut, M., Vila, G., Falissard, B., Naja, W., et al. (2003). Binge eating and psychopathology in severely obese adolescents. *International Journal of Eating Disorders, 34*, 235–243.

Istavan, J., Zavela, K., & Weidner, G. (1992). Body weight and psychological distress in NHANES 1. *International Journal of Obesity and Related Metabolic Disorders, 16*, 999–1003.

Johnson, J. G., Spitzer, R. L., & Williams, J. B. (2001). Health problems, impairment and illnesses associated with bulimia nervosa and binge eating disorder among primary care and obstetric gynaecology patients. *Psychological Medicine, 31*, 1455–1466.

Johnson, W. G., Grieve, F. G., Adams, C. D., & Sandy, J. (1999). Measuring binge eating in adolescents: Adolescent and parent versions of the questionnaire of eating and weight patterns. *International Journal of Eating Disorders, 26,* 301–314.

Kimm, S., Barton, B., Obarzanek, E., McMahon, R., Sabry, Z., & Waclawiw, M., et al. (2001). Racial divergence in adiposity during adolescence: The NHLBI growth and health study. *Pediatrics, 107,* E34.

Kuczmarski, R. J., & Flegal, K. M. (2000). Criteria for definition of overweight in transition: Background and recommendations for the United States. *American Journal of Clinical Nutrition, 72*(5), 1067–1068.

Kuczmarski, R. J., Ogden, C. L., Grummer-Strawn, L. M., Flegal, K. M., Guo, S. S., Wei, R., et al. (2000). CDC growth charts: United States. *Advance Data, 314,* 1–27.

Lamertz, C. M., Jacobi, C., Yassouridis, A., Arnold, K., & Henkel, A. W. (2002). Are obese adolescents and young adults at higher risk for mental disorders? A community study. *Obesity Research, 10,* 1152–1160.

Lamerz, A., Kuepper-Nybelen, J., Bruning, N., Wehle, C., Trost-Brinkhues, G., Brenner, H., et al. (2005). Prevalence of obesity, binge eating, and night eating in a cross-sectional field survey of 6-year-old children and their parents in a German urban population. *Journal of Child Psychology and Psychiatry, 46,* 385–393.

Levine, M. D., Ringham, R. M., Kalarchian, M. A., Wisniewski, L., & Marcus, M. D. (2001). Is family-based behavioral weight control appropriate for severe pediatric obesity? *International Journal of Eating Disorders, 30,* 318–328.

Levine, M. D., Ringham, R. M., Kalarchian, M. A., Wisniewski, L., & Marcus, M. D. (2006). Overeating among seriously overweight children seeking treatment: Results of the children's eating disorder examination. *International Journal of Eating Disorders, 39,* 135–140.

Lingswiler, V. M., Crowther, J. H., & Stephens, M. A. P. (1989). Affective and cognitive antecedents to eating episodes in bulimia and binge eating. *International Journal of Eating Disorders, 8*(5), 533–539.

Maloney, M. J., McGuire, J. B., & Daniels, S. R. (1988). Reliability testing of children's version of the eating attitude test. *Journal of the American Academy of Child and Adolescent Psychiatry, 27,* 541–543.

Marcus, M. D., & Kalarchian, M. A. (2003). Binge eating in children and adolescents. *International Journal of Eating Disorders, 34,* S47–S57.

Marcus, M. D., Moulton, M. M., & Greeno, C. G. (1995). Binge eating onset in obese patients with binge eating disorder. *Addictive Behaviors, 20,* 747–755.

McGuire, M. T., Wing, R. R., Klem, M. L., Lang, W., & Hill, J. O. (1999). What predicts weight regain in a group of successful weight losers? *Journal of Consulting and Clinical Psychology, 67,* 177–185.

Morgan, C. M., Yanovski, S. Z., Nguyen, T. T., McDuffie, J., Sebring, N. G., Jorge, M. R., et al. (2002). Loss of control over eating, adiposity, and psychopathology in overweight children. *International Journal of Eating Disorders, 31,* 430–441.

Mustillo, S., Worthman, C., Erkanli, A., Keeler, G., Angold, A., & Costello, E. J. (2003). Obesity and psychiatric disorder: Developmental trajectories. *Pediatrics*, *111*, 851–859.

Needham, B. L., & Crosnoe, R. (2005). Overweight status and depressive symptoms during adolescence. *Journal of Adolescent Health*, *36*, 48–55.

Neumark-Sztainer, D., Falkner, N., Story, M., Perry, C., Hannan, P. J., & Mulert, S. (2002). Weight-teasing among adolescents: Correlations with weight status and disordered eating behaviors. *International Journal of Obesity and Related Metabolic Disorders*, *1*, 123–131.

Newman, D. L., Moffitt, T. E., Caspi, A., Magdol, L., Silva, P. A., & Stanton, W. R. (1996). Psychiatric disorder in a birth cohort of young adults: Prevalence, comorbidity, clinical significance, and new case incidence from ages 11 to 21. *Journal of Consulting and Clinical Psychology*, *64*, 552–562.

Ogden, C. L., Carroll, M. D., Curtin, L. R., McDowell, M. A., Tabak, C. J., & Flegal, K. M. (2006). Prevalence of overweight and obesity in the United States, 1999–2004. *JAMA*, *295*, 1549–1555.

Onyike, C. U., Crum, R. M., Lee, H. B., Lyketsos, C., & Eaton, W. W. (2003). Is obesity associated with major depression? Results from the Third National Health and Nutrition Examination Survey. *American Journal of Epidemiology*, *158*, 1139–1147.

Pine, D. S., Cohen, P., Brook, J., & Coplan, J. D. (1997). Psychiatric symptoms in adolescence as predictors of obesity in early adulthood: A longitudinal study. *American Journal of Public Health*, *87*, 1303–1310.

Pine, D. S., Goldstein, R. B., Wolk, S., & Weissman, M. M. (2001). The association between childhood depression and adulthood body mass index. *Pediatrics*, *107*, 1049–1056.

Pinhas-Hamiel, O., Singer, S., Pilpel, N., Fradkin, A., Modan, D., & Reichman, B. (2006). Health-related quality of life among children and adolescents: Associations with obesity. *International Journal of Obesity*, *30*, 267–272.

Richardson, L. P., Davis, R., Poulton, R., McCauley, E., Moffitt, T. E., Caspi, A., et al. (2003). A longitudinal evaluation of adolescent depression and adult obesity. *Archives of Pediatrics & Adolescent Medicine*, *157*, 739–745.

Roberts, R. E., Deleger, S., Strawbridge, W. J., & Kaplan, G. A. (2003). Prospective association between obesity and depression: Evidence from the Alameda County study. *International Journal of Obesity and Related Metabolic Disorders*, *27*, 514–521.

Rosen, D. (2003). Eating disorders in children and adolescents: Etiology, classification, clinical features, and treatment. *Adolescent Medicine*, *14*, 49–59.

Ross, C. (1994). Overweight and depression. *Journal of Health and Social Behavior*, *35*, 63–79.

Roth, D. A., Coles, M. E., & Heimberg, R. G. (2002). The relationship between memories for childhood teasing and anxiety and depression in adulthood. *Anxiety Disorders*, *16*, 149–164.

Schwimmer, J. B., Burwinkle, T. M., & Varni, J. W. (2003). Health-related quality of life of severely obese children and adolescents. *JAMA, 289,* 1813–1819.

Shapiro, J. R., Woolson, S. L., Hamer, R. M., Kalarchian, M. A., Marcus, M. D., & Bulik, C. M. (2007). Evaluating binge eating in children: Development of the Children's Binge Eating Disorder Scale (C-BEDS). *International Journal of Eating Disorders, 40,* 82–89.

Sheslow, D., Hassink, S., Wallace, W., & DeLancey, E. (1993). The relationship between self-esteem and depression in obese children. In C. L. Williams & S. Y. S. Kimm (Eds.), *Annals of the New York Academy of Sciences: Vol. 699. Prevention and treatment of childhood obesity* (pp. 289–291). New York: New York Academy of Sciences.

Shisslak, C. M., Crago, M., McKnight, K. M., Estes, L. S., Gray, N., & Parnaby, O. G. (1998). Potential risk factors associated with weight control behaviors in elementary and middle school girls. *Journal of Psychosomatic Research, 44,* 301–313.

Smith, D. E., Marcus, M. D., Lewis, C. E., Fitzgibbon, M., & Schreiner, P. (1998). Prevalence of binge eating disorder, obesity, and depression in a biracial cohort of young adults. *Annals of Behavioral Medicine, 20,* 227–232.

Spitzer, R. L., Devlin, M., Walsh, B. T., Hasin, D., Wing, R., Marcus, M., et al. (1992). Binge eating disorder: A multisite field trial of the diagnostic criteria. *International Journal of Eating Disorders, 11,* 191–203.

Stice, E., Agras, W. S., & Hammer, L. D. (1999). Risk factors for the emergence of childhood eating disturbance: A five-year prospective study. *International Journal of Eating Disorders, 25,* 375–387.

Stice, E., & Bearman, S. (2001). Body-image and eating disturbances prospectively predict increases in depressive symptoms in adolescent girls: A growth curve analysis. *Developmental Psychology, 37,* 597–607.

Stice, E., Martinez, E. E., Presnell, K., & Groesz, L. M. (2006). Relation of successful dietary restriction to change in bulimic symptoms: A prospective study of adolescent girls. *Health Psychology, 25,* 274–281.

Stice, E., Presnell, K., Shaw, H., & Rohde, P. (2005). Psychological and behavioral risk factors for obesity onset in adolescent girls: A prospective study. *Journal of Consulting and Clinical Psychology, 73,* 195–202.

Stunkard, A. J. (1959). Eating patterns and obesity. *Psychiatric Quarterly, 33,* 284–292.

Stunkard, A., Faith, M., & Allison, K. (2003). Depression and obesity. *Biological Psychiatry, 54,* 330–337.

Sullivan, M., Karlsson, J., Sjostrom, L., Backman, L., Bengtsson, C., Bouchard, C., et al. (1993). Swedish obese subjects (SOS): An intervention study of obesity: Baseline evaluation of health and psychosocial functioning in the first 1743 subjects examined. *International Journal of Obesity and Related Metabolic Disorders, 17,* 503–512.

Swallen, K. C., Reither, E. N., Haas, S. A., & Meier, A. M. (2005). Overweight, obesity, and health-related quality of life among adolescents: The national longitudinal study of adolescent health. *Pediatrics, 115,* 340–347.

Tanofsky-Kraff, M., Cohen, M. L., Yanovski, S. Z., Cox, C., Theim, K. R., Keo, M., et al. (2006). A prospective study of psychological predictors of body fat gain among children at high risk for adult obesity. *Pediatrics, 117,* 1203–1209.

Tanofsky-Kraff, M., Theim, K. R., Yanovski, S. Z., Bassett, A. M., Burns, N. P., Ranzenhofer, L. M., et al. (2007). Validation of the emotional eating scale adapted for use in children and adolescents (EES-C). *International Journal of Eating Disorders, 40,* 232–240.

Tanofsky-Kraff, M., Yanovski, S. Z., Wilfley, D. E., Marmarosh, C., Morgan, C. M., & Yanovski, J. A. (2004). Eating-disordered behaviors, body fat, and psychopathology in overweight and normal weight children. *Journal of Consulting and Clinical Psychology, 72*(1), 53–61.

Testa, M. A., & Simonson, D. C. (1996). Assessment of quality of life outcomes. *New England Journal of Medicine, 334,* 833–840.

Theodoro, M., Talebizadeh, Z., & Butler, M. G. (2006). Body composition and fatness patterns in Prader-Willi syndrome: Comparison with simple obesity. *Obesity, 14,* 1685–1690.

Vila, G., Zipper, E., Dabbas, M., Bertrand, C., Robert, J. J., Ricour, C., et al. (2004). Mental disorders in obese children and adolescents. *Psychosomatic Medicine, 66,* 387–394.

Vitousek, K., & Manke, F. (1994). Personality variables and disorders in anorexia nervosa and bulimia nervosa. *Journal of Abnormal Psychology, 103,* 137–147.

Wadden, T., & Stunkard, A. (1987). Psychopathology and obesity. In *Annals of the New York Academy of Sciences: Vol. 499. Human obesity* (pp. 55–65). New York: New York Academy of Sciences.

Wallace, W., Sheslow, D., & Hassink, S. (1993). Obesity in children: A risk for depression. In C. L. Williams & S. Y. S. Kimm (Eds.), *Annals of the New York Academy of Sciences: Vol. 699. Prevention and treatment of childhood obesity* (pp. 301–303). New York: New York Academy of Sciences.

Wardle, J., & Cooke, L. (2005). The impact of obesity on psychological well-being. *Best Practice & Research. Clinical Endocrinology & Metabolism, 19*(3), 421–440.

Wardle, J., Williamson, S., Johnson, F., & Edwards, C. (2006). Depression in adolescent obesity: Cultural moderators of the association between obesity and depressive symptoms. *International Journal of Obesity, 30,* 634–643.

Williams, J., Wake, M., Hesketh, K., Maher, E., & Waters, E. (2005). Health-related quality of life of overweight and obese children. *JAMA, 293,* 70–76.

Zeller, M. H., Roehrig, H. R., Modi, A. C., Daniels., S. R., & Inge, T. H. (2006). Health-related quality of life and depressive symptoms in adolescents with extreme obesity presenting for bariatric surgery. *Pediatrics, 117,* 1155–1161.

III

ASSESSMENT, INTERVENTION, AND PREVENTION

7

ASSESSMENT OF OVERWEIGHT CHILDREN AND ADOLESCENTS

LINDSAY VARKULA AND LESLIE J. HEINBERG

The ultimate goals of assessment in overweight youth are to guide treatment targets, identify optimal treatment interventions, and help provide a better understanding of the role that behavior and psychosocial factors may play in this condition. This chapter focuses on interviewing strategies and psychometric measures for the behavioral, psychological, and psychosocial assessment of overweight children. Behavioral assessment of obesity in adults relies primarily on interviewing the patient in conjunction with self-report instruments and self-monitoring (Phelan & Wadden, 2004). This method also is appropriate for pediatric populations, although the inclusion of parents or primary caregivers in interviewing, self-report assessment, and monitoring is key for both children and adolescents.

It is useful to clarify in which settings and for which type of professionals the various elements of assessment apply. We base our discussion in this chapter on a comprehensive assessment to be made by a mental health professional on a patient presenting for weight loss treatment in a specialty clinic. In many cases, it is also recommended that the mental health professional collaborate with other professionals (e.g., physicians, dieticians, exercise physiologists) to ensure the best assessment and treatment of the patient. Overweight patients may present with psychological problems, behavioral problems, school problems, or other issues. In such cases, overweight and obesity can be significant in patients' lives, so in addition to being useful in specialty clinic situations, the techniques described and topics discussed may be important for mental health professionals in other settings to include in an assessment of an overweight patient.

The assessment techniques described in this chapter can also be tailored to assist a variety of other professionals working with overweight children, including primary care physicians and dieticians. Some of the techniques and topics are beyond the scope of assessments in those areas, but professionals could modify them to meet their needs. Health professionals could also use this chapter as a grounding point for things to keep in mind when doing a more specialty-appropriate assessment.

BEGINNING THE BEHAVIORAL ASSESSMENT

Meeting with a new patient may be routine for a therapist; however, for an overweight child, this type of meeting can be terrifying. In many instances, this is the first encounter the child or adolescent has ever had with a mental health professional. Furthermore, many youths will be visiting primarily as a result of parental concerns or a physician's recommendation rather than because of their own concerns. Thus, early rapport building and a nonjudgmental demeanor are of utmost importance, especially given the negative stereotypes that some people may hold about being seen by a mental health practitioner.

As with any interaction with children, it is important to keep in mind the patient's developmental level and to tailor the interview accordingly. For more information on how to perform developmentally appropriate interviews for each age group, see *Interviewing Children and Adolescents: Skills and Strategies for the Effective* DSM–IV *Diagnosis* (Morrison & Anders, 1999).

Review of Medical Assessment

No assessment of pediatric overweight is complete without an assessment of physical status. It is vital that possible medical etiologies for the overweight or medical comorbidities resulting from overweight be identified before treatment planning. Therefore, although in this chapter we focus on assessment techniques used by mental health professionals, we must emphasize that a collaborative relationship with a child's or adolescent's pediatrician or family practitioner is necessary for ideal assessment and management. A number of excellent reviews regarding medical assessment for overweight and obesity have been written and may be of interest to the reader (Hatahet & Dhurandhar, 2004; Hill & Pomeroy, 2001; Whitlock, Williams, Gold, Smith, & Shipman, 2005).

A medical evaluation usually includes a physical examination, a review of the patient's medical history and family history, and a full panel of blood work. From this, the physician will be able to identify any health conditions contributing to or causing the overweight. If this is the case, patients should be medically stabilized and have physicians' approval before starting any kind of weight management program. If the results of the medical assessment indicate that there is no underlying medical condition causing the overweight, such feedback may be helpful in convincing patients and their families that non-optimal energy balance (i.e., consuming more calories than the body burns) is the likely cause of children's overweight, and that by changing their lifestyle, they will be able to combat their problems with overweight.

Anthropometric Assessment

Although the child will likely have been assessed for weight and stature by the physician, regular weighing and measuring should be an essential part of each visit. Many youth are self-conscious or anxious about weighing, but weighing children consistently at each visit in a matter-of-fact manner will usually result in quick desensitization. In our hospital-based clinical practice, we follow the protocol recommended by the Centers for Disease Control and Prevention (2000). Office scales should be calibrated against standard weights.

The following steps are performed to assess stature:

1. Position the child on the footplate of the stadiometer without shoes.
2. Position the child with heels close together, legs straight, arms at sides, shoulders relaxed.
3. Ask the child to inhale deeply and to stand fully erect without changing the position of the heels.
4. Ensure that the heels do not rise off the foot plate and that the child's head is in the Frankfort plane.
5. Lower the perpendicular headpiece snugly to the crown of the head with sufficient pressure to compress the hair (hair ornaments, buns, braids, etc., must be removed to obtain an accurate measurement).
6. To ensure an accurate reading, the measurer's eyes must be parallel with the headpiece.
7. Read the measure to the nearest ⅛ inch if using English system or 0.1 centimeter if using metric system.
8. Reposition the child and remeasure; the measures should agree within ¼ inch if using English system or 1.0 centimeter if using metric system.

The following steps are performed to assess weight:

1. The child should wear only lightweight garments or gown.
2. Position the child on the center of the platform of the scale.
3. Record the child's weight to the nearest ½ oz (0.01 kilogram).
4. Reposition the child and repeat the weight measure; the measures should agree within ¼ pound (0.10 kilogram).

For both stature and weight, if the difference between the measures exceeds the tolerance limit, the child should be repositioned and remeasured a third time. The average of the two measures in closest agreement will be recorded. *Body mass index* (BMI; weight in kilograms/height in meters^2) can then be calculated. Because BMI cut-offs for underweight, normal weight, at-risk for overweight, and overweight vary according to age and sex, BMI percentiles should be used. These can plotted and charted on growth curves. These charts can be downloaded from the CDC Web site (http://www.cdc.gov/growthcharts/).

Parent-and-Child Interviews Versus Child-Only Interviews

Parent-and-child or caregiver-and-child assessment interviews can provide invaluable insight into family dynamics. A perspective on the patient from the viewpoint of more than one person can be helpful. Therefore, if possible, perform at least the initial part of the assessment interview with one or both parents or primary caregiver present. In the case of younger children, the participation of parents is a necessity because children are unable to convey all of the basic assessment information and because parents will likely be the major agent of lifestyle change.

There may be patients, however, especially adolescents, who are unable to be open with the therapist in the presence of parents. It may be helpful to have the parent leave the room for part of the interview so that an accurate assessment can be made.

Starting the Assessment

When meeting an overweight child and his or her family, telling them what to expect during the interview can ease anxiety. It is crucial to emphasize that the conversation will center on familiar topics such as home and school, and knowing what to expect quickly helps most patients feel more comfortable. Explain that you will be asking about such topics by conveying the message that overweight and its related issues can permeate many aspects of a person's life.

A semistructured interview is usually the best technique for gathering information about overweight children and adolescents. There are some topics (e.g., weight history, family history, school performance, social skills, diet, activity level) that must be covered with all overweight patients and some mental health concerns (e.g., psychosocial stressors, binge eating symptoms, and depressive symptoms) for which all overweight patients need to be screened. The order of the topics and questions does not necessarily need to be fixed. More sensitive topics, however, can be much easier to discuss nearer to the end of the interview once rapport has been built with the patient and family. The order of topics in this chapter can serve as a blueprint for the interview.

A good place to start the assessment is to ask the patient or family why they came to see a mental health professional. Patients will often respond that they are unhappy with the way they look, they need help, their family physicians or pediatricians recommended coming, or they wish to be healthier.

It is then helpful to ask how the patient feels about the visit. Many patients will convey excitement, but some will express reluctance. In many cases, the children and parents have different expectations and interests in addressing the problem of overweight. The parent often will have scheduled the visit without the approval of the child or adolescent. This line of questioning also becomes the first step in assessing the patient's and family's readiness for change, which is something to revisit later in the interview.

Weight History

A patient's weight history gives the interviewer a basic understanding of the duration and impact of the patient's overweight. The phrasing of the initial question about weight history is extremely important, especially because it occurs before rapport has been fully established. Take cues from the patient and the family. For example, if the patient has already described himself or herself as "overweight," then it is usually permissible, and often even helpful, to use the patients' own words when asking about it. For example, "You just described yourself as being overweight. How old were you when that first became a problem for you?" If, however, the parents have been hesitant to label a child as "overweight" or "obese," then it is important to avoid those labels when asking about weight history. In these cases, questions to the child such as, "When did you start to notice that you were bigger than other kids (in your grade at school, or your age, etc.)?" or to the parent, "When did you [or the pediatrician] first become concerned about his [her] size?" tend to be an effective way to start covering this topic.

Parents can sometimes be much more helpful than children in reporting weight history. In many cases, children were very young when the overweight began and may have had varying levels of awareness of their status as "larger than others." Parents can often provide an age estimate. The onset of weight gain is such an emotionally charged issue that it can be difficult for patients to describe it at the beginning of an interview. However, in other cases, parents may be defensive about their child's weight, particularly when they are being seen solely on the basis of a physician's strong recommendation. Family members may assert that everyone in their family is big, that their child is big boned, or that he or she will grow out of it. It is important to be sensitive to these perceptions, but remind the family that it will benefit everyone to gather as much information as possible at the evaluation.

Other children and adolescents, however, are fully able to give a time frame regarding when their weight started to be a concern. This is particularly true when pronounced weight gain occurred during puberty or when the children reached adolescence.

After establishing the age at which a patient started being overweight, the therapist should query whether there were any key life changes (e.g., birth of a sibling, parent's marriage, a move to a new home), important losses (e.g., death, divorce, imprisonment), medical diagnoses (of the patient or a close family member), changes in medications, or other marked changes to the patient's life at those times. Asking about these events not only can give the clinician a better grasp on the weight history but also can establish major topics that need to be revisited later in the interview.

In addition, patients and families can usually provide some ideas regarding what they believe are the major factors in the weight gain or maintenance of overweight. Does the patient or family believe overweight is a problem because of genetics? Does the patient or family attribute the overweight problem to a medical condition? Is the patient eating too much food? Is the patient eating unhealthy foods? Does the patient not get enough exercise? Does the patient spend too much time watching TV, playing video games, and doing computer work? Is there some other cause to which they attribute the overweight? These questions can help identify some of the areas of weakness in a patient's lifestyle and can also give the interviewer insight into the patient's and family's understanding of the overweight.

Finally, it is important to ask whether and how the patient has attempted to lose weight in the past. Often children and adolescents have not been on a specific diet (e.g., South Beach, Weight Watchers). Rather, family members will note changes that they tried to make, such as reducing soda consumption, switching from fried foods to baked foods, starting a physical activity program, and so on. The clinician should ask whether a change resulted in a loss or slowing of weight gain; how long the change was maintained; and, if stopped, what led to the resumption of previous behavioral patterns. Furthermore, it is helpful to determine whether the patient has a good idea of his or her personal barriers to weight loss. Why did one intervention work and another not work? What was involved in the behavioral change, and what were the goals? Did any weight loss result from exercise, diet, behavior, or some combination of these? Did the patient gain back any lost weight after the end of the program? Why or why not?

SPECIFIC CONTENT AREAS IN THE INTERVIEW AND FOR PSYCHOMETRIC ASSESSMENT

In this section, we review areas that are likely relevant for an overweight child or adolescent, with specific suggestions on queries and areas of exploration. We also review recommended measures for use with overweight youth.

Family History

Morrison and Anders (1999) have provided guidelines for general content of family history interviews with children and adolescents. In the case of overweight children and adolescents, however, several components of the general family history need special attention. As with the rest of the interview, while taking a family history, it is important to investigate the bidirectional relationship between the patient's overweight and the major psychosocial issues in a patient's life.

To open discussion of the patient's family life, it is helpful to ask the patient to list and describe the people who live in his or her household. Make sure to pay attention to the ages of siblings and the birth position of the patient. Are the siblings overweight? Ask the patient how well he or she gets along with parents and siblings. A brief assessment can help establish whether the patient's interactions with important others are within normal limits. It may also be necessary (especially if there are not many other family members present) to ask about the approximate height and weight of the patient's parents. It is helpful to know how ubiquitous the issue of overweight is in the patient's family.

The clinician should also obtain an understanding of the family's status and major family events. For example, are the patient's parents married and living together? Has there been a divorce or recent death? If the child is being raised by a single parent, what is the patient's relationship with his or her other biological parent? Are there any current legal battles or involvement with the law, social services, children's services, juvenile justice, or similar agencies? Again, any of these major events, changes, or stressors can be significant components in the onset or maintenance of overweight. It is also important to determine whether the child spends significant time in another household (e.g., that of a grandparent who provides after school care) or whether anyone besides the caregiver attending the interview is largely responsible for grocery shopping, cooking, or feeding the child.

The assessment of the family routine is also essential. For example, is there a reliable routine? Is the routine strict or relaxed? When does the patient wake up, get home from school, and go to bed? When is his or her curfew? When is mealtime? Is the day usually chaotic or is it calm? What are the differences in routine between school days and weekends? These characteristics give the interviewer an idea of the contents of the patient's day, what it is like to live in that patient's home, and potential points of intervention when altering the family's dietary intake or physical activity.

In establishing the patient's routine, the clinician can ask how being overweight affects this routine. Does the patient have problems at school, at play, in sports, with friends, or with family because of overweight? Does being overweight limit the patient's participation in activities such as school gym class, strenuous activities (e.g., running fast, playing hard), moderate activities (e.g., riding a bike, climbing stairs), or mild activities (e.g., walking)? Has the family ever changed plans or trips or avoided activities or places because of the patient's overweight?

Discipline in the home is another area to assess when learning about the patient's family. An understanding of this aspect of family life can help illuminate the limit-setting capabilities of the parents. In many cases, the more successful the parents can be in setting limits for their children, the easier it is to implement lifestyle changes at home. Ask whether the patient gets into trouble at home or at school and what happens because of it. Does it seem that the disciplinary measures at home, provided that they exist at all, are consistent or inconsistent? Are appropriate discipline techniques used? How severe is punishment? How often does the patient get into trouble? What does he or she usually do to get in trouble? Are the offenses minor, like failing to clean his or her room, or are major behavioral problems occurring? Any reports of unusual behavior need to be revisited when screening patients for psychopathology later in the interview.

The final component of family history is the question of the family's mental health history. Ask for specific diagnoses made by mental health professionals for any family members. It often seems more appropriate to ask this question of the patient or family toward the middle or end of the interview after some rapport has been built.

Several validated, written measures can be used during assessment to evaluate the patient and his or her relationship with the family. One useful measure is the Family Relationship Inventory (FRI), which is based on the Family Environment Scale (Moos & Moos, 1981). The three subscales of the FRI include Cohesion, which measures the degree to which family members are perceived as supportive, connected to other members, and helpful; Emotional Expressiveness, which measures the degree to which families openly express both positive and negative emotions; and Conflict, which measures the extent of discord and conflict exhibited within the family environment. A second measure is the Family Ritual Questionnaire: Dinner Time Subscale (Fiese & Kline, 1993), which looks at the family environment during dinnertime. Both of these measures can give the clinician a standardized view of the family, and both cover a comprehensive array of topics within family functioning. More information on these measures and all subsequent instruments described in this chapter may be found in Table 7.1.

TABLE 7.1

Validated, Written Assessment Measures

Name of instrument	Authors	Description	Psychometrics: IC and TR	Standardization sample
		Body image		
Self-Image Questionnaire for Young Adolescents—Body Image subscale	Petersen, Schulenberg, Abramowitz, Offer, and Jarcho (1984)	For 10- to 15-year-olds; 11-item Body Image subscale assesses positive feelings toward the body	IC: boys (−.81), girls (−.77) TR: 1 year (.60); 2 years (.44)	335 sixth-grade students who were followed through the eighth grade
Sociocultural Attitudes Towards Appearance Scale	Heinberg, Thompson, and Stormer (1995)	14-item scale assessing recognition and acceptance of societal standards of appearance; two subscales: Awareness and Internalization	IC: Awareness (.71), Internalization (.88)	College students (344 female)
		Teasing		
Perception of Teasing Scale	Thompson, Cattarin, Fowler, and Fisher (1995)	12 items indexing general weight teasing and competency teasing	IC: general weight (.94), competency (.78)	227 female undergraduates
Physical Appearance Related Teasing Scale	Thompson, Fabian, Moulton, Dunn, and Altabe (1991)	18-item scale assessing history of weight/size and general appearance teasing	IC: weight/size scale, −.91; appearance scale, −.87 TR: 2 weeks (weight/size, −.86; appearance scale, −.87)	Female undergraduates
		Depression		
Center for Epidemiological Studies Depression Scale	Radloff (1977)	Used in adolescents, looks at depressive symptoms during the past week	IC: 0.75 TR: 0.51–0.57	High school students
Center for Epidemiological Studies Depression Scale, Child Version	Weissman, Orvaschel, and Pedian (1980)	Used in children and adolescents under 16, looks at depressive symptoms during the past week	IC: 0.84–0.89 TR: 0.51–0.57	Children and adolescents at risk of depression, inpatient populations

(continues)

TABLE 7.1
Validated, Written Assessment Measures *(Continued)*

Name of instrument	Authors	Description	Psychometrics: IC and TR	Standardization sample
Children's Depression Inventory	Kovacs (1985)	27-item symptom-oriented scale, self-report	IC: 0.59–0.88 TR: 0.38–0.87	Healthy children and adolescents; obese children
Child Behavior Checklist	Achenbach and Ruffle (2000)	Parent report; includes behavioral and emotional problems and competence items	IC: 0.78–0.97 TR: 0.95–1.00	Children ages 4–18
Self-esteem				
Rosenberg Self-Esteem Scale	Rosenberg (1965)	10 items, measures self-satisfaction, self-worth, self-respect, and personal pride	IC: 0.76–0.87 TR: 0.85	5,024 junior and senior high school students
Perceived Competence Scale for Children	Harter (1982)	Reliably assesses both general and dimensional (cognitive, social, and physical) self-esteem		Multiple samples of obese children and adolescents
Weight Efficacy Life-Style Questionnaire	Clark, Abrams, Niaura, Eaton, and Rossi (1991)	20 items, describes self-efficacy in weight loss in terms of situational factors: negative emotions, availability, social pressure, physical discomfort, positive activities		$n = 382$ in clinical treatment studies
Anxiety				
State–Trait Anxiety Inventory	Spielberger, Edwards, Montuori, and Lushene (1973)	Assesses global anxiety that varies with situations (state) and that is stable across time and situations (trait)	IC: 0.82–0.87 TR: 0.31–0.71	Community samples of children and teenagers

Instrument	Author	Description	Reliability/Validity	Population
		Activity		
Baecke Physical Activity Questionnaire	Baecke, Burema, and Frijters (1982)	Assesses work activity, sports activity, and nonsports leisure activity	TR: 0.80–0.90	167 females 139 males Late teens–20's
		Family/environment		
Family Relationship Index	Holahan and Moos (1983)	27 items, three subscales looking at cohesion, expressiveness, conflict		Children with and without chronic health conditions
Family Ritual Questionnaire	Fiese and Kline (1993)	Assesses family rituals across 8 dimensions	IC: 0.52–.90 TR: 0.88	109 female undergraduates 105 male undergraduates Mean age=18 years
		Eating disorders		
Eating Attitudes Test-26	Garner Olmstead, Bohr, and Garfinkel (1982)	Assesses eating disordered cognitions and behaviors	Correlated .98 with EAT IC: .94 TR: .84	Valid in children 12 and older
Children's Eating Attitude Test	Maloney, McGuire, and Daniels (1988)	Assesses eating disordered cognitions and behaviors in children	IC: .76 (.68–.80 when stratified by grade level) TR: .81 (3 weeks)	Valid in children as young as 8
Three-factor eating questionnaire	Stunkard and Messick (1985)	51 items: three subscales assessing cognitive restraint, disinhibition, and hunger	IC: >.80 TR: .93	Spectrum of individuals with extreme dietary restraint to lack of restraint
		Dietary		
Rapid Eating Assessment for Patients	Gans, Foss, Barner, Wylie-Roset, McMurray, and Eaton (2003)	27 questions, screen for consumption related to the current food guide pyramid and 2000 U.S. dietary guidelines	TR: 0.86	105 medical students 110 consumers

Note. Empty cells indicate no data. IC = internal consistency; TR = test–retest reliability; EAT = Eating Attitudes Test.

Dietary Patterns

When trying to establish the patient's eating habits, several primary areas need to be addressed. These topics include food intake, daily eating routine, family meal habits, snacking habits, and any conflict regarding food.

From a dietary perspective, it is important to get an accurate idea of what the patient usually eats, something that can be attempted with tools such as a 3-day food record or a 24-hour food recall. In the former, the patient and family keep a detailed log of everything that the patient eats and drinks for a 3-day period. It is usually suggested that at least one of these days include a weekend. In the latter, an interviewer queries the patient on all food and beverages consumed in the past 3 days. Although this is a self-report or parent-report measure that can easily be imprecise, it does help the interviewer establish an approximation of daily caloric intake. The Rapid Eating Assessment for Patients can be used for a quick look at a patient's dietary intake and a patient's readiness to make dietary changes (Gans et al., 2003). This measure may be easier to interpret for a professional who is not a dietician. Other important topics to review include the family's food shopping habits, how many meals are eaten away from home, meals that are frequently skipped, number of snacks, and the patient's and family's basic nutrition knowledge. With younger children, it can be helpful to use toy food models during the assessment. It is always best to collaborate with a registered dietician to assess (and later treat) patients, but when this is not possible, the clinician can gain a good sense of the patient's dietary strengths and weaknesses through these measures.

Of equal importance are questions regarding the patient's behaviors concerning food intake. Patients should be queried regarding where they eat (e.g., in the car, in front of the TV), who eats with them (e.g., family, peers, no one), and what is happening while they are eating (e.g., watching TV, socializing, using the computer). Similar questions should be asked regarding snacks. Also, are any of these eating times particularly distressing or particularly enjoyable for patients? For example, is dinnertime a relaxing time of family interaction, a time of family conflict, or a time when a patient is upset that he or she is forced to eat alone in front of the television?

Another vital topic to assess is whether there is any conflict concerning food. Often, parents and children will argue about things like portion sizes, second helpings, snacks, and desserts. It is important to determine the frequency and usual results of those conflicts. Is the parent successful in his or her attempts to set limits? Is the parent disparaging in these attempts? How upset does the patient become when these arguments occur? Do other family members tease or insult the patient, especially by calling the patient "fat" or a similar derogatory term? Does the patient display any atypical behaviors such as throwing objects out of anger or crying uncontrollably? The goal is to assess the severity of these conflicts and the patient's and family's reactions to them. Conflict over food can be a serious issue for the patient and family and can interfere with subsequent intervention strategies.

After assessing all of these areas, the interviewer should have a reasonable overview of the patient's current practices with regard to food and diet. Sometimes, during this dietary discussion, parents or patients will bring up behaviors that are symptomatic of binge eating disorder (BED; see chap. 6, this volume). These behaviors will be further queried in the assessment of eating disorders (see the Eating Disorders section of this chapter).

Physical and Sedentary Activities

Because of the importance of energy balance to optimal weight maintenance, it is crucial to examine not only dietary intake for each patient but also his or her caloric expenditure during the day. Calories in excess of one's resting energy expenditure can be expended through several types of activity. The most are burned off during vigorous activity (this is when the patient's heart rate increases and he or she sweats; examples include running fast or swimming fast), many calories are burned during more moderate physical activity (e.g., walking, most playing), and the fewest calories are burned when the patient is at rest (e.g., watching television, sleeping). To get an accurate idea of the patient's energy balance, it is important to ask about the amount of time usually spent in physical and sedentary activities. The Baecke Activity Questionnaire (Baecke, Burema, & Frijters, 1982), which looks at the activities in which the patients engage and the amount of time spent in physical activity, is a brief, effective written measure to use to assess this topic.

Physical and sedentary activities can also be assessed by queries regarding the patient's daily routine. Most children who spend a lot of time playing outside will mention that activity when asked what they do after school or in the evening. Individuals who watch television, play video games, or use the computer frequently will mention these activities when asked that same question. These sorts of questions will give the interviewer a good idea of the frequency of physical activities and of *global screen time* (i.e., total time spent watching TV, using the computer, and playing electronic games) and other sedentary activities. Knowing how long a patient spends in sedentary global screen time activities is fundamental in understanding his or her general sedentary practices.

In addition, it can be helpful to ask patients what kinds of sports they like to play, whether they enjoy engaging in any special activity with their family (especially on weekends), and whether there are any other ways they find to fit activity into their lives. Many patients will mention gym class and recess at school as key times during the day for activity. Be sure to ask specific questions as to the types of activities and the intensity of the activities that they do during those times to get an idea of the amount of vigorous activity they are getting versus the amount of regular moving time. For more information on sedentary behaviors, see chapter 2 of this volume.

School Performance

Overweight children are at risk of school-performance deficits and reduced school-related quality of life (Gortmaker, Must, Perrin, Sobol, & Dietz, 1993; Schwimmer, Burwinkle, & Varni, 2003). The clinician should ask the patient and family about his or her performance in school. This helps establish the extent to which the patient is successfully able to concentrate and will also identify any difficulties with following directions or responding to limit setting. The interviewer should query where the patient attends school, grade level, approximate grades, and the patient's strong and weak subjects. How does he or she get along with teachers? Ask how the patient likes school and whether learning in that patient's school is an inviting experience.

It is also important to ask whether the patient has an individualized education program (commonly referred to by the acronym "IEP") through their school. If so, what is the reason the IEP was created? Is the patient in regular classrooms, in special education, or in special education inclusion settings? Does the patient have any sort of classroom aide or special tutoring in any subject? Is he or she able to pay attention in a classroom setting and for how long? A better understanding of the child's cognitive capabilities can help clinicians tailor interventions to the child's strengths and weaknesses and prescribe the appropriate amount of parental involvement.

Peer Difficulties

Overweight children are at risk for increased victimization by bullies, engaging in bullying behavior, teasing (Janssen, Craig, Boyce, & Pickett, 2004), and social difficulties (Schwimmer et al., 2003). The best way to first query the social aptitude of overweight patients is to ask them about their interactions at school. Ask patients who their friends are at school. Do they have a few friends or a group of friends? When do they see these friends? Do they only spend time with them at school or do they spend time with them outside of school? Then ask about other networks of friends outside of school, such as people the patient might know from their neighborhood, clubs, religious groups, or other organizations in which he or she is involved.

It is also important to establish whether patients are ever teased or bullied by any of their peers at school. Are there one or two peers in particular who are a problem, or does it seem like participation is more universal? What happens as a result of the teasing or bullying? How does the patient respond? How do parents and teachers respond? Does teasing occur every day, or is it only an occasional problem? Ask specifically what patients are teased about; not all teasing centers on weight. Remember that overweight children can also use their size to bully others. Questions about physical fights and altercations at school can be informative. Encourage patients to discuss this topic so that a clear description of the extent of the teasing and the way it affects them can be obtained. Finally, ask whether the patient feels safe going to school. There is a significant difference between children who experience some teasing at school and children who are fearful of attending school because of more extreme instances of bullying, harassment, or physical assault.

In addition to interview questions on this topic, written measures can be useful in assessing teasing and bullying. The Physical Appearance Related Teasing Scale assesses history of the patient's weight, size, and general appearance teasing (Thompson, Fabian, Moulton, Dunn, & Altabe, 1991). The Perception of Teasing Scale is a shorter measure that can be used to quantify their experience with general teasing as well as teasing related to weight and competency (Thompson, Cattarin, Fowler, & Fisher, 1995).

Psychopathology

To begin the discussion of psychological functioning, it is useful to ask how the patient copes with difficulties. What kind of coping strategies does the patient choose? Do they appear to be healthy or unhealthy means of coping? A patient's awareness of adverse events, reactions to them, and determination of ways to cope with them can be indications of maturity, self-esteem, general intellect, self-awareness, judgment, and insight.

The interviewer then needs to find out whether the patient has had any history of psychiatric or mental health problems. For example, is there a history of mental illness, trauma, or adjustment difficulty? Have any specific diagnoses been made? When were they made, and who made them (e.g., pediatrician, school counselor, psychologist, social worker)? If the patient has seen any kind of therapist or counselor, it is important to find out who, when, and for what reasons. How did the patient respond to therapy, and how did he or she get along with that particular mental health professional? If patients have been seen by a mental health professional, it is helpful to ask specifically whether their overweight or related topics (such as body image or teasing) were addressed. Finally, we typically ask permission to contact practitioners to obtain their assessment of the patient and their appropriateness for lifestyle intervention. These consultations are valuable because these practitioners have a much better understanding of the patient and his or her family than what can be gained in a brief, one-visit evaluation.

Because of the possible increased risk of particular psychological difficulties in overweight children and adolescents (see chap. 6, this volume), it is important to screen all overweight children and adolescents as part of psychological assessment. For example, we screen for the symptoms of depression based on *Diagnostic and Statistical Manual of Mental Disorders* (4th ed. [*DSM–IV*]; American Psychiatric Association, 1994) criteria during the interview and use written measures to assess depressive symptomatology. Independent of depressive illness, negative self-evaluation is common in this population, especially concerning body image (see chap. 5, this volume, and the Body Image section of this chapter).

There are several validated, written tools to assess depression in children and adolescents. One of the most common measures is the Children's Depression Inventory, which is a self-report measure completed by the child or adolescent (Kovacs, 1985). The Child Behavior Checklist is a parent-report measure that can be a useful supplement (Achenbach & Ruffle, 2000). The Child Version of the Center for Epidemiological Studies Depression Scale assesses depressive symptoms including affective, cognitive, and motivational symptoms experienced within the past week (Weissman, Orvaschel, & Padian, 1980).

The possible presence of an adjustment disorder should be assessed, particularly if during the course of the interview a patient has mentioned any key life changes (e.g., birth of a sibling, parent's marriage, a move to a new home), important losses (e.g., death, divorce, imprisonment), trauma or assault, medical diagnoses (e.g., of the patient or a close family member), or other formidable changes in the patient's life. In addition, on the basis of the patient's behavior or reported academic or psychiatric history during the interview, symptoms of other common childhood disorders (e.g., attention-deficit/ hyperactivity disorder, mood disorders, disruptive or oppositional behaviors, thought disturbances, or other behavioral problems) should be queried carefully in order to determine whether a *DSM–IV* diagnosis may be warranted.

Written measures for specific disorders can also be informative. For example, if the patient presents with symptoms of anxiety, validated written measures such as the State–Trait Anxiety Inventory can be helpful (Spielberger, Edwards, Montuori, & Lushene, 1973).

For more information on psychopathology, see chapter 6 of this volume.

Eating Disorders

BED is much more common in the population of overweight children and adolescents than in children and adolescents with average BMIs. Because of the high incidence of BED in the former population, we recommend screening all patients for BED using the *DSM–IV* research criteria during the initial assessment (see chap. 6, this volume).

Families and patients often have interesting responses to questions about BED symptoms. Many of them show surprise at the accuracy of the questions in describing their particular feelings and behaviors toward food. On the one hand, many patients and families are grateful that someone finally understands their struggles with food. On the other hand, as with several of the topics already mentioned in this chapter, BED symptoms can be highly problematic and troublesome for the patient (and the patient's family) and therefore can be difficult to discuss. It may be useful to present questions about symptoms in a way that normalizes them. For example, "Some kids tell me that they sometimes eat food even when they are not hungry. Do you ever eat when you're not hungry?" This normalization can help children and adolescents who are more timid about this topic to answer the questions honestly.

Another issue that often comes up is that the parent and the patient may disagree with each other in regard to the presence or absence of BED symptoms. This happens especially when discussing whether a patient ever engages in the behaviors of sneaking or hiding food. The patient may deny ever having done so, whereas the parent may insist that these behaviors have occurred. Sometimes arguments may erupt between the patient and parent because of these issues. Again, to encourage honesty, it is useful to normalize some of these behaviors and say that many other kids also engage in them.

To complement the interview, several validated, written measures are available for assessing eating disordered behaviors. The 26-item Eating Attitudes Test (known as "EAT-26") can be used in children over the age of 12 and assesses behaviors including dietary restraint, binge eating, and purging (Garner, Olmstead, Bohr, & Garfinkel, 1982). The Children's Eating Attitudes Test (Maloney, McGuire, & Daniels, 1988) is a version of the Eating Attitudes Test modified for younger populations and has been validated in children as young as 8. The Three-Factor Eating Questionnaire assesses the areas of cognitive restraint, disinhibition, and hunger (Stunkard & Messick, 1985). These tools can also assess the presence of disordered eating symptoms such as restricting, binge eating, and purging.

Correlates of Psychosocial Functioning

A number of other psychosocial factors that may be associated with psychological functioning or success with treatment are an important part of the assessment. As described in chapter 4 of this volume, self-esteem is an important correlate to risk and treatment success in overweight youth. To shed light on a child's view of himself or herself, it can be helpful to use a written, validated measure. One of the most common is the Rosenberg Self-Esteem Inventory (Rosenberg, 1965), which is especially helpful because of its brevity and ease of understanding. Its questions assess the extent to which a patient feels a sense of worth, pride, and self-respect. Another validated measure is the Perceived Competence Scale for Children (Harter, 1982), which assesses how competently children describe themselves in physical, cognitive, and social dimensions. Further evaluation should be part of the clinician's interview. A patient who is able to list his or her good qualities, seems proud of accomplishments, and seems to take a positive attitude toward him or herself likely has a more positive self-image. For further details on the components of self-esteem, see chapter 4 of this volume.

Although research on body image in overweight children and adolescents is relatively scarce (see chap. 5, this volume), it can be assumed that many overweight children's and adolescents' body image has been affected by their size. In some cases, the effects can be minimal, but as seen in many clinical situations, overweight patients can have a wide range of problems related to body image.

The following interview questions may be helpful in assessing the degree of body image dissatisfaction that is experienced and the effect it has on behavior. How does the patient feel about his or her body? If the patient's response indicates negative feelings toward his or her body, how severe are those negative feelings? Does the patient dislike a certain part of his or her body or is the dissatisfaction more global? How much time does the patient spend thinking about or worrying about his or her body? When the patient is unhappy about something unrelated to body image, does he or she tend to blame those other problems on the fact that he or she is "ugly" or "fat" in appearance? Is this dissatisfaction with body appearance causing the patient to change behaviors or avoid certain situations (e.g., going swimming, going shopping for clothes)? Does the patient engage in any extreme behaviors to "punish" his or her body or offending body parts? And, finally, can the patient identify any aspects of his or her appearance that are positive? For more information on body image, see chapter 5.

Several validated written measures are also helpful in assessing body image in children. The Self-Image Questionnaire for Young Adolescents—Body Image Subscale assesses positive feelings patients have toward their bodies (Petersen, Schulenberg, Abramowitz, Offer, & Jarcho, 1984). To assess the amount of pressure adolescents may be feeling through general societal influences, the media in particular, the Sociocultural Attitudes Toward Appearance Questionnaire gives internalization and awareness subscale measures (Heinberg, Thompson, & Stormer, 1995). A version for middle-school-aged boys and girls has also been developed with good psychometric properties (Smolak, Levine, & Thompson, 2001).

Self-efficacy, as described in chapter 4 of this volume, is a person's level of confidence in his or her ability to make changes. In relation to problems connected with being overweight or obese, evaluation for a sense of self-efficacy can be a determination of how well a patient believes he or she can deal with the challenges, pressures, and barriers surrounding weight loss. In part, this is a look at the level of motivation of the patient and the resources that are available to the patient. Does the patient believe that he or she can be successful in weight loss? One written measure that is particularly convenient for assessing self-efficacy in weight loss is the Weight Efficacy Life-Style Questionnaire

(Clark, Abrams, Niaura, Eaton, & Rossi, 1991). This instrument examines the availability, social pressure, physical discomfort, negative emotions, and positive activities for each patient in regard to weight loss efforts. Similarly, the Self-Efficacy Questionnaire: Physical Activities (Motl et al., 2000) is an eight-item measure of respondents' perceptions of the degree to which they feel able to make changes in their physical activity level. The measure has been validated for use with adolescent females (Motl et al., 2000). These measures and similar tools can help the clinician gain a comprehensive idea of the abilities of the patient and supplement the somewhat vague questions that may have been asked in the interview about motivation and a patient's level of faith in his or her abilities to make changes.

SUMMARY

The intent of assessment of overweight children and adolescents is not only to screen for psychopathology but also to determine how overweight has affected the patient's life and how psychosocial factors may influence or impede treatment. As discussed in other chapters in this volume, the issue of overweight may bring with it a collection of unique psychosocial, environmental, and societal stressors that are not often experienced by children and adolescents who are not overweight. The first meeting with a patient of this kind is particularly important because of the connection that is established with the patient and because of the opportunity to gain a comprehensive idea of these issues and problems as the patient sees them. Because these issues and problems vary greatly by patient, assessing a new patient is always a distinctive experience.

REFERENCES

Achenbach, T. M., & Ruffle, T. M. (2000). The Child Behavior Checklist and related forms for assessing behavioral/emotional problems and competencies. *Pediatrics in Review, 21*, 265–271.

American Psychiatric Association. (1994). *Diagnostic and statistical manual of mental disorders* (4th ed.). Washington, DC: Author.

Baecke, J. A. H., Burema, J., & Frijters, J. E. R. (1982). A short questionnaire for the measurement of habitual physical activity in epidemiological studies. *American Journal of Clinical Nutrition, 36*, 936–942.

Centers for Disease Control and Prevention. (2000). *National Health and Nutrition Examination Survey: Anthropometry procedures manual.* Retrieved July 31, 2008, from http://www.cdc.gov/nchs/data/nhanes/bm.pdf

Clark, M. M., Abrams, D. B., Niaura, R. S., Eaton, C. A., & Rossi, J. S. (1991). Self-efficacy in weight management. *Journal of Consulting and Clinical Psychology, 59*(5), 739–744.

Fiese, B. H., & Kline, C. A. (1993). Development of the Family Ritual Questionnaire: Initial reliability and validation studies. *Journal of Family Psychology, 6*(3), 290–299.

Gans, K. M., Ross, E., Barner, C. W., Wylie-Rosett, J., McMurray, J., & Eaton, C. (2003). REAP and WAVE: New tools to rapidly assess/discuss nutrition with patients. *Journal of Nutrition, 133,* 556–562.

Garner, D. M., Olmstead, M. P., Bohr, Y., & Garfinkel, P. E. (1982). The Eating Attitudes Test: Psychometric features and clinical correlates. *Psychological Medicine, 12*(4), 871–878.

Gortmaker, S. L., Must, A., Perrin, J. M., Sobol, A. M., & Dietz, W. H. (1993). Social and economic consequences of overweight in adolescence and young adulthood. *New England Journal of Medicine, 329,* 1008–1012.

Harter, S. (1982). The Perceived Competence Scale for Children. *Child Development, 53*(1), 87–97.

Hatahet, M. A., & Dhurandhar, N. V. (2004). Assessment of medical status and physical features. In J. K. Thompson (Ed.), *Handbook of eating disorders and obesity* (pp. 372–392). Hoboken, NJ: Wiley.

Heinberg, L. J., Thompson, J. K., & Stormer, S. (1995). Development and validation of the Sociocultural Attitudes Toward Appearance Questionnaire (SATAQ). *International Journal of Eating Disorders, 17,* 81–89.

Hill, K., & Pomeroy, C. (2001). Assessment of physical status of children and adolescents with eating disorders and obesity. In J. K. Thompson & L. Smolak (Eds.), *Body image, eating disorders, and obesity in youth: Assessment, prevention, and treatment* (pp. 171–191). Washington, DC: American Psychological Association.

Holahan, C. J., & Moos, R. H. (1983). The quality of social support: Measures of family and work relationships. *British Journal of Clinical Psychology, 22*(3), 157–162.

Janssen, I., Craig, W. M., Boyce, W. F., & Pickett, W. (2004). Associations between overweight and obesity with bullying behaviors in school-aged children. *Pediatrics, 113,* 1187–1194.

Kovacs, M. (1985). The Children's Depression Inventory (CDI). *Psychopharmacology Bulletin, 21,* 995–998.

Maloney, M. J., McGuire, J. B., & Daniels, S. R. (1988). Reliability testing of a children's version of the Eating Attitudes Test. *Journal of the American Academy of Child and Adolescent Psychiatry, 5,* 541–543.

Moos, R. H., & Moos, B. S. (1981). *Family Environment Scale manual.* Palo Alto, CA: Consulting Psychologists Press.

Morrison, J., & Anders, T. F. (1999) *Interviewing children and adolescents: Skills and strategies for effective DSM–IV diagnosis.* New York: Guilford Press.

Motl, R. W., Dishman, R. K., Trost, S. G., Saunders, R. P., Dowda, M., Felton, G., et al. (2002). Factorial validity and invariance of questionnaires measuring social–cognitive determinants of physical activity among adolescent girls. *Preventive Medicine, 31,* 584–594.

Petersen, A. C., Schulenberg, J. E., Abramowitz, R. H., Offer, D., & Jarcho, H. D. (1984). The Self-Image Questionnaire for Young Adolescents (SIQYA): Reliability and validity studies. *Journal of Youth and Adolescence, 13,* 93–11.

Phelan, S., & Wadden, T. A. (2004). Behavioral assessment of obesity. In J. K. Thompson (Ed.), *Handbook of eating disorders and obesity* (pp. 393–420). Hoboken, NJ: Wiley.

Radloff, L. (1977). The CES-D scale: A self-report depression scale for research in the general population. *Applied Psychological Measurement, 1,* 385–401.

Rosenberg, M. (1965). *Society and the adolescent self-image* (Rev. ed.). Middletown, CT: Wesleyan University Press.

Schwimmer, J. B., Burwinkle, T. M., & Varni, J. W. (2003). Health-related quality of life of severely obese children and adolescents. *JAMA, 289,* 1813–1819.

Smolak, L., Levine, M. P., & Thompson, J. K. (2001). The use of the sociocultural attitudes towards appearance questionnaire with middle school boys and girls. *International Journal of Eating Disorders, 29,* 216–233.

Spielberger, C. D., Edwards, C. D., Montuori, J., & Lushene, R. (1973). *State–Trait Anxiety Inventory for Children.* Palo Alto, CA: Consulting Psychologists Press.

Stunkard, A. J., & Messick, S. (1985). The Three-Factor Eating Questionnaire to measure dietary restraint, disinhibition and hunger. *Journal of Psychosomatic Research, 29*(1), 71 83.

Thompson, J. K., Cattarin, J., Fowler, B., & Fisher, E. (1995). The Perception of Teasing Scale (POTS): A revision and extension of the Physical Appearance Related Teasing Scale (PARTS). *Journal of Personality Assessment, 65,* 146–157.

Thompson, J. K., Fabian, L. J., Moulton, D., Dunn, M., & Altabe, M. N. (1991). Development and validation of the Physical Appearance Related Teasing Scale. *Journal of Personality Assessment, 56,* 513–521.

Weissman, M. M., Orvaschel, H., & Padian, N. (1980). Children's symptom and social functioning self-report scales: Comparison of mothers' and children's reports. *Journal of Nervous and Mental Disease, 168,* 736–740.

Whitlock, E. P., Williams, S. B., Gold, R., Smith, P. R., & Shipman, S. A. (2005). Screening and interventions for childhood overweight: A summary of evidence for the U.S. Preventive Services Task Force. *Pediatrics, 116,* e125–e144.

8

INTERVENTION: STRATEGIES DESIGNED TO AFFECT ACTIVITY LEVEL, INTAKE PATTERNS, AND BEHAVIOR

MYLES S. FAITH AND BRIAN H. WROTNIAK

Behavioral intervention strategies intended to improve the dietary intake and physical activity levels of overweight children to help them restore energy balance and lose excess body weight are reviewed in this chapter. Our focus is on intervention (chap. 9, this volume, addresses pediatric obesity prevention), and particularly family-based approaches, because the efficacy of these interventions, compared with individual treatments in youth, is backed by decades of empirical evidence (Epstein, Myers, Raynor, & Saelens, 1998; Faith, Fontaine, Cheskin, & Allison, 2000). We begin by providing an overview of ways to help determine which youth are the most appropriate candidates for weight loss. Second, we review the fundamental components of behavior change techniques for weight control (e.g., self-monitoring, role modeling, functional analysis of behavior, stimulus control) along with a discussion of social and family support. Third, we discuss dietary intervention components of weight loss in youth. Fourth, we discuss the role of physical activity in family-based interventions. Fifth, we briefly review the evidence for the efficacy of family-based behavioral interventions and future research needs. We conclude with a list of Web sites and readings that provide practical resource materials for health care professionals, parents, and youth.

WHICH CHILDREN SHOULD RECEIVE TREATMENT?

An important preliminary question involves the determination of which children should receive treatment. An expert panel consensus report offered guidelines to parents and health professionals on this topic (Barlow & Dietz, 1998). Figure 8.1 presents an overview of these guidelines, which include a two-stage screening process.

The initial screen focuses on the child or adolescent's body mass index (BMI). For children whose BMI is equal to or exceeds the 95th percentile (age-and sex-specific), an in-depth medical assessment is recommended. These children are considered to be "obese" according to the most recent guidelines

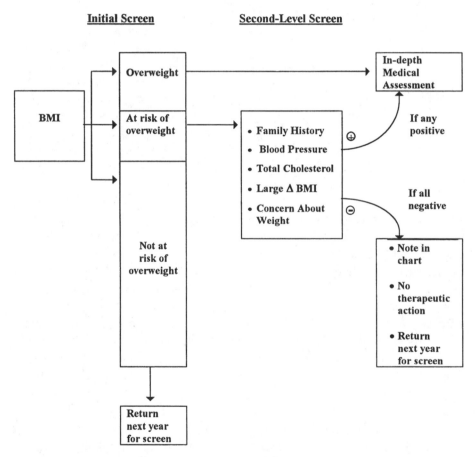

Figure 8.1. Guidelines for screening of overweight in children and adolescents. From "Guidelines for Overweight in Adolescent Preventive Services: Recommendations From an Expert Committee. The Expert Committee on Clinical Guidelines for Overweight in Adolescent Preventive Services," by J. H. Himes and W. H. Dietz, 1994, *American Journal of Clinical Nutrition, 59,* p. 312. Copyright 1994 by the American Society for Nutrition. Reprinted with permission.

of the American Medical Association (AMA). For any child whose BMI falls between the 85th and 94th percentiles (i.e., "overweight" according to the AMA guidelines), a second-level screen determines whether an in-depth medical assessment is warranted. This second-level screen focuses on the following five domains, with additional medical assessment recommended for children who exhibit any of these characteristics:

- Family history of cardiovascular disease, parental hypercholesterolemia; family history of diabetes mellitus or parental obesity, or unknown family history;
- High blood pressure (Report of the Second Task Force, 1987);
- Elevated total cholesterol (i.e., $\geq$ 5.2 mmol/L or $\geq$ 200 mg/dL; National Heart, Lung, and Blood Institute, 1991);
- A large recent increase in BMI (e.g., annual increase of 3–4 BMI units); and
- Child or adolescent concerns about weight or display of any emotional or psychological manifestations possibly related to overweight or perceptions of overweight.

Expert guidelines recommend an in-depth medical examination for any child who is at risk for overweight and scores positive on any of these criteria. In contrast, medical examination is not indicated for children who are at risk for overweight but score negative on all of these criteria.

BMI growth charts can be downloaded from the Centers for Disease Control and Prevention (http://www.cdc.gov/growthcharts). These charts include BMI-for-age percentile curves, which offer age- and gender-specific charts for specifying a child's BMI percentile. An international set of guidelines for defining overweight and obesity in children and adolescents also has been proposed (Cole, Bellizzi, Flegal, & Dietz, 2000). Using data from Brazil, Great Britain, Hong Kong, the Netherlands, Singapore, and the United States, growth curves were constructed for each age group to identify the BMI scores that would "project" to a BMI of 25 (i.e., overweight) or 30 (i.e., obese) at 18 years of age. For additional information on BMI percentiles and BMI percentile cutoffs, please see the Introduction chapter in this volume.

One of the major considerations in the determination of treatment prospects is whether the child has *metabolic syndrome*, which refers to a cluster of risk factors for cardiovascular disease and Type 2 diabetes, including abdominal obesity, dyslipidemia, glucose intolerance, and hypertension (Duncan, Li, & Zhou, 2004; Monzavi et al., 2006). Recently, the International Diabetes Federation (Zimmet et al., 2007) proposed criteria for defining at-risk status and the presence of metabolic syndrome in children and adolescents. Separate criteria were proposed for children 6 to less than 10 years, 10 to 16 years, and older than 16 years of age. Among children ages 6 to 10 years of age, for example, the following criteria for metabolic syndrome were proposed:

(a) obesity ≥ 90th percentile (or adult cut-off if lower) as assessed by waist circumference, (b) triglycerides ≥ 1.7 mm/L, (c) HDL cholesterol < 1.03 mmol/L, (d) blood pressure ≥ 130 mm Hg systolic or ≥ 85 mm Hg diastolic, (e) glucose ≥ 5.6 mmol/L (oral glucose tolerance test recommended) or known Type 2 diabetes mellitus. Children or adolescents who meet these criteria may be particularly appropriate candidates for weight loss interventions, given that they may be at risk for future cardiovascular disease or Type 2 diabetes.

As described earlier, many children who present for treatment often seek help not because of the medical complications of obesity but because of psychosocial issues such as weight teasing (Puhl & Brownell, 2001, 2003, 2006). In addition, weight discrimination and teasing surrounding sports and physical activity may be important reasons why certain overweight youth avoid sports in gyms or other social settings (Faith, Leone, Ayers, Heo, & Pietrobelli, 2002). Therefore, attention must be paid not only to weight status and medical comorbidities but also to issues of peer relations, body image, and teasing history. These children may derive benefit from hearing a professional talk about these issues in a caring and supportive manner. A more thorough discussion of weight bias and teasing may be found in chapter 4 of this volume.

BEHAVIOR MODIFICATION BASICS

The nuts and bolts of behavior change strategies for weight control strive to (a) enhance awareness of targeted behavior, (b) modify the antecedent situations or consequences associated with the targeted behavior, and (c) reinforce changes in the targeted behavior. These aims are achieved through a series of processes that are based on operant conditioning and social learning theories (Bandura, 1977, 1986). These processes include self-monitoring, functional analysis of behavior, goal setting, feedback, stimulus control, and reinforcement procedures (Wadden, Crerand, & Brock, 2005). These behavioral strategies are the hallmark of pediatric obesity treatment because achieving negative energy balance relies on changing dietary and physical activity behaviors. Each process is explained in the following sections.

Self-Monitoring

A critical step for initiating, and ultimately maintaining, individual behavior change is self-monitoring (Foreyt & Goodrick, 1991). The main purpose of self-monitoring is to provide feedback on the frequency with which the target behavior typically occurs, something that individuals can be notoriously poor at estimating. When children are challenged to estimate how much television they watch during a typical week or how many servings of fruits and vegetables they consume each day, estimates are often inaccurate despite the best of intentions. Self-monitoring addresses this problem by requiring one to record each time a targeted behavior occurs during an observation period (Korotitsch & Nelson-Gray, 1999). The situation in which the target behavior occurs can also be monitored to raise awareness of the contextual cues that relate to the target behavior and to allow for a functional analysis of behavior (see the following section). A variety of target behaviors can be monitored, including the intake of specific foods (e.g., fruits and vegetables, energy-dense foods), total food intake, minutes of physical activity, and television or screen viewing time. Therefore, precisely defining the target behavior is a key part of self-monitoring.

A variety of diaries, forms, logs, and formats can be used for self-monitoring. In addition, the mere action of tracking one's behavior can promote behavior change and therefore can be an effective intervention (Kazdin, 2001). The frequency with which individuals self-monitor is a reliable predictor of weight loss in obese children and adults (Berkowitz, Wadden, Tershakovec, & Cronquist, 2003; Wadden, Berkowitz, et al., 2005) and is associated with long-term weight loss maintenance (Wing & Hill, 2001). At the same time, successful weight loss, increased feelings of control, and enhanced weight control are often powerful reinforcements that can enhance the act of monitoring. Finally, self-monitoring can provide an objective benchmark against which goal setting (described later) can be determined and behavior change can be evaluated. Hence, the first step to self-monitoring is to identify a specific behavior to be changed.

Functional Analysis of Behavior

Understanding the functions or purposes that behaviors serve is important for behavior change. To this end, a functional analysis of behavior (FAB) can be used to determine the situational circumstances that promote a target behavior and the consequences that sustain it. Self-monitoring strategies can raise awareness of these relations and allow for an FAB. Specifically, FAB involves a detailed analysis of the antecedents of the target behavior (i.e., What factors or contexts precede behavior change?), the target behavior itself, and the consequences of the behavior (e.g., What reactions does the behavior elicit from others that might sustain behavior change?). When successfully implemented, an FAB can highlight environmental changes that might be helpful in facilitating behavior changes among individuals who are exposed to the environments in question. For example, children often eat high-fat snack foods when sitting at home watching television or playing video games (i.e., the antecedent event), and such snacking becomes associated with positive feelings or satisfaction (i.e., the consequence). This suggests that efforts to modify snacking behavior—in this example—would either need to change the antecedent event (e.g., restrict allotted television viewing time) or change the consequence (e.g., provide snack foods that are less desirable and therefore less likely to be overconsumed).

Goal Setting

Goal setting is a well-established individual behavior change strategy. On the basis of the learning principle of successive approximation, children are encouraged to set small, attainable goals that build up to a larger goal. Smaller goals are more likely to be attained, thereby providing children a sense of mastery that can support additional behavior change (Wadden & Foster, 2000). Reappraisal of goals, a common strategy for behavior change, involves setting new goals when initial goals were not achieved and revisiting or revising goals that have not yet been achieved. An important consideration is the establishment of achievable goals. It has been well documented, for example, that many obese adults hold weight loss goals that are unlikely to be achieved even with superior behavior modification programs (Foster, Wadden, Vogt, & Brewer, 1997; Wadden et al., 2003). This may lead to frustration and hinder behavior change. When working with obese children, it is especially important that goals are set that are achievable, relatively immediate (e.g., focus on a changed behavior rather than losing 10 pounds), and can promote feelings of accomplishment and self-efficacy. Goals that are unrealistic (e.g., completely give up soda or desserts) can lead to frustration. Small, progressive, and sustainable goals are the ideal.

Stimulus Control

Increasing the frequency of more healthy behaviors (e.g., fruit and vegetable intake) is easier when environmental cues for less healthy behaviors are removed or limited (Heatherton & Nichols, 1994), a concept known as *stimulus control*. Examples of stimulus control for reducing intake of undesirable foods include restricting the locations where eating takes place (e.g., limiting eating at home to the kitchen and dining room), the people with whom social eating occurs (e.g., friends who regularly go for ice cream), the activities associated with undesirable food choices (e.g., television viewing), or the times when eating occurs out of the home (e.g., on the way home from work). As another example, Robinson (1999) demonstrated that altering the home environment to limit television access was associated with increased physical activity and prevention of weight gain in children. Television watching may influence both physical activity or inactivity and eating behavior (Robinson, 2001).

Stimulus control not only involves the removal of cues that prompt undesirable behaviors but also includes the provision or amplification of cues that prompt desirable behaviors. A case in point is the literature on food provision in the context of weight loss interventions for adult obesity. Behavioral interventions that provided obese patients with healthier foods to take home generally achieved greater weight loss success than comparable behavioral interventions that did not incorporate food provision (Jeffery et al., 1993; Wing et al., 1996). In a similar manner, providing a home-based exercise bicycle to obese children that interfaced with their televisions promoted child weight loss (Faith et al., 2001).

Feedback

Feedback is a critical component of behavior change and is typically achieved through careful self-monitoring of behavior. For example, feedback on weight control can be achieved by regularly weighing oneself (e.g., weekly), which appears to be important for longer term maintenance of weight loss (Wing & Hill, 2001).

Positive Reinforcement Strategies

Positive reinforcement is an important component of individual behavior change, especially when it can help offset the discomfort of giving up less healthy behaviors (Wadden, Crerand, et al., 2005). Praise and recognition can be among the strongest strategies, which may explain why weight loss is enhanced when peers and family members are supportive. This is especially true for childhood obesity prevention and treatment strategies (Epstein et al., 1998). As described later, training caregivers in "positive parenting" techniques is associated with enhanced child weight loss. This involves training parents to avoid punitive or overly critical interactions with their children and, instead, to focus on rewarding any and all positive behaviors.

An interesting concept related to positive reinforcement is that of displacement or substitution. There is some evidence that reinforcing, and thereby increasing, fruit and vegetable intake can lead to the "natural" displacement of energy-dense foods (Epstein et al., 2001; Goldfield & Epstein, 2002). This has been documented in at least one randomized clinical trial of children who were at risk for obesity and whose parents were trained either to reward increased fruit and vegetable intake or reduced energy-dense food intake by their children (Epstein et al., 2001). Results indicated that both groups showed comparable reductions in percentage overweight, suggesting that increasing fruit and vegetable intake may have displaced fat or sugar intake.

Social Support and the Role of Family

Social learning theory underscores the importance of social support for facilitating individual behavior change. Indeed, studies indicate that family members play pivotal roles in facilitating weight control by other family members. Brownell, Heckerman, Westlake, Hayes, and Monti (1978) conducted one of the first studies to document the role of family support for enhancing weight control. They studied the 8-month weight loss of obese adults assigned to one of three behavioral weight loss treatment conditions: (a) cooperative spouse–couples training, in which both the obese patient and his or her spouse attended all training sessions; (b) cooperative spouse–subject alone training, in which only the obese patient received treatment despite having a spouse who was willing to attend treatment; and (c) noncooperative spouse training, in which the obese patient received treatment alone because his or her spouse was unwilling to attend. Participants and their spouses were randomized to the first two conditions but not to the third condition. The behavioral training program was consistent for all patients. Results indicated that weight loss was significantly greater among subjects in the first group (13.6 kilograms) than for subjects in the second and third groups (8.8 kilograms and 6.8 kilograms, respectively). Similar to Brownell et al.'s results, other studies also found that weight loss is enhanced when spouses are included in treatment (Pearce, LeBow, & Orchard, 1981); however, not all studies found that including spouses in treatment improved weight loss for the target obese patient (Wing, Marcus, Epstein, & Kupfer, 1983; also see chap. 3, this volume).

More consistent evidence for the role of family support comes from family-based intervention studies for pediatric obesity. Reviews of this literature have been provided elsewhere (Epstein et al., 1998), and there is compelling evidence that obese children lose more weight when their parents are actively involved in treatment than when they are not. Epstein, Valoski, Wing, and McCurley (1994) provided 10-year follow-up data on obese children and their parents who were randomly assigned to one of three family-based behavioral weight loss interventions: (a) an intervention that targeted the parent and child together; (b) an intervention that just targeted the child; or (c) a nonspecific intervention that reinforced the families for attendance. Parents in the first group were trained actively in the behavioral change strategies (see next section) that could be applied to their children to help them achieve better lifestyle changes. Results indicated that 43% of the children in this first group reduced their percentage overweight by at least 20% (a relatively large treatment effect) in comparison with only 22% of the children in the second group and 29% of the children in the third group. The mean reduction in percentage overweight over 10 years also was significantly greater for the first group than the other groups (see Figure 8.2).

Golan, Weizman, Apter, and Fainaru (1998) compared the effects of a behavioral weight control intervention for obese children ages 6 to 11 years that targeted either the parent or the obese child as the active agent of behavior change. Both interventions used the same behavior change principles, includ-

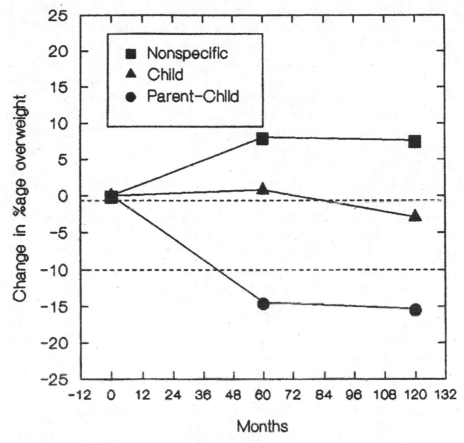

Figure 8.2. Reduction in child percentage overweight over 10 years is significantly greater among children whose parents were actively involved and reinforced for initial treatment participation compared with children whose parents were not reinforced for participation. From "Ten-Year Outcomes of Behavioral Family-Based Treatment for Childhood Obesity," by L. H. Epstein, A. Valoski, R. R Wing, and J. McCurley, 1994, *Health Psychology, 13*(5), p. 378. Copyright 1994 by the American Psychological Association.

ing self-monitoring, stimulus control, and reinforcement (see later discussion). After 1 year, reduction in child percentage overweight was significantly greater among the intervention targeting parents (mean reduction = 14.6%) compared with the intervention targeting children (mean reduction = 8.1%). After 7 years, the superior outcome of the parent intervention group remained significant (mean reductions = 29.0% vs. 20.2% in the two groups, respectively, *p* < .05; Golan & Crow, 2004).

The key behavior modification strategies in parent skills training include behavioral contracting, stimulus control, and positive reinforcement (Dietz & Robinson, 2005). *Behavioral contracting* refers to an explicit contract among family members that stipulates the behavioral goals that family members will attempt to reach and the reinforcements they will receive for attaining such goals. Rewards other than food and money are used and include family-based and interpersonal rewards (e.g., praise, family trips, sports equipment). *Stimulus control* refers to practical restructuring of the physical home environment described earlier in the chapter. Positive reinforcement strategies for families form the foundation for treatment as parents are trained to move away from punitive parenting strategies to more positive parenting strategies. Additional strategies for parents were provided by Barlow and Dietz (1998).

Finally, we note that there is increasing evidence that pharmacotherapy can be a viable adjunctive component of conventional behavioral modification strategies. Berkowitz, Wadden, Tershakovec, and Cronquist (2003) found that weight loss was approximately doubled among youth who received behavioral therapy plus the drug sibutramine (brand name Meridia; a serotonin and norepinepherine reuptake inhibitor) compared with youth who received only behavioral therapy. Sibutramine helps to reduce appetite, and the efficacy of the medication was recently replicated in a large scale multisite randomized clinical trial (Berkowitz et al., 2006). However, it must be taken under physician care because of the possibility of increased blood pressure side effects.

DIETARY COMPONENTS OF WEIGHT CONTROL

Dietary modification is a powerful and necessary component for child weight loss. Treatments focusing solely on dietary modification have achieved short-term (Epstein, Wing, Penner, & Kress, 1985; Rocchini et al., 1988) and long-term (Epstein et al., 1994) weight losses. Short-term interventions lacking a dietary component achieved mixed results (Blomquist, Borjeson, Larsson, Persson, & Sterky, 1965), but there is no evidence for long-term efficacy of treatments lacking a dietary component.

Many programs have used Epstein's StopLight Diet (Epstein & Squires, 1978; Ludwig, 2000) or a variant for dietary prescriptions. Using the Food Guide Pyramid of the U.S. Department of Agriculture as a foundation, children are encouraged to increase intake of low-fat, nutrient-rich "Green" foods (e.g., fruits and vegetables); to consume moderate-calorie "Yellow" foods in moderation (e.g., certain grain foods); and to minimize if not eliminate high-fat, high-sugar "Red" foods (e.g., candies). Detailed lists of food alternatives and their corresponding calories are provided to families, who are encouraged to try new and varied Green and Yellow foods. Most behavioral programs initially strive to reduce children's total daily caloric intake providing recommendations for increasing physical activity gradually (e.g., 10 minutes at a time) until the child is physically active for 60 minutes or more each day. Providing families with information on local community centers and organizations that offer physical activity for youth, such as the YMCA, can help promote physical activity.

Providing children with suggestions for decreasing sedentary behaviors can help encourage greater engagement in physical activity. Reducing children's sedentary behaviors can be a more effective weight management strategy than providing an exercise program (Epstein et al., 1995). Therefore, asking how much time children spend watching television, using the computer, and playing video games, and suggesting ways to reduce children's exposure to these sedentary activities (e.g., have a television turn-off day; limit the number of hours of television, computer, and video game use; remove televisions from children's bedrooms) can help to increase physical activity and lead to healthier outcomes. (For more information on assessment issues, see chap. 7, this volume.)

One strategy to help children become more physically active is the use of pedometers. Pedometers can help motivate youth to engage in physical activity. They are relatively inexpensive, easy to use, and provide an objective measure of physical activity. A baseline level of physical activity can be determined by having the child wear the pedometer for a week to determine the average number of steps per day. Depending on their average daily steps, individuals are classified as *very inactive* (≤ 2,500 steps), *inactive* (2,501–5,000 steps), *moderately active* (5,001–7,500 steps), *active* (7,501–10,000 steps), or *very active* (>10,000 steps; CORE Tools and Patient Information, 2005). Once a baseline activity level is determined, an appropriate goal could be achieving the next activity level by increasing average steps per day by 2,000 (about 1 mile). Physical activity goals can then be progressed until the child averages 10,000 to 15,000 steps per day (Tudor-Locke et al., 2004). The Web site "America on the Move" (see list of Web sites at the end of this chapter) provides information on using a pedometer and ways for increasing physical activity. Individuals can also sign up to receive a free daily e-mail tip for increasing physical activity.

Physical activity goals for youth should be established on the basis of each child's current amount of physical activity engagement and gradually increased to meet recommendations. Research with adults shows that physical activity does not have to be completed all at once to obtain health benefits but can be accumulated in smaller bouts throughout the day (Jakicic, Wing, Butler, & Robertson, 1995).

When developing exercise goals, the child should be encouraged to choose activities that are enjoyable and realistic. Parental involvement is also necessary (Wrotniak, Epstein, Paluch, & Roemmich, 2004). Parental support through transportation and behavioral modification techniques such as

while maintaining adequate nutrition for development and growth. A recommended first step is increasing children's awareness of eating habits through self-monitoring, with parental help. With appropriate reductions of total calories and fat intake, children can meet their nutritional needs through increasing the nutrient density of foods eaten, shift toward negative energy balance, and gradually substitute for unhealthy food choices. There is no evidence to date that carefully controlled behavioral programs promote disordered eating or formal eating disorders among child participants (Epstein et al., 1998). Few studies have evaluated different nutrition plans or tested particular aspects of the overall dietary component.

Expert consensus suggests that a lifestyle approach to changing overweight children's eating habits can gradually decrease overall caloric intake, minimize the risk of youths' failing to meet recommended nutrient intake, and maximize long-term weight control (Barlow & Dietz, 1998). This may be especially true for children who are mildly to moderately obese (i.e., a BMI falling between the 85th and 95th percentiles according to the Centers for Disease Control and Prevention growth charts). More restrictive approaches, such as protein-sparing modified fasts and very-low-calorie diets, have been less frequently investigated. Those studies suggest long-term outcomes similar to those induced by moderate caloric restrictive diets among moderately overweight adolescents (Figueroa-Colon, von Almen, Franklin, Schuftan, & Suskind, 1993). These more restrictive dietary plans have been recommended in combination with careful physician monitoring for severely obese adolescents or less overweight adolescents with major health complications secondary to obesity (Stallings, Archibald, Pencharz, Harrison, & Bell, 1988).

Finally, research by Ludwig and colleagues tested the effects of a lower glycemic index (GI) diet compared with traditional reduced-fat diets for weight loss in obese children and adolescents (Ludwig, 2000). The GI of a food or beverage reflects characteristics of its carbohydrate content, specifically, the effects on blood glucose levels following consumption of the item relative to a "standard" food (typically white bread). Foods with a higher GI are more rapidly digested and are associated with marked fluctuations in blood sugar levels. Low-GI foods are more slowly digested and absorbed, produce gradual rises in blood glucose and insulin levels, and are associated with greater feelings of fullness (Ludwig et al., 1999). Lower GI diets are not necessarily lower in dietary fat, at least in comparison with traditional lower fat diets recommended by the U.S. Department of Agriculture. Results of some studies suggest that diets promoting reduced-GI foods are more effective for weight loss than those promoting reduced-fat foods (Ebbeling, Leidig, Sinclair, Hangen, & Ludwig, 2003). On the one hand, it may be that the lower GI diet feels less restrictive for adolescents and therefore leads to greater weight loss. On the other hand, a more recent study failed to find differences between a low-GI diet and a low-fat diet for adolescent weight loss (Ebbeling, Leidig, Feldman, Lovesky, & Ludwig, 2007). This is a controversial issue (Sheard et al., 2004), and teaching youth to understand and monitor the GI of foods may be challenging.

PHYSICAL ACTIVITY

Physical activity (i.e., any bodily movement produced by skeletal muscle that yields increased energy expenditure) can create negative energy balance and thereby facilitate weight loss. Indeed, the most successful pediatric obesity programs have included a physical activity component (Epstein, Wing, Penner, et al., 1985), but physical activity components have not always augmented the effects of dietary modification (Epstein, Wing, Koeske, & Valoski, 1984; Hills & Parker, 1988). There appear to be consistent short-term effects of physical activity interventions on both children's weight status as well as cardiorespiratory fitness and other cardiovascular health benefits (Becque, Katch, Rocchini, Marks, & Moorehead, 1988; Rocchini et al., 1988; Sasaki, Shindo, Tanaka, Ando, & Arakawa, 1987). Exercise programs that stress planned aerobic sessions seem to be more beneficial for children's weight loss than lower energy expenditure calisthenics programs (Epstein, Wing, Penner, et al., 1985). However, for long-term weight maintenance, data suggest that the best results are achieved through lifestyle approaches that attempt to weave physical activity into day-in day-out everyday living (Epstein et al., 1994). Lifestyle interventions work to integrate more physical activity into daily activities (e.g., climbing stairs instead of taking the elevator, parking one's car at a distance from a supermarket, walking to the grocery store).

It should be noted that several clinical studies attempted to improve the metabolic profile of overweight youth via resistance training. Kang et al. (2002) showed that intensive physical training interventions for obese adolescents (i.e., 5 days a week over 8 months) improved insulin resistance syndrome markers in these youth. A series of uncontrolled studies by Sothern et al. (2000) tested a multidisciplinary obesity treatment program that included moderate-intensity progressive exercises. The researchers found that treatment participation was associated with improvements in weight status and lipid profile in adolescents. Shaibi et al. (2006) randomized 22 overweight Latino adolescent males to either a twice per week exercise resistance training (RT) program or a nonexercising control group for 16 weeks. There was a trend for greater reductions in percentage body fat in the RT group than in the control group, and insulin sensitivity showed significantly greater improvements in the RT than the control group.

Weight loss can also be achieved by targeting reductions in sedentary activities (e.g., television viewing) rather than targeting increased physical activity per se (Epstein et al., 1995; Epstein, Paluch, Gordy, & Dorn, 2000).

Although children who reduce targeted sedentary activities redistribute of their time to other sedentary activities, data indicate that children nonetheless redistribute and allocate enough time to increased physical a ities to facilitate weight management. Hence, targeting reduced seden activity (e.g., television viewing, video games, computers) has become a v treatment strategy. See chapter 2 of this volume for additional discussion these issues.

Being physically active also leads to improved fitness and helps prever. obesity-related disease in youth. Children who are physically active have improved aerobic endurance and muscular strength (Sallis, McKenzie, & Alcaraz, 1993). Physical activity may also reduce healthy children's risk factors for Type 2 diabetes, certain types of cancers, and cardiovascular disease (Chakravarthy, Joyner, & Booth, 2002; Sallis, Patterson, Buono, & Nader, 1988). In children with chronic disease, regular physical activity in children who are overweight increases physical fitness (Ignico & Mahon, 1995) and reduces body weight (Epstein, Valoski, Wing, & McCurley, 1990).

Conversely, sedentary activity increases the prevalence of many chronic health conditions, including obesity. Obese children can have pulmonary complications including decreased exercise tolerance (Deforche et al., 2003), asthma (Epstein, Wu, Paluch, Cerny, & Dorn, 2000), and sleep problems (Barlow & Dietz, 1998). Inactivity may also result in decreased muscle strength and impair motor function, making it more difficult to participate in daily activities (Hills, Hennig, Byrne, & Steele, 2002; Wearing, Hennig, Byrne, Steele, & Hills, 2006).

Although the benefits of physical activity are often recognized by parents and children, implementing these changes can be challenging. Because of the value placed on physical appearance and prejudices against obese individuals, children who are overweight may feel embarrassed and ashamed (Pierce & Wardle, 1997). Communication must occur in ways that express feelings of compassion and caring and not of blame. It is important to inform families that obesity is a chronic medical condition that can be treated. Questions about physical activity should be framed to focus on behaviors rather than on the characteristics of the individual. For example, ask a child "Do you find daily physical activity sometimes difficult to do?" instead of "Do you lack willpower?" (Barlow & Dietz, 1998). By taking the time to understand each family's particular situation, treatment recommendations can be refined and empathetic support provided.

Educating families on healthy behaviors and strategies to attain goals that can be implemented immediately and continued over the long term is an essential component of weight control. Children and their families should be educated on age-appropriate physical activity, dietary considerations, and behavioral modification techniques. A discussion of physical activity begins by asking how much physical activity the child is currently doing and then

parental modeling and positive reinforcement can help the child with making healthy physical activity changes. For weight loss and weight maintenance, lifestyle- and age-appropriate activities such as bicycling, dancing, swimming, and roller-skating may be better choices for children than traditional exercise like walking on a treadmill and doing sit-ups (Epstein et al., 1994). Physical activity goals should be matched to children's fitness levels. Encouraging and providing opportunities for children to be physically active because it is fun, challenging, and can improve motor skills (Wrotniak, Epstein, Dorn, Jones, & Kondilis, 2006) rather than focusing on weight loss may also help to motivate youth and to promote lifelong physical activity behaviors. There are many active games on the "Eat Smart. Play Hard" Web site (see list of Web sites at the end of this chapter) that can be useful in helping establish a program for children.

THE EFFICACY OF BEHAVIORAL TREATMENT FOR CHILDHOOD OBESITY

Family-based behavioral treatment programs have been the most extensively studied interventions to date and have reliably produced the best short- and long-term results. Compared with the treatment of adult obesity, the treatment of pediatric obesity has achieved much better outcomes over short- and long-term periods (Epstein et al., 1994; Wilson, 1994). Family behavioral modification appears to be more effective for younger children (i.e., younger than 10 years of age) than for older children, and for girls than for boys, when examined up to 24 months after treatment (Epstein, Paluch, Roemmich, & Beecher, 2007). More than 20 years ago, Epstein, Wing, Woodall, et al. (1985) demonstrated the efficacy of family-based methods compared with nutrition education for weight loss among a sample of overweight 5- to 8-year-olds. Family-based methods reduced mean percentage overweight from 41.9% to 15.6%, whereas nutrition education resulted in a smaller reduction in percentage overweight from 39.2% to 28.0%. Efficacy of family behavioral modification has been documented in a number of other studies with young children (Aragona, Cassady, & Drabman, 1975; Graves, Meyers, & Clark, 1988; Senediak & Spence, 1985; Wheeler & Hess, 1976), and there is increasing support for its efficacy with adolescents (Berkowitz et al., 2003, 2006).

Not all reviews have reached such favorable conclusions. A comprehensive review by Summerbell et al. (2003) of 18 randomized clinical trials for childhood and adolescent obesity, in which treatment lasted at least 6 months, could not reach any conclusions because of methodological limitations and heterogeneity of the literature. They concluded that "there is a limited amount of quality data on the components of programs to treat childhood obesity that favour one program over another. . . . We conclude that no direct conclusions can be drawn from this review with confidence" (p. 1). Ideas for future research suggested by the authors include identification of family factors, culture and religion, and the broader physical environment in predicting success in child weight loss.

CONCLUSION

Family-based treatments for childhood obesity have been empirically tested and supported over the past 3 decades. Behavioral principles of self-monitoring, goal-setting, reinforcement, and positive parenting practices provide the foundation. As the prevalence of childhood obesity increases nationwide, there will likely be a need to develop more efficacious treatments (for heavier children) to address the comorbidities of childhood obesity (especially metabolic syndrome and Type 2 diabetes) and to make existing interventions more disseminable. There is also a great need to test existing behavioral intervention programs with families who are more ethnically and economically diverse than have been examined to date. In addition, there is a need to test behavioral interventions in more geographically diverse settings, especially rural communities that often have limited health care access.

SUGGESTED WEB SITES AND READINGS

We recommend the following organizations, publications, and Web sites for materials on family-based behavioral treatment for childhood obesity:

America on the Move. Web site designed to promote physical activity through pedometer strategies and challenges: http://aom.americaonthemove.org/site/c.krLXJ3PJKuG/b.1524889/k.BFFA/Home.htm

CalorieKing.com Food Database. Nutritional information for more than 50,000 American generic and brand name foods (including over 260 fast-food chains): http://www.calorieking.com/foods/category.php?cat=21

Centers for Disease Control and Prevention. *Body and mind.* Web site offering general health information and aimed at young people: http://www.bam.gov/

Epstein, L., & Squires, S. (1978). *StopLight diet for children.* New York: Little, Brown. (Available from used book vendors such as http://www.albris.com)

Ludwig, D. (2007). *Ending the food fight.* New York: Houghton Mifflin.

National Heart Lung and Blood Association. *We Can: Ways to enhance children's activity and nutrition.* Web site with information on preventing overweight and increasing activity in children: http://www.nhlbi.nih.gov/health/public/heart/obesity/wecan/whats-we-can/resources_parents.htm#new

National Institute of Diabetes, Digestive, and Kidney Disorders. Weight-Control Information Network. Web site with information on weight control and nutrition for health professionals and the general public: http://win.niddk.nih.gov/index.htm or http://win.niddk.nih.gov/publications/over_child.htm

Nemours Foundation. *KidsHealth*. Interactive BMI calculator with tutorial: http://www.kidshealth.org/kid/stay_healthy/weight/bmi.html

Sothern, M., Von Almen, K., & Schumacher, H. (2001). *TrimKids*. New York: HarperCollins.

U.S. Department of Agriculture. *MyPyramid.gov*. Nutrition information for adults: http://www.mypyramid.gov/

U.S. Department of Agriculture. *MyPyramid Blastoff Game*. Interactive game for children with nutrition information: http://www.mypyramid.gov/kids/kids_game.html

U.S. Department of Agriculture. *Eat Smart. Play Hard*. Interactive tool for children with nutrition information: http://www.fns.usda.gov/eatsmartplayhardkids/

U.S. Department of Health and Human Services. *Dietary guidelines for Americans*. Web site with links to publications on diet, published every 5 years since 1980: http://www.health.gov/dietaryguidelines/

U.S. Department of Health and Human Services. *Verb*. Web site with a physical activity interactive program: http://www.verbnow.com/

REFERENCES

Aragona, J., Cassady, J., & Drabman, R. S. (1975). Treating overweight children through parental training and contingency contracting. *Journal of Applied Behavior Analysis, 8*(3), 269–278.

Bandura, A. (1977). *Social learning theory*. Englewood Cliffs, NJ: Prentice-Hall.

Bandura, A. (1986). *Social foundations of thought and action: A social cognitive theory*. Englewood Cliffs, NJ: Prentice-Hall.

Barlow, S. E., & Dietz, W. H. (1998). Obesity evaluation and treatment: Expert Committee recommendations. The Maternal and Child Health Bureau, Health Resources and Services Administration and the Department of Health and Human Services. *Pediatrics, 102*(3), E29.

Becque, M. D., Katch, V. L., Rocchini, A. P., Marks, C. R., & Moorehead, C. (1988). Coronary risk incidence of obese adolescents: Reduction by exercise plus diet intervention. *Pediatrics, 81*(5), 605–612.

Berkowitz, R. I., Fujioka, K., Daniels, S. R., Hoppin, A. G., Owen, S., Perry, A. C., et al. (2006). Effects of sibutramine treatment in obese adolescents: A randomized trial. *Annals of Internal Medicine, 145*(2), 81–90.

Berkowitz, R. I., Wadden, T. A., Tershakovec, A. M., & Cronquist, J. L. (2003). Behavior therapy and sibutramine for the treatment of adolescent obesity: A randomized controlled trial. *JAMA, 289*(14), 1805–1812.

Blomquist, B., Borjeson, M., Larsson, Y., Persson, B., & Sterky, G. (1965). The effect of physical activity on the body measurements and work capacity of overweight boys. *Acta Paediatrica Scandinavica, 54*, 566–572.

Brownell, K. D., Heckerman, C. L., Westlake, R. J., Hayes, S. C., & Monti, P. M. (1978). The effect of couples training and partner co-operativeness in the behavioral treatment of obesity. *Behavior Research and Therapy, 16*(5), 323–333.

Chakravarthy, M. V., Joyner, M. J., & Booth, F. W. (2002). An obligation for primary care physicians to prescribe physical activity to sedentary patients to reduce the risk of chronic health conditions. *Mayo Clinic Proceedings, 77*(2), 165–173.

Cole, T. J., Bellizzi, M. C., Flegal, K. M., & Dietz, W. H. (2000). Establishing a standard definition for child overweight and obesity worldwide: International survey. *British Medical Journal, 320*(7244), 1240–1243.

CORE tools and patient information: Using step counters to increase physical activity. (2005). *Obesity Management, 1*(2), 70–72. doi:10.1089/obe.2005.1.70

Deforche, B., Lefevre, J., De Bourdeaudhuij, I., Hills, A. P., Duquet, W., & Bouckaert, J. (2003). Physical fitness and physical activity in obese and nonobese Flemish youth. *Obesity Research, 11*(3), 434–441.

Dietz, W. H., & Robinson, T. N. (2005). Clinical practice. Overweight children and adolescents. *New England Journal of Medicine, 352*(20), 2100–2109.

Duncan, G. E., Li, S. M., & Zhou, X. H. (2004). Prevalence and trends of a metabolic syndrome phenotype among U.S. adolescents, 1999–2000. *Diabetes Care, 27*(10), 2438–2443.

Ebbeling, C. B., Leidig, M. M., Feldman, H. A., Lovesky, M. M., & Ludwig, D. S. (2007). Effects of a low-glycemic load vs low-fat diet in obese young adults: A randomized trial. *JAMA, 297*(19), 2092–2102.

Ebbeling, C. B., Leidig, M. M., Sinclair, K. B., Hangen, J. P., & Ludwig, D. S. (2003). A reduced-glycemic load diet in the treatment of adolescent obesity. *Archives of Pediatrics and Adolescent Medicine, 157*(8), 773–779.

Epstein, L. H., Gordy, C. C., Raynor, H. A., Beddome, M., Kilanowski, C. K., & Paluch, R. (2001). Increasing fruit and vegetable intake and decreasing fat and sugar intake in families at risk for childhood obesity. *Obesity Research, 9*(3), 171–178.

Epstein, L. H., Myers, M. D., Raynor, H. A., & Saelens, B. E. (1998). Treatment of pediatric obesity. *Pediatrics, 101*(3, Pt 2), 554–570.

Epstein, L. H., Paluch, R. A., Gordy, C. C., & Dorn, J. (2000). Decreasing sedentary behaviors in treating pediatric obesity. *Archives of Pediatrics and Adolescent Medicine, 154*(3), 220–226.

Epstein, L. H., Paluch, R. A., Roemmich, J. N., & Beecher, M. D. (2007). Family-based obesity treatment, then and now: Twenty-five years of pediatric obesity treatment. *Health Psychology, 26*(4), 381–391.

Epstein, L. H., & Squires, S. (1978). *The Stoplight Diet for Children.* Boston: Little, Brown.

Epstein, L. H., Valoski, A., Wing, R. R., & McCurley, J. (1990). Ten-year follow-up of behavioral, family-based treatment for obese children. *JAMA, 264*(19), 2519–2523.

Epstein, L. H., Valoski, A., Wing, R. R., & McCurley, J. (1994). Ten-year outcomes of behavioral family-based treatment for childhood obesity. *Health Psychology, 13*(5), 373–383.

Epstein, L. H., Valoski, A. M., Vara, L. S., McCurley, J., Wisniewski, L., Kalarchian, M. A., et al. (1995). Effects of decreasing sedentary behavior and increasing activity on weight change in obese children. *Health Psychology, 14*(2), 109–115.

Epstein, L. H., Wing, R. R., Koeske, R., & Valoski, A. (1984). Effects of diet plus exercise on weight change in parents and children. *Journal of Consulting and Clinical Psychology, 52*(3), 429–437.

Epstein, L. H., Wing, R. R., Penner, B. C., & Kress, M. J. (1985). Effect of diet and controlled exercise on weight loss in obese children. *Journal of Pediatrics, 107*(3), 358–361.

Epstein, L. H., Wing, R. R., Woodall, K., Penner, B. C., Kress, M. J., & Koeske, R. (1985). Effects of family-based behavioral treatment on obese 5- to-8-year-old children. *Behavior Therapy, 16*, 205–212.

Epstein, L. H., Wu, Y. W., Paluch, R. A., Cerny, F. J., & Dorn, J. P. (2000). Asthma and maternal body mass index are related to pediatric body mass index and obesity: Results from the Third National Health and Nutrition Examination Survey. *Obesity Research, 8*(8), 575–581.

Faith, M. S., Berman, N., Heo, M., Pietrobelli, A., Gallagher, D., Epstein, L. H., et al. (2001). Effects of contingent television on physical activity and television viewing in obese children. *Pediatrics, 107*(5), 1043–1048.

Faith, M. S., Fontaine, K. R., Cheskin, L. J., & Allison, D. B. (2000). Behavioral approaches to the problems of obesity. *Behavior Modification, 24*(4), 459–493.

Faith, M. S., Leone, M. A., Ayers, T. S., Heo, M., & Pietrobelli, A. (2002). Weight criticism during physical activity, coping skills, and reported physical activity in children. *Pediatrics, 110*(2, Pt 1), e23.

Figueroa Colon, R., von Almen, T. K., Franklin, F. A., Schuftan, C., & Suskind, R. M. (1993). Comparison of two hypocaloric diets in obese children. *American Journal of Disabled Children, 147*(2), 160–166.

Foreyt, J. P., & Goodrick, G. K. (1991). Factors common to successful therapy for the obese patient. *Medicine and Science in Sports and Exercise, 23*(3), 292–297.

Foster, G. D., Wadden, T. A., Vogt, R. A., & Brewer, G. (1997). What is a reasonable weight loss? Patients' expectations and evaluations of obesity treatment outcomes. *Journal of Consulting and Clinical Psychology, 65*(1), 79–85.

Golan, M., & Crow, S. (2004). Targeting parents exclusively in the treatment of childhood obesity: Long-term results. *Obesity Research, 12*(2), 357–361.

Golan, M., Weizman, A., Apter, A., & Fainaru, M. (1998). Parents as the exclusive agents of change in the treatment of childhood obesity. *American Journal of Clinical Nutrition, 67*(6), 1130–1135.

Goldfield, G. S., & Epstein, L. H. (2002). Can fruits and vegetables and activities substitute for snack foods? *Health Psychology, 21*(3), 299–303.

Graves, T., Meyers, A. W., & Clark, L. (1988). An evaluation of parental problem-solving training in the behavioral treatment of childhood obesity. *Journal of Consulting and Clinical Psychology, 56*(2), 246–250.

Heatherton, T. F., & Nichols, P. A. (1994). Personal accounts of successful versus failed attempts at life change. *Personality and Social Psychology Bulletin, 20,* 664–675.

Hills, A. P., Hennig, E. M., Byrne, N. M., & Steele, J. R. (2002). The biomechanics of adiposity—Structural and functional limitations of obesity and implications for movement. *Obesity Reviews, 3*(1), 35–43.

Hills, A. P., & Parker, A. W. (1988). Obesity management via diet and exercise intervention. *Child: Care, Health and Development, 14*(6), 409–416.

Himes, J. H., & Deitz, W. H. (1994). Guidelines for overweight in adolescent preventive services: Recommendations from an expert committee. The Expert Committee on Clinical Guidelines for Overweight in Adolescent Preventive Services. *American Journal of Clinical Nutrition, 59*(2), 307–316.

Ignico, A. A., & Mahon, A. D. (1995). The effects of a physical fitness program on low-fit children. *Research Quarterly in Exercise and Sports, 66*(1), 85–90.

Jakicic, J. M., Wing, R. R., Butler, B. A., & Robertson, R. J. (1995). Prescribing exercise in multiple short bouts versus one continuous bout: Effects on adherence, cardiorespiratory fitness, and weight loss in overweight women. *International Journal of Obesity, 19*(12), 893–901.

Jeffery, R. W., Wing, R. R., Thorson, C., Burton, L. R., Raether, C., Harvey, J., et al. (1993). Strengthening behavioral interventions for weight loss: A randomized trial of food provision and monetary incentives. *Journal of Consulting and Clinical Psychology, 61*(6), 1038–1045.

Kang, H. S., Gutin, B., Barbeau, P., Owens, S., Lemmon, C. R., Allison, J., et al. (2002). Physical training improves insulin resistance syndrome markers in obese adolescents. *Medicine and Science in Sports and Exercise, 34*(12), 1920–1927.

Kazdin, A. (2001). *Behavior modification in applied settings* (6th ed.). Belmont, CA: Wadsworth/Thomson Learning.

Korotitsch, W. J., & Nelson-Gray, R. O. (1999). An overview of self-monitoring research in assessment and treatment. *Psychological Assessment, 11,* 415–425.

Ludwig, D. S. (2000). Dietary glycemic index and obesity. *Journal of Nutrition, 130*(2S Suppl.), 280S–283S.

Ludwig, D. S., Majzoub, J. A., Al-Zahrani, A., Dallal, G. E., Blanco, I., & Roberts, S. B. (1999). High glycemic index foods, overeating, and obesity. *Pediatrics, 103*(3), E26.

Monzavi, R., Dreimane, D., Geffner, M. E., Braun, S., Conrad, B., Klier, M., et al. (2006). Improvement in risk factors for metabolic syndrome and insulin resistance in overweight youth who are treated with lifestyle intervention. *Pediatrics, 117*(6), e1111–e1118.

National Heart, Lung, and Blood Institute. (1991). *Report of the Expert Panel on Blood Cholesterol Levels in Children and Adolescents* (NIH Publication No. 91-2732). Bethesda, MD: Author.

Pearce, J. W., LeBow, M. D., & Orchard, J. (1981). Role of spouse involvement in the behavioral treatment of overweight women. *Journal of Consulting and Clinical Psychology, 49*(2), 236–244.

Pierce, J. W., & Wardle, J. (1997). Cause and effect beliefs and self-esteem of overweight children. *Journal of Child Psychology and Psychiatry, 38*(6), 645–650.

Puhl, R., & Brownell, K. D. (2001). Bias, discrimination, and obesity. *Obesity Research, 9*(12), 788–805.

Puhl, R. M., & Brownell, K. D. (2003). Psychosocial origins of obesity stigma: Toward changing a powerful and pervasive bias. *Obesity Reviews, 4*(4), 213–227.

Puhl, R. M., & Brownell, K. D. (2006). Confronting and coping with weight stigma: An investigation of overweight and obese adults. *Obesity, 14*(10), 1802–1815.

Report of the Second Task Force on Blood Pressure Control in Children 1987. Task Force on Blood Pressure Control in Children. National Heart, Lung, and Blood Institute, Bethesda, Maryland. (1987). *Pediatrics, 79*(1), 1–25.

Robinson, T. N. (1999). Reducing children's television viewing to prevent obesity: A randomized controlled trial. *JAMA, 282*(16), 1561–1567.

Robinson, T. N. (2001). Television viewing and childhood obesity. *Pediatric Clinics of North America, 48*(4), 1017–1025.

Rocchini, A. P., Katch, V., Anderson, J., Hinderliter, J., Becque, D., Martin, M., et al. (1988). Blood pressure in obese adolescents: Effect of weight loss. *Pediatrics, 82*(1), 16–23.

Sallis, J. F., McKenzie, T. L., & Alcaraz, J. E. (1993). Habitual physical activity and health-related physical fitness in fourth-grade children. *American Journal of Disabled Children, 147*(8), 890–896.

Sallis, J. F., Patterson, T. L., Buono, M. J., & Nader, P. R. (1988). Relation of cardiovascular fitness and physical activity to cardiovascular disease risk factors in children and adults. *American Journal of Epidemiology, 127*(5), 933–941.

Sasaki, J., Shindo, M., Tanaka, H., Ando, M., & Arakawa, K. (1987). A long-term aerobic exercise program decreases the obesity index and increases the high density lipoprotein cholesterol concentration in obese children. *International Journal of Obesity, 11*(4), 339–345.

Senediak, C., & Spence, S. H. (1985). Rapid versus gradual scheduling of therapeutic contact in a family based behavioural weight control programme for children. *Behavioral Psychotherapy, 13,* 265–287.

Shaibi, G. Q., Cruz, M. L., Ball, G. D., Weigensberg, M. J., Salem, G. J., Crespo, N. C., et al. (2006). Effects of resistance training on insulin sensitivity in overweight Latino adolescent males. *Medicine and Science in Sports and Exercise, 38*(7), 1208–1215.

Sheard, N. F., Clark, N. G., Brand-Miller, J. C., Franz, M. J., Pi-Sunyer, F. X., Mayer-Davis, E., et al. (2004). Dietary carbohydrate (amount and type) in the prevention and management of diabetes: A statement by the American Diabetes Association. *Diabetes Care, 27*(9), 2266–2271.

Sothern, M. S., Despinasse, B., Brown, R., Suskind, R. M., Udall, J. N., Jr., & Blecker, U. (2000). Lipid profiles of obese children and adolescents before and after significant weight loss: Differences according to sex. *Southern Medical Journal, 93*(3), 278–282.

Stallings, V. A., Archibald, E. H., Pencharz, P. B., Harrison, J. E., & Bell, L. E. (1988). One-year follow-up of weight, total body potassium, and total body nitrogen in obese adolescents treated with the protein-sparing modified fast. *American Journal of Clinical Nutrition, 48*(1), 91–94.

Summerbell, C. D., Ashton, V., Campbell, K. J., Edmunds, L., Kelly, S., & Waters, E. (2003). Interventions for treating obesity in children. *Cochrane Database of Systematic Reviews* (3), CD001872. doi: 10.1002/14651858.cd001872

Tudor-Locke, C., Pangrazi, R. P., Corbin, C. B., Rutherford, W. J., Vincent, S. D., Raustorp, A., et al. (2004). BMI-referenced standards for recommended pedometer-determined steps/day in children. *Preventive Medicine, 38*(6), 857–864.

Wadden, T. A., Berkowitz, R. I., Womble, L. G., Sarwer, D. B., Phelan, S., Cato, R. K., et al. (2005). Randomized trial of lifestyle modification and pharmacotherapy for obesity. *New England Journal of Medicine, 353*(20), 2111–2120.

Wadden, T. A., Crerand, C. E., & Brock, J. (2005). Behavioral treatment of obesity. *Psychiatric Clinics of North America, 28*(1), 151–170, ix.

Wadden, T. A., & Foster, G. D. (2000). Behavioral treatment of obesity. *Medical Clinics of North America, 84*(2), 441–461, vii.

Wadden, T. A., Womble, L. G., Sarwer, D. B., Berkowitz, R. I., Clark, V. L., & Foster, G. D. (2003). Great expectations: "I'm losing 25% of my weight no matter what you say." *Journal of Consulting and Clinical Psychology, 71*(6), 1084–1089.

Wearing, S. C., Hennig, E. M., Byrne, N. M., Steele, J. R., & Hills, A. P. (2006). Musculoskeletal disorders associated with obesity: A biomechanical perspective. *Obesity Reviews, 7*(3), 239–250.

Wheeler, M. E., & Hess, K. W. (1976). Treatment of juvenile obesity by successive approximation control of eating. *Journal of Behavior Therapy and Experimental Psychiatry, 7*, 235–241.

Wing, R. R., & Hill, J. O. (2001). Successful weight loss maintenance. *Annual Review of Nutrition, 21*, 323–341.

Wing, R. R., Jeffery, R. W., Burton, L. R., Thorson, C., Nissinoff, K. S., & Baxter, J. E. (1996). Food provision vs structured meal plans in the behavioral treatment of obesity. *International Journal of Obesity, 20*(1), 56–62.

Wing, R. R., Marcus, M. D., Epstein, L. H., & Kupfer, D. (1983). Mood and weight loss in a behavioral treatment program. *Journal of Consulting and Clinical Psychology, 51*(1), 153–155.

Wilson, G. T. (1994). Behavioral treatment of childhood obesity: Theoretical and practical implications. *Health Psychology, 13*(5), 371–372.

Wrotniak, B. H., Epstein, L. H., Dorn, J. M., Jones, K. E., & Kondilis, V. A. (2006). The relationship between motor proficiency and physical activity in children. *Pediatrics, 118*(6), e1758–e1765.

Wrotniak, B. H., Epstein, L. H., Paluch, R. A., & Roemmich, J. N. (2004). Parent weight change as a predictor of child weight change in family-based behavioral obesity treatment. *Archives of Pediatrics and Adolescent Medicine, 158*(4), 342–347.

Zimmet, P., Alberti, G., Kaufman, F., Tajima, N., Silink, M., Arslanian, S., et al. (2007). The metabolic syndrome in children and adolescents. *Lancet, 369*(9579), 2059–2061.

9

PREVENTION: CHANGING CHILDREN'S DIET AND PHYSICAL ACTIVITY PATTERNS VIA SCHOOLS, FAMILIES, AND THE ENVIRONMENT

RUSSELL JAGO, DEBBE THOMPSON, SHARON O'DONNELL,
KAREN CULLEN, AND TOM BARANOWSKI

This chapter identifies intervention approaches to the prevention of childhood obesity. As noted in other chapters in this volume, childhood obesity results from an energy imbalance whereby the energy consumed (diet) exceeds the energy expended (resting metabolic rate and physical activity). Therefore, obesity prevention relies on understanding the factors that influence that imbalance, such as healthy diet and physical activity. This chapter focuses on approaches to changing children's diet and physical activity behaviors as a means of preventing childhood obesity.

The mediating variable model (Figure 9.1) is an effective way of understanding the factors that influence children's diet and physical activity patterns. The model outlines how interventions can affect outcomes such as fruit and vegetable (FV) consumption. In this case, the child's self-efficacy is the mediating variable, and self-efficacy is targeted by the intervention

This work is a publication of the U.S. Department of Agriculture (USDA) Agricultural Research Service (ARS) Children's Nutrition Research Center, Department of Pediatrics, Baylor College of Medicine and Texas Children's Hospital, Houston, TX. This project has been funded in part by federal funds from the USDA/ARS under cooperative agreement 58-6250-6001. The contents of this publication do not necessarily reflect the views or polices of the USDA, nor do mentions of trade names, commercial products, or organizations imply endorsement by the U.S. Government.

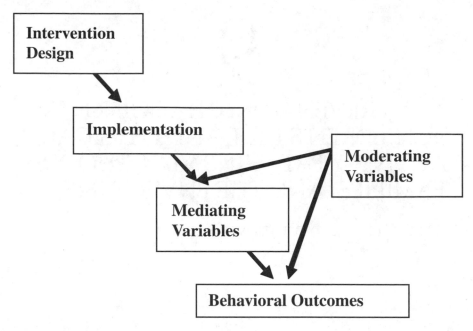

Figure 9.1. The mediating variable model.

to improve the behavioral outcome of eating fruit and vegetables. The model provides a framework for understanding the factors that influence diet and physical activity patterns as well as how both behaviors can be changed (Baranowski & Jago, 2005). The model suggests that interventions that change diet or physical activity behaviors work by changing mediating variables.

The second key component of the model is the moderators; that is, variables that do not change, such as participant demographics or baseline psychosocial characteristics. For example, a physical activity intervention might focus on increasing students' enjoyment of physical education (PE), but analysis of the intervention might indicate that the program only worked among boys. In this instance, student gender is the moderator (enjoyment is the mediator). Identifying moderators of prevention policies increases the likelihood that the prevention policies can be tailored to specific groups.

This chapter provides a brief review of the field of obesity prevention among youth by examining the diet and physical activity literature from three areas: schools, families, and environmental–economic influences. We review each domain, identify successful policies, identify strategies that hold promise but might not have been fully examined, and highlight any key mediators or moderators of successful programs.

SCHOOLS AND OBESITY PREVENTION

Nutrition education is conducted in schools, and school food environments provide opportunities for children to choose and eat healthy foods. For example, FV availability in the school cafeteria was a significant predictor of FV consumption following a 2-year intervention (Perry et al., 2004). However, not all school food was regulated, and the presence of snack vending machines was negatively related to daily fruit consumption among middle school youth (Kubik, Lytle, Hannan, Perry, & Story, 2003). Improvement in middle school student lunch consumption was found after a local school district enacted a snack bar food policy change (Cullen, Watson, Zakeri, & Ralston, 2006). Moreover, a statewide school nutrition policy to improve school food provision resulted in increased consumption of vegetables, decreased consumption of sweetened beverages and snack chips, and decreased energy from dietary fat among middle school students (Cullen, Watson, & Zakeri, 2008). Similarly, many schools provide regularly scheduled PE lessons. Schools, therefore, are logical partners in changing children's diet and physical activity patterns (Story, Kaphingst, & French, 2006).

School-Based Nutrition Interventions

Although a number of obesity prevention studies have included a nutrition component, the majority of these studies have been implemented in elementary schools, so there is a lack of data for other children (Baranowski, Cullen, Nicklas, Thompson, & Baranowski, 2002). A recent review of school-based interventions that included body composition as an outcomes measure (Thompson, Baranowski, Zakeri, Jago, & Cullen, 2006) found 11 studies that met the authors' rigorous methodological inclusion criteria.

The multicomponent Planet Health intervention targeted increasing FV intake and decreasing consumption of high-fat foods (Gortmaker et al., 1999). After 2 years, the prevalence of obesity was lower among intervention school girls than among control school girls. Dietary changes included a significant increase in FV consumption and a significantly smaller increase in estimated energy intake per day among the intervention girls than among the control girls. The lack of a change among the boys indicates that gender moderated the effect and alternative strategies might be needed for boys.

Two other middle school studies did not measure anthropometric outcomes. One 2-year intervention targeted increasing FV and low-fat foods but did not achieve dietary change (Lytle et al., 2004). Alternatively, a 2-year intervention that included family (three newsletters a year), student–environmental (more fruit and water at school plus nutrition information), and individual (1-hour computer-tailored intervention each year) components was successful

(Haerens et al., 2006). At the end of this 2-year study, girls in the intervention had significantly lower increases in body mass index z-scores than those in the control condition group, but diet was not measured.

We found three high school nutrition interventions. A social marketing intervention had no significant impact on FV intake (Nicklas, Johnson, Myers, Farris, & Cunningham, 1998). An environmental intervention increased the availability of low-fat foods in the cafeteria, and the researchers reported a higher percentage of low-fat food sales in intervention compared with control condition schools; individual student intake, however, was not measured (French, Story, Fulkerson, & Hannan, 2004). An intervention in a high school in the Zuni Pueblo replaced soft drinks in vending machines with sugar-free beverages and provided water coolers as well as nutrition and diabetes education (Ritenbaugh et al., 2003). No individual dietary data were collected, but no soft drinks were sold by Year 3, and plasma insulin values declined (Ritenbaugh et al., 2003).

Several school-based programs with both curriculum and cafeteria modifications targeting dietary fat consumption were successful at achieving reductions in student total and saturated fat consumption (Luepker et al., 1996; Simons-Morton, Parcel, Baranowski, Forthofer, & O'Hara, 1991), kilocalories and fat consumption (Caballero et al., 2003), and total-fat-only consumption (Hooper, Munoz, Gruber, & Nguyen, 2005). Programs have also achieved reductions in the fat content of school meals (Luepker et al., 1996; Simons-Morton et al., 1991), and all of the FV interventions achieved small but significant increases in fruit or vegetable consumption (Anderson et al., 2005; Baranowski, Baranowski, Cullen, Marsh, et al., 2003; Gortmaker et al., 1999; Horne et al., 2004; Perry et al., 1998).

In terms of policy, as of July 2006, all school districts in the United States that participate in the National School Lunch Program must have a local wellness policy as mandated by the Child Nutrition Improvement and Integrity Act of 2004. Mandates include goals for nutrition education, physical activity, and other school-based activities as well as nutrition guidelines for all foods and beverages available on school campuses. Recent data indicate that school food wellness policies improve student consumption at lunch (Cullen et al., 2006); however, full evaluations of these programs have not been performed (School Nutrition Association, 2006). Such evaluations should be a priority for future research. These studies should include measures of energy intake and expenditure for the entire day and for discrete time periods (e.g., intake by meals, energy expended in the afternoon or at school). A particularly important area of research is whether students eat more foods or become more sedentary after improvements in school food and physical activity environments.

Although dietary psychosocial variables are likely mediators, there is a relative shortage of information in this area. Significant increases in knowledge were found in several studies (Baranowski et al., 2000; Caballero et al.,

2003; Luepker et al., 1996). Changes in dietary self-efficacy, social norms (Reynolds et al., 2000), perceived support (Luepker et al., 1996; Perry et al., 1998), increasing *asking skills* (i.e., the ability to ask for a food of choice; Perry et al., 1998), and verbal encouragement from cafeteria workers have also been reported (Perry et al., 2004).

Overall, the literature suggests that school-based interventions can be used to change children's dietary intake by implementing new policies that limit high-fat, high-sugar foods and provide more FV and water options. Because knowledge, self-efficacy, increasing asking skills, and encouragement from food workers are likely mediators of dietary change, programs that focus on targeting these concepts will likely help prevent childhood obesity.

Changing Physical Education Lessons

Preintervention data from the Child and Adolescent Trial for Cardiovascular Health (CATCH) showed that elementary school children engaged in moderate to vigorous physical activity (MVPA) for fewer than 36% of their regularly scheduled PE lessons (McKenzie et al., 2001). Similarly, fewer than 17 minutes of MVPA were reported during regularly scheduled middle school PE (McKenzie et al., 2004). These low levels of MVPA are disconcerting because the number of PE lessons has been reduced to provide curriculum time for core subjects such as math and English. Therefore, maximizing activity in PE should be a focus of school-based interventions.

CATCH focused on training elementary school staff, both specialist and nonspecialist teachers, in PE instruction techniques and behavior and provided equipment to facilitate increased activity by enabling smaller group sizes (McKenzie et al., 2001). The intervention resulted in a 2.5-minute increase in the minutes of MVPA per lesson (McKenzie et al., 2001). Moreover, the program resulted in a greater increase in the MVPA in the lessons taught by nonspecialists (although overall more activity was achieved in classes taught by specialist PE teachers). Thus, PE lessons can be changed to increase physical activity, but the amount of activity obtained was moderated by teacher expertise, with lessons taught by specialists providing more MVPA.

The Middle School Physical Activity & Nutrition (M-SPAN) study included both diet and physical activity components (McKenzie et al., 2004). The PE component focused on increasing time spent in physical activity during the lesson and increasing student enjoyment (mediator) of the lesson. The program trained staff to improve classroom management and instruction skills and helped the teachers to design and implement new PE curricula. Direct observation of classes revealed a significant increase in MVPA in the intervention schools; however, this difference was only significant among the boys (gender as a moderator), and there was no significant effect on the student enjoyment (no mediation). Collectively, these studies indicate that PE lessons can be changed by training PE teachers in techniques that maximize activity time and by implementing more active curricula, but more work is needed to find ways to increase activity among girls.

FAMILIES AND OBESITY PREVENTION

Families provide both the genes and primary environment (Maes, Neale, & Eaves, 1997) for children. Families are thus a major influence on weight and associated knowledge, attitudes, and behaviors in youth (Dietz & Gortmaker, 2001).

Families, Diet, and Obesity Prevention

Few family-based youth obesity prevention interventions have been reported in the literature. Most have emphasized both nutrition and physical activity (Baranowski, Baranowski, Cullen, Thompson, et al., 2003; Beech et al., 2003; Fitzgibbon et al., 2005; Rodearmel et al., 2006; Story et al., 2003) but have demonstrated only limited success. A recent meta-analysis of youth obesity prevention programs concluded that parental involvement was not associated with significantly greater effectiveness (Stice, Shaw, & Marti, 2006). A review of family involvement in weight management programs concluded that uncertainty exists regarding how best to design family-based interventions but that there appears to be a positive correlation between the number of behavior change techniques taught and the effects on parent and child weight (McLean, Griffin, Toney, & Hardeman, 2003). Given the shortage of proven successful interventions, examining family correlates of children's diet likely offers the best available insights into potentially important but untested means of using families to change children's dietary behavior.

Family Correlates of Youth Dietary Intake

The home environment is a critical factor in the development of a child's dietary habits and subsequent obesity risk (Davison, Francis, & Birch, 2005). A recent review concluded that consumption appears to be influenced by home availability of foods, particularly FV (Jago, Baranowski, & Baranowski, 2007). Although conclusions regarding causality were not possible, a postulated mechanism of influence was that availability increased consumption through increased exposure that in turn influenced preference. Food preference has been correlated with consumption (Drewnowski, Henderson, Levine, & Hann, 1999), and parents play a key role in the development of food preference. A review of factors influencing early food preferences (Birch, 1998) reported that *neophobia*, or fear of new things, is a developmentally appropriate reaction in young children. Repeated exposure and tastings can overcome neophobic reactions (Birch, 1998). The social context within which food is offered was also reported to be important in the development of food preferences. A negative social context such as offering a reward for consuming a disliked food has been shown to result in a decreased preference for that food (Birch, 1998; Birch, Marlin, & Rotter, 1984). Helping parents understand the importance of making healthy foods available and how to address neophobic responses in children has the potential to enhance preferences, and, ultimately, consumption. Modeling by others, particularly mothers, has also been shown to influence food preferences (Birch & Fisher, 1998).

Meal structure may also be an influencing factor. Evidence suggests that youth who eat dinner with their families have higher quality diets (Gillman et al., 2000) and a lower risk of obesity (Veugelers & Fitzgerald, 2005). Use of controlling or restrictive parental feeding strategies (i.e., restricting certain foods while encouraging others) has been associated with reduced development of self-control eating mechanisms in youth, which may result in greater risk of obesity, particularly in girls (Birch, 1998).

Developmental differences in parental influence over youth dietary practices need to be considered when designing family-based youth obesity interventions (Lindsay, Sussner, Kim, & Gortmaker, 2006). From gestation through adolescence, parents have increasingly less influence over youth dietary practices (Lindsay et al., 2006), and as a result, family-based interventions should be tailored to the differences in parental influence during each period. Family interventions early in development are more likely to be effective because of stronger family influences. New strategies that focus on modifying parenting style, provision of healthy foods, and making family meal times fun and enjoyable (all mediators) seem to hold the most promise for family-based obesity prevention efforts.

Families, Physical Activity, and Obesity Prevention

In the most comprehensive review of correlates of physical activity (102 published articles), different patterns of findings in regard to how parents influenced physical activity were found among children (4–12 years old) versus adolescents (13–18 years old, Sallis, Prochaska, & Taylor, 2000). Among children, no parent-related variables were consistently related to physical activity; among adolescents, parental support was consistently strongly related, direct help was consistently weakly related, and having opportunities to exercise (a variable influenced by parent choices) was consistently weakly related to physical activity. Similarly conflicting results in regard to parental or family influences have recently appeared. Part of the inconsistency appears to have resulted from the diversity in measures of family influences (almost every study used unique measures of family influence) as well as of physical activity that were used. However, parental provision of transportation was related to total physical activity and participation in sports or activity lessons among both boys and girls (Hoefer, McKenzie, Sallis, Marshall, & Conway, 2001) and may be an important mediator to target in future interventions.

Intervention Studies With Families to Increase Children's Physical Activity

The task force for reviewing physical activity interventions for the U.S. *Guide to Community Prevention Service* (Kahn et al., 2002) reviewed the interventions involving family-based social support. They identified 11 acceptable studies and concluded that they "generally indicated no change, with some studies showing increases in activity and others showing decreases" (Kahn et al., 2002, p. 83). Alternatively, hope was resurrected for family interventions when a more recent review (Timperio, Salmon, & Ball, 2004) of interventions promoting physical activity among children and adolescents concluded that interventions "that included contact with families generally appeared to be most effective" (p. 20). The Council on Sports Medicine and Fitness and Council on School Health (2006) of the American Academy of Pediatrics encouraged interventions with parents to find ways to overcome problems of neighborhood safety, encouraged parents to be physical activity role models, and provided more social support for physical activity for their children. However, no guidance was provided on how these goals might be achieved.

Public policy in regard to physical activity could encourage parents to more actively support their child's physical activity (e.g., provide incentives for lower health insurance premiums for children who meet some minimum level of physical activity) or preempt parent action when parents do not appear to be taking appropriate actions (e.g., increase the school day to 8:00 a.m. to 6:00 p.m. and require some minimum level of PE and after school activity in that time period, as is being done in the United Kingdom [Department for Education and Skills, 2005]). Some states have increased the daily school time devoted to PE, but there has been no obvious effect on body mass index (Cawley, Meyerhoefer, & Newhouse, 2005), which is likely due to various restraints on resulting levels of physical activity.

Conceptual Models of Families and Child Physical Activity

Several models address how families might influence youth physical activity. The health-promoting family model (Christensen, 2004) proposes that family members can reciprocally influence each others' health behaviors, with children also influencing parents' behaviors. Trost et al.'s (2003) model places a central emphasis on parental support for child physical activity. A third model emphasizes the importance of *family rules* (a form of parenting style) and family support with regard to physical activity within alternative types of families (Soubhi, Potrim, & Paradis, 2004). Because these models lack consistency, a new conceptual model that integrates multiple family variables would likely provide the best promise for understanding familial influence on children's physical activity.

The original findings among correlates of child and adolescent physical activity suggest that the greatest promise for promoting physical activity through interventions with parents would involve enhancing family support (informational and emotional) for physical activity and encouraging families to provide direct help (e.g., provide material support by transporting to physical activity events or paying for sports participation). The literature is not clear on procedures for enhancing the abilities or motivations of families to do so; thus, this would seem to be a priority area for research and evaluated action.

ENVIRONMENT, ECONOMY, AND OBESITY PREVENTION

The relatively recent nature of the childhood obesity problem implies that it is not the result of a change in the genetic makeup of children. How environmental factors and the decisions made by policymakers and community leaders can affect and possibly help in the prevention of childhood obesity is a rapidly changing and evolving area of research. One facet of this research originates from the field of economics and assesses spatial and economic influences on food choices and provision.

Environment, Economy, and Dietary Patterns

In a market environment, there are multiple suppliers of food. The locations of food stores and the variety and prices of food offered are decided by individual owners or corporations. Locational disparities exist when neighborhoods are heterogeneous with respect to population density and neighborhood resources (O'Donnell & Baranowski, 2007). Price competition among local stores and restaurants and the presence of low-price warehouse stores may lead to variations in food prices and variations in the availability of food.

Given the complexity of the market environment, cross-sectional research has examined the presence of disparities, in the form of locational, price, or price and locational disparities in low-income communities. With the exception of one national study (Powell, Slater, Mirtcheva, Bao, & Chaloupka, 2007), results are based on local environments specific to a study group (Morland, Wing, & Diez Roux, 2002) or market (Zenk, Schulz, Israel, et al., 2005). Most studies have examined the concentration of food stores, but a small number have examined the presence of fast food establishments (Macintyre, McKay, Cummins, & Burns, 2005).

The Food Desert Literature

Food deserts are low-income communities with limited access to affordable and healthy food (Cummins & Macintyre, 2002). The term implies the absence of large food stores and a small selection of foods that are priced above local market prices. The existence of food deserts is somewhat controversial. Low-income families without vehicular access in Northern Ireland were found to be excluded from large food stores (Furey, Strugnell, & McIlveen, 2001). However, in Glasgow, Scotland, a measure of socioeconomic deprivation indicated that more food chain outlets tended to be located in the poorest areas of the city (Cummins & Macintyre, 1999), and a similar finding was reported in London (Donkin, Dowler, Sevenson, & Turner, 1999). Some cities that experienced a decentralization of large food stores also experienced a reduction in the concentration of stores in the older section of the city (Clarke, Eyre, & Guy, 2002; Cummins & Macintyre, 1999). This might suggest that forward planning of store locations could be used to resolve disparities. This was tested in a natural experiment in the United Kingdom in which participants who used smaller food stores as their main source of FV switched their source to a newly constructed large food store (Wrigley, Warm, Margetts, & Whelan, 2002). Two potential problems have been identified: (a) Construction of a new food store to resolve the disparity in access may be a costly, temporary fix if the community cannot support the store (Shaffer, 2002), and (b) the addition of a new store may result in the closure of existing stores, thus shifting the location of the disparity (Clarke et al., 2002).

Locational Disparities

Food deserts usually involve the absence of large grocery stores. The smaller stores in such neighborhoods sell their goods at higher than average prices. Locational disparity literature includes analyses of food resources within all neighborhoods in a city. This literature has examined spatial variations in the concentration of large food stores. On the basis of a multistate sample of the neighborhoods of survey participants, research has found that predominantly African American neighborhoods had fewer supermarkets but more small grocery stores and convenience stores (Moore & Diez Roux, 2006; Morland et al., 2002). In single-market studies, this same finding was reported in African American neighborhoods in Atlanta, Georgia (Helling & Sawicki, 2003), Chicago (Alwitt & Donley, 1997; Gallagher, 2003), Detroit, Michigan (Zenk, Schulz, Israel, et al., 2005), and Houston, Texas (O'Donnell & Baranowski, 2007) and in African American and Hispanic neighborhoods in Los Angeles (Shaffer, 2002). A national study found that chain supermarkets were less available in African American and Hispanic neighborhoods (Powell et al., 2007). Further research should consider that differences in concentration by race may result from other demographic differences, consumption patterns (primarily differences in nonfood consumption patterns and frequency of shopping), institutional discrimination (e.g., mortgage lending practices that lead to racial segregation), or racially biased business practices of grocery store owners (Helling & Sawicki, 2003). Support for the concept of demographic pressures is provided from population research that reported a negative bivariate association between the level of income in the neighborhood and large food store accessibility (Morland et al., 2002; Powell et al., 2007; Zenk, Schulz, Hollis-Neely et al., 2005). When characteristics of the neighborhood and workforce population density were added to the analysis, neighborhood income level was not associated with the concentration of chain supermarkets and superstores, but the presence of physical neighborhood characteristics that are associated with low-income communities was negatively associated with the concentration of these stores (O'Donnell & Baranowski, 2007).

Price Disparities

Research has examined price variation of food within an urban market using the total cost of food plans. The Thrifty Food Plan (TFP) is a low-cost, nutritionally adequate meal plan that is the basis for the maximum food stamp allocation in the United States (U.S. Department of Agriculture, 2004). Chain grocery stores in the Minneapolis–St. Paul area had significantly lower prices for TFP meats, dairy, dry and canned goods, and bread and grain than did smaller independent stores, with mixed results for TFP produce (Chung & Meyers, 1999). Only 23% of the 324 grocery stores in the Washington, DC, area had the complete list of TFP items. Independent stores had the highest prices ($103.30 for all TFP items) and were missing an average of seven items. The average cost of all TFP items at chain supermarkets was $100.54, with only one bundle item missing. Discount food stores had the lowest prices ($85.86), but the average number of missing items was 15 (Andrews, Kanter, Lino, & Rippinger, 2001). Food prices at larger grocery stores tended to be lower than prices at smaller stores, but in markets where large chain stores can exercise their monopoly power, larger stores had higher prices (Aalto-Setälä, 2002, 2003).

Collectively, the literature suggests that locational and price factors moderate the food available to children and their families. Strategies that focus on resourcing affordable healthy foods such as FV in low-income, high-minority neighborhoods are likely to be key in dietary efforts to prevent childhood obesity.

Environment and Youth Physical Activity

The study of environmental influences on youth physical activity is still in its infancy, but a recent review grouped these studies around three themes:

(a) recreational infrastructure, (b) transport infrastructure, and (c) local conditions (Davison & Lawson, 2006). Two consistent predictors of youth activity were access to home activity equipment and having equipment or play structures in schools (Davison & Lawson, 2006). The number of exercise-related pieces of equipment was a significant predictor of physical activity among 10- to 11-year-old Missouri girls but not boys (Stuckey-Ropp & DiLorenzo, 1993), indicating a moderating effect for gender. The presence of equipment in school playgrounds was related to physical activity among U.S. middle school students (Sallis et al., 2001). Painting school playgrounds with designs that encourage traditional playground games resulted in increased physical activity among elementary school students (Stratton & Mullan, 2005). These studies suggest that enhancing home activity equipment and ensuring that schools provide space for physical activity are two relatively simple environmental changes that could be implemented to increase physical activity.

Aspects of the transportation infrastructure that have been associated with physical activity among youth include the presence of good-quality sidewalks (Jago, Baranowski, Zakeri, & Harris, 2005), suitable road crossings (Boarnet, Anderson, Day, McMillan, & Alfonzo, 2005), and easy access by foot or bicycle to destinations such as shops and recreation centers (Mota, Almeida, Santos, & Ribeiro, 2005). The local condition that seems most likely to be associated with physical activity is aesthetics and particularly whether the neighborhood is clean and tidy (Mota et al., 2005). Turning these findings into policies to increase physical activity is inherently difficult because changing the physical environment is expensive. Nevertheless, local advocacy efforts to keep streets clean and tidy, improve sidewalks, and install crossings in existing neighborhoods or ensure that these facilities are incorporated into future developments are likely to be fruitful.

The most studied environmental intervention has been walk-to-school initiatives. The Marin County (northern California) Safe Routes to School initiative worked with local traffic engineers and school volunteers to identify safe routes to school and then encouraged school teams to promote walking and cycling among students. Participating schools reported a 64% increase in walking trips to school and a 114% increase in cycling over a 2-year period (Staunton, Hubsmith, & Kallins, 2003). This study therefore provides support for promoting walking to school and finding safe routes to school as key environmental policies that can be implemented to increase physical activity among youth.

CONCLUSION

We have provided a review of the childhood obesity prevention literature by focusing on strategies that could be implemented to influence children's diet and physical activity patterns. Research discussed in this chapter suggests that strategies to limit high-fat/high-sugar foods and modify PE provision could be implemented in schools to prevent obesity, and families could make healthy foods available at home, model healthy eating, and increase family support for physical activity. At the policy level, there is a need to make healthy foods available at affordable prices and to develop advocacy groups to campaign for clean and safe environments that are conducive to physical activity. Some strategies, such as making healthy foods available at home, appear easier than providing low-cost healthy foods in low-income communities. However, the evidence demonstrates that changing human behavior is complex and requires innovative and advanced strategies. More information is needed about the ways in which interventions work, the extent to which mediators work as planned, and whether there are any moderator effects. Such knowledge will enable the development of more targeted interventions that are increasingly likely to achieve behavior change and prevent obesity among youth. The strategies outlined in this chapter are a starting point for prevention efforts, but a great deal more needs to be done. Researchers need to identify methods to facilitate healthy eating and physical activity among children, develop and test new strategies to facilitate behavior change, and continue to reflect on progress until we find successful means of preventing childhood obesity.

REFERENCES

Aalto-Setälä, V. (2002). The effect of concentration and market power on food prices: Evidence from Finland. *Journal of Retailing, 78,* 207–216.

Aalto-Setälä, V. (2003). Explaining price dispersion for homogeneous grocery products. *Journal of Agricultural & Food Industrial Organization, 1*(1), Article 9. Available at http://www.bepress.com/jafio/vol1/iss1/art9

Alwitt, L., & Donley, T. (1997). Retail stores in poor urban neighborhoods. *Journal of Consumer Affairs, 31,* 139–164.

Anderson, A. S., Porteous, L. E., Foster, E., Higgins, C., Stead, M., Hetherington, M., et al. (2005). The impact of a school-based nutrition education intervention on dietary intake and cognitive and attitudinal variables relating to fruits and vegetables. *Public Health Nutrition, 8*(6), 650–656.

Andrews, M., Kanter, L., Lino, M., & Rippinger, D. (2001). *Using USDA's Thrifty Food Plan to assess food availability and affordability (Food Review)*. Washington, DC: Economic Research Services, U.S. Department of Agriculture.

Baranowski, T., Baranowski, J., Cullen, K. W., Marsh, T., Islam, N., Zakeri, I., et al. (2003). Squire's Quest! Dietary outcome evaluation of a multimedia game. *American Journal of Preventive Medicine, 24*(1), 52–61.

Baranowski, T., Baranowski, J. C., Cullen, K. W., Thompson, D. I., Nicklas, T., Zakeri, I. E., et al. (2003). The Fun, Food, and Fitness Project (FFFP): The Baylor GEMS pilot study. *Ethnicity & Disease, 13*(1, Suppl. 1), S30–S39.

Baranowski, T., Cullen, K. W., Nicklas, T., Thompson, D., & Baranowski, J. (2002). School-based obesity prevention: A blueprint for taming the epidemic. *American Journal of Health Behavior, 26*(6), 486–493.

Baranowski, T., Davis, M., Resnicow, K., Baranowski, J., Doyle, C., Lin, L. S., et al. (2000). Gimme 5 fruit, juice, and vegetables for fun and health: Outcome evaluation. *Health Education & Behavior, 27*(1), 96–111.

Baranowski, T., & Jago, R. (2005). Understanding mechanisms of change in children's physical activity programs. *Exercise and Sport Science Reviews, 33*(4), 163–168.

Beech, B. M., Klesges, R. C., Kumanyika, S., Murray, D. M., Klesges, L., McClanahan, B., et al. (2003). Child and parent targeted interventions: The Memphis GEMS pilot study. *Ethnicity & Disease, 13*(Suppl. 1), S40–S53.

Birch, L. L. (1998). Development of food acceptance patterns in the first years of life. *Proceedings of the Nutrition Society, 57*(4), 617–624.

Birch, L., & Fisher, J. O. (1998). Development of eating behaviors among children and adolescents. *Pediatrics, 101*, 539–549.

Birch, L., Marlin, D. W., & Rotter, J. (1984). Eating as a "means" activity in a contingency: Effects on young children's food preferences. *Child Development, 55*, 432–439.

Boarnet, M. G., Anderson, C. L., Day, K., McMillan, T., & Alfonzo, M. (2005). Evaluation of the California Safe Routes to School legislation: Urban form changes and children's active transportation to school. *American Journal of Preventive Medicine, 28*(2 Suppl. 2), 134–140.

Caballero, B., Clay, T., Davis, S. M., Ethelbah, B., Rock, B. H., Lohman, T. G., et al. (2003). Pathways: A school-based, randomized controlled trial for the prevention of obesity in American Indian school-children. *American Journal of Clinical Nutrition, 78*(5), 1030–1038.

Cawley, J., Meyerhoefer, C., & Newhouse, D. (2005). *The impact of physical education requirements on youth physical activity and overweight.* Retrieved May 12, 2006, from http://www.nber.org/papers/w11411

Child Nutrition Improvement and Integrity Act of 2004, H.R. 3873, 108th Congress (2004).

Christensen, P. (2004). The health promoting family: A conceptual framework for future research. *Social Science & Medicine, 59*, 377–387.

Chung, C., & Meyers, S. (1999). Do the poor pay more for food? *Journal of Consumer Affairs, 33*, 276–296.

Clarke, G., Eyre, H., & Guy, C. (2002). Deriving indicators of access to food retail provision in British cities: Studies of Cardiff, Leeds and Bradford. *Urban Studies, 39*, 2041–2060.

Council on Sports Medicine and Fitness and Council on School Health. (2006). Active healthy living: Prevention of childhood obesity through increased physical activity. *Pediatrics, 117*(5), 1834–1842.

Cullen, K. W., Watson, K., & Zakeri, I. (2008). Improvements in middle school student dietary intake after implementation of the Texas Public School Nutrition Policy. *American Journal of Public Health, 98*(1), 111–117.

Cullen, K. W., Watson, K., Zakeri, I., & Ralston, K. (2006). Exploring changes in middle-school student lunch consumption after local school food service policy modifications. *Public Health Nutrition, 9*(6), 814–820.

Cummins, S., & Macintyre, S. (1999). The location of food stores in urban areas: A case study in Glasgow. *British Food Journal, 101,* 545–553.

Cummins, S., & Macintyre, S. (2002). "Food deserts"—Evidence and assumption in health policymaking. *British Medical Journal, 325,* 436–438.

Davison, K. K., Francis, L., & Birch, L. (2005). Re-examining obesigenic families: Parents' obesity-related behaviors predict girls' change in BMI. *Obesity Research, 13,* 1980–1990.

Davison, K. K., & Lawson, C. T. (2006). Do attributes in the physical environment influence children's physical activity? A review of the literature. *International Journal of Behavioral Nutrition and Physical Activity, 3,* 19. doi:10.1186/1479-5868-3-19

Department for Education and Skills. (2005). *Extended schools: Access to opportunities and services for all: A prospectus.* London: Department for Education and Skills.

Dietz, W. H., & Gortmaker, S. L. (2001). Preventing obesity in children and adolescents. *Annual Review of Public Health, 22,* 337–353.

Donkin, A., Dowler, E., Sevenson, S., & Turner, S. (1999). Mapping access to food at a local level. *British Food Journal, 101,* 554–564.

Drewnowski, A., Henderson, S. A., Levine, A., & Hann, C. (1999). Taste and food preferences as predictors of dietary practices in young women. *Public Health Nutrition, 2*(4), 513–519.

Fitzgibbon, M. L., Stolley, M. R., Schiffer, L., Van Horn, L., Kaufer Christoffel, K., & Dyer, A. (2005). Two-year follow-up results for Hip-Hop to Health Jr.: A randomized controlled trial for overweight prevention in preschool minority children. *Journal of Pediatrics, 146*(5), 618–625.

French, S. A., Story, M., Fulkerson, J. A., & Hannan, P. (2004). An environmental intervention to promote lower-fat food choices in secondary schools: Outcomes of the TACOS Study. *American Journal of Public Health, 94*(9), 1507–1512.

Furey, S., Strugnell, C., & McIlveen, H. (2001). An investigation of the potential existence of food deserts in rural and urban areas of Northern Ireland. *Agriculture and Human Values, 18,* 447–457.

Gallagher, M. (2003). *Race and place matter for major Chicago area grocers* (Community Development Policy Paper). Chicago: Metro Chicago Information Center.

Gillman, M. W., Rifas-Shiman, S. L., Frazier, A. L., Rockett, H. R., Camargo, C. A., Jr., Field, A. E., et al. (2000). Family dinner and diet quality among older children and adolescents. *Archives of Family Medicine, 9*(3), 235–240.

Gortmaker, S. L., Peterson, K., Wiecha, J., Sobol, A. M., Dixit, S., Fox, M. K., et al. (1999). Reducing obesity via a school-based interdisciplinary intervention among youth. *Archives of Pediatric and Adolescent Medicine, 153,* 409–418.

Haerens, L., Deforche, B., Maes, L., Stevens, V., Cardon, G., & De Bourdeaudhuij, I. (2006). Body mass effects of a physical activity and healthy food intervention in middle schools. *Obesity, 14*(5), 847–854.

Helling, A., & Sawicki, D. (2003). Race and residential accessibility to shopping and services. *Housing Policy Debate, 14*, 69–101.

Hoefer, W. R., McKenzie, T. L., Sallis, J. F., Marshall, S. J., & Conway, T. L. (2001). Parental provision of transportation for adolescent physical activity. *American Journal of Preventive Medicine, 21*(1), 48–51.

Hooper, C. A., Munoz, K. D., Gruber, M. B., & Nguyen, K. P. (2005). The effects of a family fitness program on the physical activity and nutrition behaviors of third grade children. *Research Quarterly for Exercise and Sport, 76*(2), 130–139.

Horne, P. J., Tapper, K., Lowe, C. F., Hardman, C. A., Jackson, M. C., & Woolner, J. (2004). Increasing children's fruit and vegetable consumption: A peer-modelling and rewards-based intervention. *European Journal of Clinical Nutrition, 58*(12), 1649–1660.

Jago, R., Baranowski, T., & Baranowski, J. (2007). Fruit and vegetable availability: A micro environmental mediating variable? *Public Health Nutrition 10*(7), 681–689.

Jago, R., Baranowski, T., Zakeri, I., & Harris, M. (2005). Observed environmental features and the physical activity of adolescent males. *American Journal of Preventive Medicine, 29*(2), 98–104.

Kahn, E. B., Ramsey, L. T., Brownson, R. C., Heath, G. W., Howze, E. H., Powell, K. E., et al. (2002). The effectiveness of interventions to increase physical activity: A systematic review. *American Journal of Preventive Medicine, 22*(4S), 73–107.

Kubik, M. Y., Lytle, L. A., Hannan, P. J., Perry, C. L., & Story, M. (2003). The association of the school food environment with dietary behaviors of young adolescents. *American Journal of Public Health, 93*(7), 1168–1173.

Lindsay, A. C., Sussner, K. M., Kim, J., & Gortmaker, S. (2006). The role of parents in preventing childhood obesity. *Future Child, 16*(1), 169–186.

Luepker, R. V., Perry, C. L., McKinlay, S. M., Nader, P. R., Parcel, G. S., Stone, E. J., et al. (1996). Outcomes of a field trial to improve children's dietary patterns and physical activity: The Child and Adolescent Trial for Cardiovascular Health (CATCH). *JAMA, 275*(10), 768–776.

Lytle, L. A., Murray, D. M., Perry, C. L., Story, M., Birnbaum, A. S., Kubik, M. Y., et al. (2004). School-based approaches to affect adolescents' diets: Results from the TEENS study. *Health Education and Behavior, 31*(2), 270–287.

Macintyre, S., McKay, L., Cummins, S., & Burns, C. (2005). Out-of-home food outlets and area deprivation: Case study in Glasgow, UK. *International Journal of Behavioral Nutrition and Physical Activity, 2*, 16.

Maes, H. H., Neale, M. C., & Eaves, L. J. (1997). Genetic and environmental factors in relative body weight and human adiposity. *Behavioral Genetics, 27*(4), 325–351.

McKenzie, T. L., Sallis, J. F., Prochaska, J. J., Conway, T. L., Marshall, S. J., & Rosengard, P. (2004). Evaluation of a two-year middle school physical education intervention: MSPAN. *Medicine and Science in Sports and Exercise, 36*(8), 1382–1388.

McKenzie, T. L., Stone, E. J., Feldman, H. A., Epping, J. N., Yang, M., Strikmiller, P. K., et al. (2001). Effects of the CATCH physical education intervention:

Teacher type and lesson location. *American Journal of Preventive Medicine*, *21*(2), 101–109.

McLean, N., Griffin, S., Toney, K., & Hardeman, W. (2003). Family involvement in weight control, weight maintenance and weight-loss interventions: A systematic review of randomised trials. *International Journal of Obesity*, *27*(9), 987–1005.

Moore, L. V., & Diez Roux, A. V. (2006). Associations of neighborhood characteristics with the location and type of food stores. *American Journal of Public Health*, *96*(2), 325–331.

Morland, K., Wing, S., & Diez Roux, A. (2002). The contextual effect of the local food environment on residents' diets: The atherosclerosis risk in communities study. *American Journal of Public Health*, *92*(11), 1761–1767.

Mota, J., Almeida, M., Santos, P., & Ribeiro, J. C. (2005). Perceived neighborhood environments and physical activity in adolescents. *Preventive Medicine*, *41*(5–6), 834–836.

Nicklas, T. A., Johnson, C. C., Myers, L., Farris, R. P., & Cunningham, A. (1998). Outcomes of a high school program to increase fruit and vegetable consumption: Gimme 5—A fresh nutrition concept for students. *Journal of School Health*, *68*(6), 248–253.

O'Donnell, S., & Baranowski, T. (2007). *Mind the (food) gap: Locational disparities of major food stores in a US city* (Working paper). Unpublished manuscript.

Perry, C. L., Bishop, D., Taylor, G. L., Davis, M., Story, M., Bishop, S. C., et al. (2004). A randomized school trial of environmental strategies to encourage fruit and vegetable consumption among children. *Health Education and Behavior*, *31*(1), 65–76.

Perry, C. L., Bishop, D. B., Taylor, G., Murray, D. M., Mays, R., Dudovitz, B. S., et al. (1998). Changing fruit and vegetable consumption among children: The 5-a-Day power plus program in St. Paul, Minnesota. *American Journal of Public Health*, *88*(4), 603–609.

Powell, L. M., Slater, S., Mirtcheva, D., Bao, Y., & Chaloupka, F. J. (2007). Food store availability and neighborhood characteristics in the United States. *Preventive Medicine*, *44*(3), 189–195.

Reynolds, K. D., Franklin, F. A., Binkley, D., Raczynski, J. M., Harrington, K. F., Kirk, K. A., et al. (2000). Increasing the fruit and vegetable consumption of fourth-graders: Results from the High 5 project. *Preventive Medicine*, *30*(4), 309–319.

Ritenbaugh, C., Teufel-Shone, N. I., Aickin, M. G., Joe, J. R., Poirier, S., Dillingham, D. C., et al. (2003). A lifestyle intervention improves plasma insulin levels among Native American high school youth. *Preventive Medicine*, *36*(3), 309–319.

Rodearmel, S. J., Wyatt, H. R., Barry, M. J., Dong, F., Pan, D., Israel, R. G., et al. (2006). A family-based approach to preventing excessive weight gain. *Obesity 14*(8), 1392–1401.

Sallis, J. F., Conway, T. L., Prochaska, J. J., McKenzie, T. L., Marshall, S. J., & Brown, M. (2001). The association of school environments with youth physical activity. *American Journal of Public Health*, *91*(4), 618–620.

Sallis, J. F., Prochaska, J. J., & Taylor, W. C. (2000). A review of correlates of physical activity of children and adolescents. *Medicine and Science in Sports and Exercise*, *32*(5), 963–975.

School Nutrition Association. (2006). *A Foundation for the Future II*. Alexandria, VA: School Nutrition Association.

Shaffer, A. (2002). *The persistence of L.A.'s grocery gap: The need for a new food policy and approach to market development* (Policy paper). Center for Food Justice, Urban and Environmental Policy Institute, Occidental College, Los Angeles.

Simons-Morton, B. G., Parcel, G. S., Baranowski, T., Forthofer, R., & O'Hara, N. M. (1991). Promoting physical activity and a healthful diet among children: Results of a school-based intervention study. *American Journal of Public Health*, *81*(8), 986–991.

Soubhi, H., Potrim, L., & Paradis, G. (2004). Family process and parent's leisure time physical activity. *American Journal of Health Behavior*, *28*, 218–230.

Staunton, C. E., Hubsmith, D., & Kallins, W. (2003). Promoting safe walking and biking to school: The Marin County success story. *American Journal of Public Health*, *93*(9), 1431–1434.

Stice, E., Shaw, H., & Marti, C. N. (2006). A meta-analytic review of obesity prevention programs for children and adolescents: The skinny on interventions that work. *Psychological Bulletin*, *132*(5), 667–691.

Story, M., Kaphingst, K. M., & French, S. (2006). The role of schools in obesity prevention. *Future Child*, *16*(1), 109–142.

Story, M., Sherwood, N., Himes, J. H., Davis, M., Jacobs, D. R., Cartwright, Y., et al. (2003). An after-school obesity prevention program for African-American girls: The Minnesota GEMS pilot study. *Ethnicity & Disease*, *13*(1 Suppl.), 54–64.

Stratton, G., & Mullan, E. (2005). The effect of multicolor playground markings on children's physical activity level during recess. *Preventive Medicine*, *41*(5–6), 828–833.

Stuckey-Ropp, R. C., & DiLorenzo, T. M. (1993). Determinants of exercise in children. *Preventive Medicine*, *22*, 880–889.

Thompson, D., Baranowski, T., Zakeri, I., Jago, R., Davis, J., & Cullen, K. (2006). Effectiveness of school-based environmental vs. individual approaches to diet, physical activity and sedentary behavior change among youth. In R. K. Flamenbaum (Ed.), *Childhood obesity and health research* (pp. 157–174). Hauppauge, NY: Nova Science Publishers.

Timperio, A., Salmon, J., & Ball, K. (2004). Evidence-based strategies to promote physical activity among children, adolescents and young adults: Review and update. *Journal of Science and Medicine in Sport*, *7*(1 Suppl.), 20–29.

Trost, S. G., Sallis, J. F., Pate, R. R., Freedson, P. S., Taylor, W. C., & Dowda, M. (2003). Evaluating a model of parental influence on youth physical activity. *American Journal of Preventive Medicine*, *25*(4), 277–282.

U.S. Department of Agriculture. (2004). *Official USDA food plans: Cost of food at home at four levels*. Washington, DC: Center for Nutrition Policy and Promotion.

Veugelers, P., & Fitzgerald, A. (2005). Prevalence of risk factors for childhood overweight and obesity. *Canadian Medical Association Journal, 173*, 607–613.

Wrigley, N., Warm, D., Margetts, B., & Whelan, A. (2002). Assessing the impact of improved retail access on diet in a "food desert": A preliminary report. *Urban Studies, 39*, 2061–2082.

Zenk, S. N., Schulz, A. J., Hollis-Neely, T., Campbell, R. T., Holmes, N., Watkins, G., et al. (2005). Fruit and vegetable intake in African Americans: Income and store characteristics. *American Journal of Preventive Medicine, 29*(1), 1–9.

Zenk, S. N., Schulz, A. J., Israel, B. A., James, S. A., Bao, S., & Wilson, M. L. (2005). Neighborhood racial composition, neighborhood poverty, and the spatial accessibility of supermarkets in metropolitan Detroit. *American Journal of Public Health, 95*(4), 660–667.

10

FUTURE DIRECTIONS IN PEDIATRIC OBESITY

J. KEVIN THOMPSON AND LESLIE J. HEINBERG

The dramatic increase in recent decades in the prevalence of childhood and adolescent obesity has spawned a parallel rise in the attention of researchers and clinicians to try to understand mechanisms, psychosocial issues, prevention options, and treatment strategies. The chapters in this book identify key themes and guidelines for future research.

Definitions of obesity and overweight in children need to be clarified and be consistent across research. Many clinicians and researchers consider the term *obesity* to be stigmatizing to children and instead prefer to consider various degrees of overweight. Many others believe that using the more precise definitions of *obesity* (with ranges from mild to severe) is more informative and more likely to engender the concern and alarm needed to address the problem.

In the area of etiology, research on the human genome—specifically, the human obesity gene map—is moving forward rapidly. A knowledge of genomic information will facilitate the detection of young individuals who may be at risk for overweight or obesity, allowing for precision in delineating subcategories on the basis of ethnicity, age, and gender. Such classifications may also assist in the prediction of which individuals develop an obesity-related comorbidity such as diabetes. Ultimately, an understanding of the human genome will help determine a more precise patient–treatment match, and specific medication and nutritional or psychological interventions can be based on an understanding of a particular patient's genetic structure.

Research funding and activity in this area must increase to bring about such an outcome. To date, much of the interest is speculative and based on research with animals and adult humans. Age-related issues may be involved in the expression of genes that affect the gene's interaction with the environment and behavioral or dietary patterns. Clearly, work in the area of genetics is exciting, but consideration must be given to developmental issues along with psychological factors (gene–behavior interactions) if this area of research is to maximize understanding of pediatric obesity. Finally, this work is in formative stages, and efficacious prevention and treatment strategies are likely to be many years in the future.

Work on the genomic structure that is linked to obesity is of enormous importance, but it is also clear that social, environmental, and interpersonal factors have contributed to the rise in prevalence rates. Clearly, genes alone cannot explain the tripling of pediatric obesity rates in one generation. Thus, although genomic factors play a role in the onset and maintenance of obesity, psychosocial and behavioral factors play a strong role in the increased prevalence rates and have direct effects on the psychological and physical health of the overweight or obese individual. The fundamental cause of obesity—for children as well as adults—is positive energy balance (i.e., consuming more calories than are expended). Thus, behaviors and behavior change remain fundamental in the etiology, prevention, and treatment of overweight and obesity. Furthermore, research has clearly demonstrated that children and adolescents who are overweight or obese receive negative social feedback (e.g., teasing, cruel comments) and that these experiences are associated with higher levels of body dissatisfaction and depression and higher rates of suicidal ideation and actual suicide. Although these connections have been documented repeatedly in the literature, only recently have programs begun to be implemented to prevent or address these types of negative social experiences. As outlined in chapter 4 of this volume, Neumark-Sztainer and colleagues have developed the V.I.K. (Very Important Kids) program to prevent weight stigmatization and promote productive weight-related behaviors and interactions. They have also developed a family-based program to encourage supportiveness from family members in the child's need to counter negative social attitudes. Both of these programs are in the initial stages of evaluation, yet the data are encouraging, and the approaches deserve widespread evaluation.

It is also obvious from several chapters in this volume that numerous social and environmental factors are currently operating, in the United States and other countries, that produce and perpetuate the obesity epidemic in young people. Technological advances and modernization have created an environment that facilitates sedentary rather than active endeavors. Research clearly and consistently demonstrates that TV viewing time is associated with elevated weight status. Physical education and recess levels have decreased over the years to provide more time for didactic, in-class instruction (and to limit the liability associated with sports participation). Most schools continue to offer poor nutritional selections (although there are unique and innovative exceptions). Activity levels and the nutritional value of meal selections degrade during the teenage years while sedentary activities increase.

This constellation of factors has no doubt contributed to the increased prevalence of overweight and obesity, and leading figures in academia and social policy have begun to call for action. Families, schools, community organizations, public corporations, the health care system, and politicians need to become involved and to address the problem. Physical activity needs to be an option for all young people, even those who live in potentially unsafe urban areas. Schools need to prioritize this issue and increase activity options rather than removing them from the curriculum. Communities, along with city and county governments, need to work to enhance the possibility of outdoor activities by designing parks, walkways, and bicycle paths that are safe and accessible. Parents and teachers must demand that healthy and affordable food choices be available in the schools. In 2003, the American Academy of Pediatrics released a policy statement on pediatric obesity that called for physicians and health professionals and their national organizations to do the following:

a. Help parents, teachers, coaches, and others who influence youth to discuss health habits, not body habitus, as part of their efforts to control overweight and obesity.
b. Enlist policy makers from local, state, and national organizations and schools to support a healthful lifestyle for all children, including proper diet and adequate opportunity for regular physical activity.
c. Encourage organizations that are responsible for health care and health care financing to provide coverage for effective obesity prevention and treatment.
d. Encourage public and private sources to direct funding toward research into effective strategies to prevent overweight and obesity and to maximize limited family and community resources to achieve healthful outcomes for youth.
e. Support and advocate for social marketing intended to promote healthful food choices and increased physical activity. (American Academy of Pediatrics, 2003, pp. 427–428)

More recently, the American Academy of Pediatrics' Council on Sports Medicine and Fitness and Council on School Health (2006) made the following recommendations for advocacy in support of physical activity by physicians, health care professionals, and related national organizations:

- Social marketing that promotes increased physical activity.
- The appropriate allocation of funding for quality research in the prevention of childhood obesity.
- The development and implementation of a school wellness counsel on which local physician representation is encouraged.
- A school curriculum that teaches children and youth the health benefits of regular physical activity.
- Comprehensive community sport and recreation programs that allow for community and school facilities to be open after hours and make physical activities available to all children and youth at reasonable costs; access to recreation facilities should be equally available to both sexes.
- The reinstatement of compulsory, quality, daily PE [physical education] classes in all schools (kindergarten through grade 12) taught by qualified, trained educators. The curricula should emphasize enjoyable participation in physical activity that helps students develop the knowledge, attitudes, motor skills, behavioral skills, and confidence required to adopt and maintain healthy active lifestyles. These classes should allow participation by all children regardless of ability, illness, injury, and developmental disability, including those with obesity and those who are disinterested in traditional competitive team sports. Commitment of adequate resources for program funding, trained PE personnel, safe equipment, and facilities is also recommended.
- The provision of a variety of physical activity opportunities in addition to PE, including the protection of children's recess time and the requirement of extracurricular physical activity programs and nonstructured physical activity before, during, and after school hours, that address the needs and interests of all students.
- The reduction of environmental barriers to an active lifestyle through the construction of safe recreational facilities, parks, playgrounds, bicycle paths, sidewalks, and crosswalks. (p. 1839)

Although we concur with these recommendations, we would also add the following, which are germane to weight bias and stigma (adapted from Puhl & Latner, 2007; see also chap. 5, this volume) and strongly suggest that psychologists and other mental health professionals interested in obesity support and advocate on their behalf:

- Carry out additional research on how stigma increases vulnerability to low self-esteem, depression, and body dissatisfaction.
- Evaluate whether different forms of weight-based victimization differentially affect emotional, social, and academic outcomes for obese youth of different ages and ethnicity.
- Examine whether reductions in weight stigma improve social, emotional, and academic outcomes.
- Perform research on whether protective factors buffer obese children from negative consequences of stigma.

- Carry out prospective and cross-cultural work to determine the developmental time course of weight bias.
- Assess and evaluate attributions about causes of obesity and how they relate to biased attitudes.
- Perform more research on the presence and remediation of weight bias among professionals, families, and peers.

More work is also needed in the area of evaluation of interventions designed to treat obesity. Well-designed protocols are needed to evaluate the effectiveness and efficacy of the interventions. Individual difference variables need to be considered as potential moderators or mediators of the success of such interventions. Along with factors such as age, socioeconomic status, gender, and ethnicity (see especially chaps. 3, 7, and 9, this volume), researchers might consider such factors as body dissatisfaction (chap. 4, this volume), self-efficacy (to make specific lifestyle changes), motivation, and barriers (presumed and real). It may also be important to consider interventions that are long term, beginning in early childhood and continuing during the adolescent and teenage years, when the risk for unhealthy eating and sedentary behaviors seems especially problematic.

Prevention of overweight and obesity is a prominent goal of those involved in this area. Intervention programs that involve the entire family system have been developed, and encouraging signs that they are effective have emerged. Family-based treatment programs, which have included a variety of behavior-oriented strategies, have also been found to be effective. However, much more evaluative work needs to be done. Although some treatment programs have been available for roughly 30 years, dissemination continues to be an issue, and in view of the vast increase in the at-risk population, it will be essential to increase the availability of treatment and prevention programs to potential participants. In addition, more research is needed on the long-term effectiveness of these programs, along with information regarding which particular factors are associated with maintenance or relapse.

The future health of children and adolescents depends on an active, well-planned, and well-funded assault on the obesity epidemic. As this book has detailed, an array of biological, social, and interpersonal variables are being explored in connection with the causes and consequences of overweight and obesity. Researchers are creating new programs to deal with stigmatization and bias as well as evaluating a variety of prevention and treatment programs. Much of this work has been recent and has evolved rapidly. Our hope is that through concerted focus and collaboration among relevant parties (public policy, researchers, communities, families), along with carefully planned and orchestrated research, great progress will be made in the next decade in our understanding and management of pediatric obesity.

REFERENCES

American Academy of Pediatrics. (2003). Policy statement: Prevention of pediatric overweight and obesity. *Pediatrics, 112,* 424–430.

American Academy of Pediatrics, Council on Sports Medicine and Fitness and Council on School Health. (2006). Active healthy living: Prevention of childhood obesity through increased physical activity. *Pediatrics, 117,* 1834–1842.

Puhl, R. M., & Latner, J. D. (2007). Stigma, obesity, and the health of the nation's children. *Psychological Bulletin, 133,* 557–580.

AUTHOR INDEX

Page numbers in italics refer to listings in the references.

Aalborg, A., 84, *94*
Aalto-Setälä, V., 193, *195*
Abramowitz, R. H., 145, 154, *157*
Abrams, D. B., 146, *155*
Abu-Abid, A., 7, *11*
Achenbach, T. M., 146, 152, *155*
Ackard, D. M., 123, *128*
Adachi-Mejia, A., 66, *72*
Adair, L., 63, *74*
Adamiak, M., 80, *97*
Adams, C. D., 127, *131*
Adeyanju, M., 84, *97*
Adler, R., 8, *12*
Adolph, A. L., 43, *54*
Agranat-Meged, A. N., 125, *128*
Agras, W. S., 124, *133*
Aickin, M. G., *199*
Ajdacic, V., *130*
Akdeniz, F., *129*
Alberti, G., 161, *180*
Alcaraz, J. E., 171, *179*
Alexander, A. M., 101, *111*
Alfonzo, M., 194, *196*
Allen, K., 7, *13*
Allison, D. B., *50*, 84, *95*, 116, *129*, 159, *177*
Allison, K., 126, *133*, *178*
Al Mamun, A., *13*
Almeida, M., 194, *199*
Almeida, M. J., 40 *54*
Al-Nakeeb, Y., 107, *110*
ALSPAC Study Team, 83, *95*
Altabe, M. N., 99, *114*, 145, 151, *157*
Alverdy, J., 126, *129*
Alwitt, L., *195*
Al-Zahrani, A., *34*, *178*
Amato, A., *35*

American Academy of Pediatrics, 6, 7, *11*, 45, 49, *50*, 205, *208*
American Academy of Pediatrics Council on Sports Medicine and Fitness and Council on School Health, 205, *208*
American Beverage Association, 69, *72*
American Medical Association, 3, *12*, 116, *128*
American Psychiatric Association, *12*, 115, 122, *128*, 152, *155*
Amy, N. K., 84, *94*
Anders, T. F., 138, 143, *156*
Andersen, R. E., 10, *50*
Anderson, A. S., 186, *195*
Anderson, C. B., 47, 48, *50*
Anderson, C. L., 194, *196*
Anderson, J., 168, *179*
Anderson, P. M., 37, 41, 43, 44, 45, 47, *50*
Anderson, S., 69, *75*
Anderson, S. E., 119, 121, *128*
Andersson, S. W., 45, *56*
Ando, M., *179*
Andrews, M., 193, *195*
Anesbury, T., 88, *94*
Aneshensel, C. S., 107, *112*
Angold, A., *132*
Aout, M., *34*
Apter, A., 166, *177*
Arakawa, K., *179*
Arcan, C., 63, *72*
Archibald, E. H., *180*
Ard, J. D., 44, *50*
Argona, J., 173, *175*
Argyropoulos, G., *35*
Arinell, H., 107, *114*

Armatas, C., 106, *112*
Arnold, K., *131*
Arslanian, S., 161, *180*
Arredondo, E. M., 46, *50*
Arveiler, D., *76*
Ashton, V., *180*
Austin, E. W., *72*
Austin, S. B., 62, 66, 67, 69, *72, 73, 74*
Ayala, G. X., *50*
Aye, T., 7, *12*
Ayers, T. S., 162, *177*

Bacino, C., 28, *33*
Backman, L., *133*
Baecke, J. A. H., 147, 149, *155*
Bagley, C., 84, *94*
Baird, J., *12*
Bajema, C. J., 6, *13*
Ball, G. D., *179*
Ball, K., 8, *12*, 46, *51*, 190, *200*
Banasiak, S. J., 107, *109*
Bandini, L. G., 125, *129*
Bandura, A., 162, *175*
Bangiwala, S. I., 38, *54*
Banis, H. T., 8, *12*
Banks, M., 83, *97*
Banyas, B., 7, *13*
Bao, S., *201*
Bao, Y., 191, *199*
Baquero, B., *50*
Baranowski, J. C., 185, 186, 188, 194,
    195, 196, 198
Baranowski, T., 40, *50, 52*, 185, 186,
    188, 191, 192, 193, 194, *195,
    198, 199, 200*
Barbeau, P., *178*
Barendregt, J. J., *13*
Barlow, S. E., 4, *12*, 160, 168, 169, 171,
    175
Barner, C. W., 147, 148, *156*
Barr-Anderson, D. J., 66, *72*
Barry, M. J., *199*
Barsh, G. S., 19, *34*
Bartlett, S. J., 40, *50*
Barton, B. A., *74, 131*
Baskin, D. G., 19, *34*
Baskin, M. L., *50*

Bassett, A. M., *134*
Baxter, J. E., *180*
Beach, M., *72*
Bearinger, L., 63, *73*
Bearman, S. K., 100, *113*, 121, *133*
Beccaria, L., *128*
Becker, J. A., 107, *114*
Becque, M. D., 170, *175*
Beddome, M., *176*
Beech, B. M., *52*, 188, *196*
Beecher, M. D., 173, *176*
Bell, C. G., 22, 23, 25, 26, 27, 30, *33*
Bell, L. E., *180*
Bell, S. K., 88, *94*
Bellis, D. B., 69, *72*
Bellizi, M. C., 161, *176*
Bengtsson, C., *133*
Beque, D., 168, *179*
Bere, E., *54*
Berenson, G. S., 6, *12, 52*
Berkey, C. S., 46, *55*, 62, 64, 67, 71,
    73, 74, 76, 110, *130*
Berkowitz, R. I., 46, *52, 73*, 163, 168,
    173, *175, 180*
Berman, N., *177*
Berridge, K. C., 22, *33*
Berry, C. C., 47, *55, 57*
Bertrand, C., *134*
Beuhring, T., 82, *95, 112, 130*
Beydoun, M. A., 3, 4, 5, 6, *14*
Biddle, S. J. H., 40, 41, *50, 53, 54*
Billington, C., 84, *98*
Binkley, D., *199*
Birch, L. L., 43, 45, 47, *50, 52*, 61, 62,
    73, 74, 76, 188, 189, *196, 197*
Birkett, D., 46, *53*
Birnbaum, A. S., *55*, 67, *73, 198*
Bishop, D. B., *199*
Bishop, S. C., *199*
Blair, S. N., 83, 84, *94, 98*
Blanco, I., *34, 178*
Blecker, U., *180*
Blimkie, C. J., *55*
Blissett, J., 45, *50*
Bloom, S., 20, *35*
Bloom, S. R., 21, 22, *33, 34*
Bloomquist, B., 168, *176*

Blum, R. W., 97, *112*

Boarnet, M. G., 194, *196*

Boergers, J., 81, 82, 97

Boerwinkle, E., 28, *33*

Bohr, Y., 147, 153, *156*

Booth, F. W., 171, *176*

Borjeson, M., 168, *176*

Borys, J. M., 28, *34*

Borzekowski, D. L. G., 43, *51*

Bosio, L., *128*

Bouatia-Naji, N., 25, 30, *34*

Bouchard, C., 17, 18, 19, 24, 25, 26, 27, *33, 34, 35, 133*

Boukaert, J., 171, *176*

Boutelle, K. N., 64, 66, *74*, 89, 95, 102, 103, *109*

Boutin, P., 25, *34*

Bowman, S. A., 44, *51*

Boyce, W. F., 8, *13*, 81, 83, 96, 150, *156*

Boyle, C., *33*

Bract, C., 123, *129*

Brambilla, P., 115, *128*

Brand-Miller, J. C., *179*

Braun, S., *178*

Bray, G. A., 6, *12*

Breen, P. A., *33*

Brener, N., 69, 70, *74, 76*

Brenner, H., *131*

Brewer, G., 164, *177*

Brewerton, T. D., 106, *110*

Briefel, R., 47, 57Britz, A., 117, *128*

Brock, J., 162, *180*

Brodersen, N. H., 42, *51*

Brodie, M., 41, *54*

Brook, J., 121, *132*

Brorge, S., 7, *12*

Brown, M., *199*

Brown, R., 46, *51, 180*

Brownell, K. D., 84, 85, 98, 101, *111*, *119, 130*, 162, 166, *176, 179*

Brownson, R. C., 56, *198*

Broyles, S. L., *55*

Brug, J., *54*

Bruning, N., *131*

Bryant-Waugh, R. J., 122, 127, *128*

Brylinsky, J. A., 80, *94*

Buch, T., 30, *35*

Bukusoglu, N., *129*

Bulik, C. M., 124, 125, *129, 133*

Bunnell, D., 107, *109*

Buono, M. J., 171, *179*

Burant, C., 68, *74*

Burdette, H. L., 42, *51*, 60, *73*

Burema, J., 147, 149, *155*

Burns, C., 191, *198*

Burns, N. P., *134*

Burrows, A., 100, *109*

Burton, L. R., *178, 180*

Burwinkle, T. M., 8, *13*, 126, *133*, 150, *157*

Butcher, K. E., 37, 41, 43, 44, 45, 47, *50*

Butler, B. A., 172, *178*

Butler, M. G., 115, *134*

Butryn, M. L., 126, 127, *129*

Butte, N., 28, *33*

Butte, N. F., 43, *54*

Byrne, N. M., 171, *178, 180*

Caballero, B., 186, *196*

Cafri, G., 8, *14*, 105, 108, *110, 114*

Cai, G., 25, 28, *33*

Cain, K. L., 38, *55*

Camargo, C. A., Jr., 52, 67, 72, 73, *74*, *110, 130, 197*

Cameron, N., 11, *50, 53*

Campbell, K. J., 46, 47, 48, *51, 180*

Campbell, R. T., *201*

Carbone, M. T., *33*

Cardon, G., *197*

Carnell, S., 47, 48, *51, 56*

Carpenter, K. M., 116, *129*

Carroll, M. D., 4, *13*, 17, *35, 62, 75, 132*

Cartwright, Y., *200*

Cash, T. F., 107, *110*

Casiday, R. E., 47, *51*

Caspersen, C. J., 38, *51*

Caspi, A., *132*

Cassady, J., 173, *175*

Catellier, D. J., *56*

Cato, R. K., *180*

Cattarin, J., 8, *12, 14*, 113, 145, 151, *157*

Cawley, J., 47, *51*, 190, *196*

Centers for Disease Control and Prevention, 65, *73*, 139, *155*

Cerny, F. J., 171, *177*

Certain, K. L., *51*

Cetin, N., *129*

Chagnon, Y. C., *35*

Chakravarthy, M. V., 171, *176*

Chaloupka, F. J., 191, *199*

Chambliss, H., 80, *95*

Chambliss, H. O., 83, 84, *94, 98*

Charles, M. A., 28, *34*

Charpentier, G., *34*

Chen, W., 25, 28, *33*

Chen, Y., *72*

Cherman, C., *112*

Cheskin, L. J., 40, *50*, 84, *95*, 159, *177*

Child Nutrition Improvement and
    Integrity Act of 2004, 186, *196*

Childress, A. C., 106, *110*

Chiumello, G., *128*

Christakis, D. A., 40, *56*

Christensen, P., 190, *196*

Christenson, G. M., 38, *51*

Chung, C., 63, *73*, 193, *196*

Cirillo, G., 25, 29, *33, 35*

Civitarese, A., 26, *33*

Clark, L., 173, *178*

Clark, M. M., 146, *155*

Clark, N. G., *179*

Clark, V. L., *180*

Clarke, G., 192, *196*

Clay, T., *196*

Clément, K., 25, 26, 27, *34*

Cohen, E., 61, *76*

Cohen, M. L., *134*

Cohen, P., 119, 121, *128, 132*

Colditz, G. A., 7, *14, 54*, 67, *72, 74, 75,
    110, 130*

Cole, S. A., 28, *33*

Cole, T. J., 161, *176*

Coles, M. E., 120, *132*

Coller, T., 80, *96*

Collins, M. E., 106, *110*

Committee on Public Education, 70, *73*

Conklin, D., 84, *94*

Conrad, B., *178*

Contento, I. R., 47, *53*

Conway, T. L., 38, 40, *54, 55*, 190, *198,
    199*

Cook, N. R., 7, *12*, 28, *33*

Cooke, L. J., 45, 46, 48, *51, 56*, 119,
    134

Coon, K. A., 41, *51*

Cooper, M., 100, 107, *109*

Cooper, P., 106, *109*

Cooper, P. J., 38, *51*, 107, *110*, 127, *128*

Coovert, M. D., 8, *14*, 101, *113*

Coplan, J. D., 121, *132*

Corbin, C. B., 40, *56*, 180

CORE Tools and Patient Information:
    Using Step Counters to Increase
    Physical Activity, *176*

Corsi, I., *35*

Costello, E. J., *132*

Council on Sports Medicine and Fitness
    and Council on School Health,
    190, *196*

Cox, C., *134*

Cox, N., 19, *35*

Crago, M., *133*

Craig, W. M., 8, *13*, 81, 83, *96*, 150,
    156

Crawford, D., 8, *12*

Crawford, D. A., 46, *51*

Crawford, P., 100, *113*

Crerand, C. E., 162, *180*

Crespo, C. J., 40, *50*

Crespo, N. C., *179*

Crick, N. R., 81, *94*

Cronquist, J. L., 163, 168, *175*

Crosby, R. B., *129*

Crosnoe, R., 119, *132*

Crossan, S., *112*

Crow, S., 46, *53*, 100, 102, *110, 177*

Crowther, J. H., *131*

Crum, R. M., 118, *132*

Cruz, M. L., *179*

Cullen, K. W., 48, *52*, 185, 186, 188,
    195, 196, 197, 200

Cummings, D. E., 19, 20, 21, 22, 23, *33,
    34*

Cummins, S., 191, 192, *197, 198*

Cunningham, A., 186, *199*

Curtin, C., 125, *129*

Curtin, L. R., 17, *35, 132*

Cuzzolaro, M., 108, *110*

Dabbas, M., *134*

Dagenais, F., 71, *75*

Dale, D., 40, *56*

Dallal, G. E., 6, *13, 34, 178*

Dalton, M., *72*

D'Angelo, S., *52*

Daniels, S. R., 7, *12, 52, 55,* 60, *73,74,*
117, 127, *131, 134,* 147, 153,
156, 175

Danner, F. W., *52*

Davidson, D., *95*

Davies, B. A., *130*

Davis, M., *196, 199, 200*

Davis, R., 117, *129, 132*

Davis, S. M., *196*

Davison, K. K., 45, *50,* 66, *73,* 188, 194,
197

Day, K., *194, 196*

de Almeida, M., *52*

De Bourdeaudhuij, I., 48, *52,* 171, *176,*
197

Decluwe, V., 123, *129*

Deforche, B., 171, *176, 197*

Deitcher, C., 125, *128*

Deitz, W. H., *178*

DeJong, W., 88, *94*

DeLancey, E., 117, *133*

Deleger, S., 117, *132*

del Giudice, E. M., 25, 29, *33, 35*

Dellinger, A. M., 38, *52*

Dellinger, E. P., *33*

Demory-Luce, D., 44, *52*

Dennison, D. A., *52,* 66, *73*

Department for Education and Skills,
190, *197*

Desmond, R. A., *50*

Desmond, S., 84, *97*

Despinasse, B., *180*

Devlin, M., *133*

DeWalt, K. M., 48, *52*

Deweirder, M., 28, *34*

de Zwann, M., 122, *129*

Dhurandhar, N. V., 138, *156*

Diego, V., 28, *33*

Dietz, W. H., 6, 7, 8, *12, 13, 14,* 150,
156, 160, 161, 167, 168, 169,
171, *175, 176,* 188, *197*

Diez Roux, A. V., 191, 192, *199*

Dillingham, D. C., *199*

DiLorenzo, T. M., 194, *200*

Dina, C., 28, *34*

Dishman, R. K., 55, *156*

Di Toro, R., *33*

Dixit, S., *53, 197*

Doll, H. A., *130*

Dong, F., *199*

Donkin, A., 188, 192, *197*

Donley, T., *195*

Donnelly, J. M., 106, *112*

Dora, C. A., 42, *52*

Dorn, J. M., *170, 173, 176, 180*

Dorn, J. P., 171, *177*

Dornbusch, S. M., 80, *98*

Dowda, M., 40 *54,* 64, *76, 156, 200*

Dowler, E., 188, 192, *197*

Downie, J., 60, *75*

Doyle, C., *196*

Drab, D. L., 108, *111*

Drabman, R. S., 173, *175*

Dreimane, D., *178*

Drewnowski, A., *52, 197*

Drotar, D., 68, *74*

Druce, M., 21, 22, *33*

Dubois, L., 60, *73*

Dubois, S., 28, *34*

Dudovitz, B. S., *199*

Due, P., *52, 54*

Duerksen, S., *50*

Duncan, G. E., 161, *176*

Duncan, M. J., 107, *110*

Dunn, M., 145, 151, *157*

Duquet, W., 171, *176*

D'Urso, L., *33*

Dyer, A., *197*

Dyer, A. R., 7, *12*

Dymek, M., 126, *129*

Eaton, C., 147, 148, *156*

Eaton, C. A., 146, *155*

Eaton, D., 70, *74*

Eaton, W. W., 118, *132*

Eaves, L. J., 188, *198*

Ebbeling, C. B., 44, *51,* 169, 170, *176*

Eddy, K. T., *130*

Edlund, B., 107, *114*

Edmunds, L., *180*
Edwards, C., 118, 119, *134*
Edwards, C. D., 146, 152, *157*
Eich, D., *130*
Eisenberg, M. E., 62, 63, 64, 66, *73, 74,*
    86, 87, *94,* 100, 101, 102, 105,
    110, 111, 112, 120, *129*
Elder, J. P., *50*
Eliakim, A., 45, *52*
Ellenberg, D., *112*
Engeland, A., 7, *12*
Engels, R., 66, 71, *76*
Engström, I., 107, *114*
Epping, J., 70, *74*
Epping, J. N., *198*
Epstein, L. H., 43, 56, 126, *129,* 159,
    166, 167, 168, 169, 170, 171,
    172, 173, *176, 177, 180, 181*
Erb, T. A., 66, *73*
Eremis, S., 117, 118, *129*
Erickson, S. J., 119, *129*
Erkanli, A., *132*
Ernst, M. M., 126, *129*
Estes, L. S., *133*
Ethelbah, B., *196*
Evens, C., 46, *53*
Expert Committee, 4, *12*
Eyre, H., 192, *196*

Fabian, L. J., 101, *110,* 145, 151, *157*
Faibisch, L., 80, *97*
Fainaru, M., 166, *177*
Fairburn, C. G., 107, *110,* 122, 124, *130*
Faith, M. S., 45, 46, 47, 48, *52,* 61, *73,*
    84, *95,* 116, 126, *129, 133,* 159,
    162, 165, *177*
Falissard, B., *130*
Falkner, N. H., 80, 82, *95,* 96, 101, 102,
    112, 119, *130, 132*
Farooqi, I. S., 24, 25, 26, 27, *33*
Farris, R. P., 186, *199*
Feldman, H. A., 69, *72,* 169, 170, *176,*
    198
Felton, G., *156*
Ferguson, A. V., 22, *34*
Field, A. E., 7, *12,* 46, *52,* 55, 62, 64, 66,
    72, 73, 74, 76, 103, *110,* 123, *130*

Fiese, B. H., 144, 147, *156*
Figueroa-Colon, R., 169, *177*
Filion, Y., 71, *75*
Finley, C. E., 83, *94*
Fisch, G., 7, *13*
Fisher, D., 7, *12*
Fisher, E., 145, 151, *157*
Fisher, J. O., 45, 46, 47, 50, *53,* 61, *74,*
    189, *196*
Fitzgerald, A., 189, *201*
Fitzgibbon, M., 122, *133*
Fitzgibbon, M. L., *197*
Fitzpatrick, S., *50*
Flegal, K. M., 4, *13,* 17, *35,* 62, *75,* 116,
    131, 132, 161, *176*
Foehr, U. G., 41, *54,* 66, 68, 70, 71, *75*
Fontaine, K. R., 84, *95,* 159, *177*
Foreyt, J. P., 162, *177*
Forthofer, R., *200*
Foster, E., *195*
Foster, G. D., 84, *95,* 164, *177, 180*
Fowler, B., 145, 151, *157*
Fox, E., 101, *114*
Fox, M. K., *53, 197*
Fradkin, A., *132*
Francis, L. A., 43, *52,* 61, 66, *73, 74,*
    188, *197*
Frank, A., 85, *95*
Frank, G. C., 47, *57*
Franklin, F. A., 169, *177, 199*
Franz, M. J., *179*
Frayo, R. S., *33*
Frazier, A. L., 46, *52,* 55, 64, *73, 74, 76,*
    110, 130, 197
Freedman, D. S., 6, 7, *12, 13*
Freedson, P. S., 64, *76, 200*
Freeman, R. J., 117, *129*
Frelut, M., *130*
French, S. A., 63, 69, 70, *74, 75, 76,* 86,
    95, 97, 112, 185, 186, *197, 200*
Fried, E., 69, *74*
Friedel, S., 28, *35*
Friedland, O., 45, *52*
Friedman, M. A., 119, *130*
Frijters, J. E. R., 147, 149, *155*
Froguel, P., 22, *33*
Fry, M., 22, *34*

Fujioka, K., *175*
Fulkerson, J. A., 63, 65, 70, *74*, *75*, 89, 95, 186, *197*
Fulton, J., 70, *74*
Furey, S., 192, *197*

Galen, B. R., 81, 95
Galili-Weisstub, E., 125, *128*
Gallagher, D., *177*
Gallagher, M., 192, *197*
Gamma, A., *130*
Gans, K. M., 147, 148, *156*
Gapinski, K. D., 85, 98
Garfinkel, P. E., 108, *110*, 147, 153, *156*
Garner, D. M., 107, *110*, 117, *129*, 147, 153, *156*
Garrison, M. M., 40, 56
Garside, D. B., 7, *12*
Geffner, M. E., *178*
Geliebter, A., 22, 35
Geller, F., 28, 30, 34, 35
Gerberding, J. L., 3, *13*
Ghaderi, A., 95
Ghorbani, S., *130*
Ghoussaini, M., 25, 30, *34*
Gibson, E. L., *51*
Gibson, J., *72*
Gidding, S. S., 49, *52*
Gillman, M., 60, *73*, *75*
Gillman, M. W., 7, *12*, 38, 46, *52*, 63, *74*, *110*, *130*, 189, *197*
Girard, M., 60, *73*
Glanz, K., 38, 55
Glasofer, D. R., 123, *130*
Gleason, J. H., 101, *111*
Glynn, N. W., *74*
Goksen, D., *129*
Golan, M., 46, 47, 53, 166, *177*
Gold, R., 138, *157*
Goldberg, J., 41, *51*
Goldfield, G. S., *177*
Goldstein, R. B., 121, *132*
Goldstone, A. P., 21, *34*
Goldzweig, G., 125, *128*
Golub, S., 84, 88, 96
Goodman, E., 120, 121, *130*
Goodman, N., 80, 98

Goodrick, G. K., 162, *177*
Goran, M. I., 6, *12*, 61, 76
Gordon-Larsen, P., 38, 43, *53*, 63, *74*
Gordy, C. C., 170, *176*
Gorely, T., 41, *50*, *53*
Gortmaker, S., *198*
Gortmaker, S. L., 8, *12*, 39, 41, 44, 48, *51*, *53*, 56, 150, *156*, 185, 186, 188, *197*
Gower, B. A., 6, *12*
Graves, T., 173, *178*
Gray, J. J., 106, *114*
Gray, N., *133*
Gray-Donald, K., 38, 54
Greenland, P., 7, *12*
Greenleaf, C., 80, 95
Greeno, C. G., 123, *131*
Greenstein, J., 44, *53*
Grieve, F. G., 127, *131*
Griffin, S., 188, *199*
Griffiths, L. J., 83, 95
Grilo, C. M., 101, *111*
Grimm-Thomas, K., *50*
Grocz, L. M., 127, *133*
Gruber, M. B., 186, *198*
Grummer-Strawn, L. M., *13*, *131*
Grunbaum, J. A., *53*
Gueorguiev, M., 29, *34*
Gunnell, D., 7, *13*
Guo, J., *112*
Guo, S. S., *131*
Gurthrie, J., 69, *75*
Gussow, J. D., 47, *53*
Gustafson, S. L., 40, *53*
Guthrie, C. A., 48, 56
Gutin, B., 55, *178*
Guy, C., 192, *196*

Haan, M., 76
Haas, S. A., 118, *134*
Haerens, L., 186, *197*
Häglöf, B., 107, *114*
Haines, J., 80, 82, 83, 86, 87, 88, 94, 95, 96, 101, 102, 105, *111*, *112*, 120, *129*
Haire-Joshu, D., 56
Hall, W., 60, *73*

Hamer, R. M., *133*

Hammer, L. D., 124, *133*

Hangen, J. P., *176*

Hann, C., *197*

Hannan, P. J., 63, 65, 70, *72, 74, 75,* 80, *95, 96, 97,* 101, 102, 105, *111, 112, 132,* 185, 186, *197, 198*

Hanson, C., 44, *57*

Hanson, N., 62, *74*

Hardeman, W., 188, *199*

Hardman, C. A., *198*

Harper, M. G., 38, *53*

Harrell, J. S., 38, *54*

Harrington, K. F., *199*

Harris, M., 194, *198*

Harris, T., 83, 90, *96*

Harrison, J. E., *180*

Harrison, K., 71, *74,* 105, *111*

Harter, S., 146, 153, *156*

Hartman, K., 67, *74*

Harvey, J., *178*

Hasin, D., *133*

Hasin, D. S., 116, *129*

Hasler, G., 117, *130*

Hassink, S., 117, *133, 134*

Hastorf, A. H., 80, *98*

Hatahet, M. A., 138, *156*

Hay, P. J., *130*

Haycraft, E., 45, *50*

Haydel, K. F., 118, *129*

Hayden-Wade, H. A., 82, *95*

Hayes, S. C., 166, *176*

He, J., 25, *35*

Heaslip, S., 80, *98*

Heath, G. W., *198*

Heatherton, T. F., 164, *178*

Hebebrand, J., 25, *34*

Hebl, M. R., 84, *95*

Heckerman, C. L., 166, *176*

Heimberg, R. G., 120, *132*

Heinberg, L. J., 99, *114,* 145, 154, *156*

Helling, A., 192, 193, *198*

Henderson, S., 60, *75*

Henderson, S. A., *197*

Hendricks, K., 44, 47, *57*

Henkel, A. W., *131*

Hennig, E. M., 171, *178, 180*

Heo, M., 162, *177*

Herbozo, S., 8, *14, 114*

Herpertz, S., *130*

Herpertz-Dahlmann, B. M., *128, 130*

Hertz, S., 107, *109*

Herva, A., 121, *130*

Heshka, S., *52*

Hesketh, K., 86, 96, 126, *134*

Hess, C., *34*

Hess, K. W., *180*

Hetherington, M., *195*

Heude, B., 25, 28, *34*

Heussen, N., *130*

Higgins, C., *195*

Higgins, D. B., 6, *12*

Hill, A. J., 81, *97*

Hill, J. O., 124, *131,* 163, *180*

Hill, K., 138, *156*

Hills, A. P., 170, 171, *176, 178, 180*

Himes, J. H., *74,* 160, *200*

Himes, S., 8, *14*

Hinderliter, J., 168, *179*

Hindin, T. J., 47, *53*

Hines, J. H., *178*

Hinney, A., 25, 29, *34*

Hirvensalo, M., 38, *55*

Hodges, E. A., 47, *53*

Hodges, E. L., 106, *110*

Hoefer, W. R., 190, *198*

Hoffman, E., 105, *113*

Hohmann, S., *34*

Holahan, C. J., 147, *156*

Hollis-Neely, T., 193, *201*

Holmes, N., *201*

Holsen, I., 100, *111*

Holtkamp, K., 125, *130*

Home, P. J., *198*

Hooper, C. A., 186, *198*

Hoppin, A. G., *175*

Horwood, J. P., 83, *95*

Houston, C., *56*

Howze, E. H., *198*

Hoyda, T. D., 22, *34*

Hu, F., 60, *75*

Hu, J., 38, *54*

Hubsmith, D., 194, *200*

Huddy, D. C., 107, *111*

Huges, S. O., 53
Hughes, S. O., 47, 50, 54
Hulthen, L., 45, 56
Hunter, G. R., 6, 12
Hunter, J. A., 83, 97
Huse, K., 30, 35

Iacono, W. G., 106, 112
Ievers-Landis, C., 68, 74
Ignico, A. A., 178
Inge, T. H., 117, 134
Ingerski, L. M., 13
Ingram, D. K., 39, 53
Ireland, M., 89, 96, 102, 111
Irving, L. M., 80, 87, 96, 97, 102, 112
Isherwood, R., 84, 94
Islam, N., 195
Isnard, J., 119, 130
Israel, B. A., 191, 192, 201
Israel, R. G., 199

Jackson, M. C., 198
Jacobi, C., 131
Jacobs, D. R., 200
Jacques, P. F., 6, 13
Jago, R. J. D., 185, 188, 194, 196, 198, 200
Jakicic, J. M., 172, 178
James, S. A., 201
Janicke, D. M., 13
Janssen, I., 8, 13, 81, 83, 96, 150, 156
Janssens, J., 66, 71, 76
Jaramillo, S. J., 44, 53
Jarcho, H. D., 145, 154, 157
Jarrell, M. P., 106, 110
Jay, S. M., 8, 12
Jebb, S. A., 40 54
Jeffrey, R. W., 82, 95, 130, 165, 178, 180
Jeffreys, M., 7, 13
Jenkins, P. L., 66, 73
Jeyaram, S., 85, 98
Joe, J. R., 199
Johnson, C. C., 186, 199
Johnson, C. L., 4, 13
Johnson, D. B., 46, 53
Johnson, F., 118, 119, 134
Johnson, J. G., 122, 130

Johnson, R. L., 107, 111
Johnson, S., 8, 14, 113
Johnson, S. L., 50
Johnson, W. G., 127, 131
Jones, E., 86, 97
Jones, K. E., 173, 180
Jorge, M. R., 131
Joukamaa, M., 130
Jouret, B., 34
Joyner, M. J., 171, 176

Kadow, K., 13
Kahn, E. B., 190, 198
Kahn, J., 72
Kahn, R. A., 51
Kalarchian, M. A., 122, 123, 126, 127, 131, 133, 166, 167, 177
Kallins, W., 194, 200
Kang, H. S., 170, 178
Kann, L., 42, 53
Kanter, L., 193, 195
Kaphingst, K. M., 185, 200
Kaplan, G. A., 117, 132
Karlsson, J., 133
Karvonen, J. T., 130
Katch, V. L., 168, 170, 175, 179
Kaufer Christoffel, K., 197
Kaufman, F., 161, 180
Kaye, W. H., 125, 129
Kazdin, A., 163, 178
Keeler, G., 132
Keery, H., 64, 66, 74, 104, 111
Keller, K. L., 52
Kelly, S., 180
Kelly, T., 25, 35
Kemper, H. C. G., 38, 56
Kenardy, J., 8, 12
Kendell, G., 60, 75
Kendler, K. S., 124, 129
Keo, M., 134
Keranen, L., 84, 94
Kerns, J., 52, 61, 73
Kessler, A., 95
Khan, L. K., 6, 7, 12
Kilanowski, C. K., 176
Killen, J. D., 71, 75, 118, 129
Kim, J., 39, 53, 69, 72, 198

Kimm, S. Y., 65, 74, 119, *131*
Kinchen, S. A., *53*
Kirk, K. A., *199*
Klausner, J., 7, *11*
Kleijnen, J., *12*
Klein-Platat, C., *76*
Klem, M. L., 124, *131*
Klepp, K. I., *52, 54*
Klesges, L., *196*
Klesges, L. M., *52*
Klesges, R. C., *196*
Klier, M., *178*
Kline, C. A., 144, 147, *156*
Koerner, J., 107, *109*
Koeske, R., 170, *177*
Kondilis, V. A., 173, *180*
Konig, I. R., 28, *35*
Konrad, K., *130*
Koplan, J. P., 37, 41, 49, *53*
Korbonits, M., 25, 29, *34*
Korotitsch, W. J., 163, *178*
Korsch, B. M., 8, *12*
Kotchen, J. M., *52*
Kovacs, M., 145, 152, *156*
Kowen, G., 45, *52*
Kraak, V. I., 37, *53*
Kraft, P., 100, *111*
Kress, M. J., *177*
Kriska, A. M., *74*
Krol, R., 84, *97*
Krolner, R., *54*
Kronsberg, S. S., *74*
Kubik, M. Y., 55, 185, *198*
Kuczmarski, R. J., 116, *131*
Kuepper-Nybelen, J., *131*
Kuester, S., 69, *76*
Kumanyika, S., *196*
Kuntz, K. M., 48, *56*
Kupfer, D., 166, *180*
Kwoh, C., 68, *74*

Laasko, L., 7, *13*
Laitinen, J., 38, *55, 130*
Laksy, K., *130*
Lamertz, C. M., 118, *128, 131*
Lamerz, A., *131*
Landsborough, L., 60, *75*

Lang, W., 124, *131*
Larson, N., 63, *72*
Larsson, Y., 168, *176*
Lask, B. D., 127, *128*
Latner, J. D., 8, *13*, 91–93, *97, 112,*
    206, 208
Latner, M. C., 81, *96*
Lau, R., 67, *74*
Laurencelle, L., 38, *56*
Law, C., *12*
Lawson, C. T., 194, *197*
Lawson, M., *51*
Lawson, M. C., 81, *96*
LeBow, M. D., 166, *179*
Lecouer, C., 29, 30, *33, 34*
Lee, H. B., 118, *132*
Lee, J., 82, *98*
Lee, S., 70, *74*
Lefevre, J., 171, *176*
le Grange, D., 126, *129*
Leibenson, L., 125, *128*
Leidig, M. M., 169, 170, *176*
Lemmon, C. R., *178*
Leone, M. A., 162, *177*
Levin, M. P., *112*
Levine, A., *197*
Levine, M. D., 123, 126, *131*
Levine, M. P., 80, 87, 95, 98, 100, 105,
    111, 113, 154, *157*
Levitsky, L. L., 7, *12*
Lewis, C. E., 122, *133*
Li, C., 61, *76*
Li, S., 28, *33*
Li, S. M., 161, *176*
Lichtenstein, A. H., *52*
Lin, L. S., *196*
Lindsay, A. C., 39, *53*, 189, *198*
Lindsay, R. S., 38, *55*
Lingswiler, V. M., *131*
Lino, M., 193, *195*
Liverman, C. T., 37, *53*
Lo, A., 100, *113*
Lobbens, S., *34*
Lohman, T. G., *196*
Longacre, M., *72*
Loos, R. J., 17, 24, 25, 26, 27, *34*
Lore, J., 40, *55*

Lovell, P., 96
Lovesky, M. M., 169, 170, *176*
Lowe, C. F., *198*
Lowry, K. W., *13*
Lowry, R., *53*, 70, *74*
Lucas, P., *12*
Ludwig, D. S., 18, *34*, 44, *51*, 168, 169, 170, *176*, *178*
Luepker, R. V., 186, 187, *198*
Lushene, R., 146, 152, *157*
Lutz, T. A., 22, *34*
Lyketsos, C., 118, *132*
Lynch, J., *63*, 76
Lyons, P., 84, *94*
Lytle, L. A., 44, *53*, *55*, *67*, *73*, 185, *198*
Lytle, L. L., *54*

Ma, M. K., *33*
Macintyre, S., 191, 192, *197*, *198*
Mackenbach, J. P., *13*
Maes, H. H., 188, *198*
Maes, L., *197*
Magdol, L., *132*
Magnusson, J., 88, *98*
Mahar, M. T., 40, *55*
Maher, E., 126, *134*
Mahon, A. D., *178*
Majzoub, J. A., *34*, *178*
Makris, A. P., *95*
Malina, R. M., *55*
Maloney, M. J., 127, *131*, 147, 153, *156*
Malspeis, S., *74*
Manke, F., 125, *134*
Manzoni, P., *128*
Marano, O., 100, *110*
Marciel, K. K., *13*
Marcus, M. D., 122, 123, 126, 127, *131*, *133*, 166, *180*
Margetts, B., 192, *201*
Markey, C. N., *50*, 61, 62, *73*
Marks, C. R., 170, *175*
Marks, J. S., 3, *13*
Marlin, D. W., 189, *196*
Marmarosh, C., *113*, *134*
Maroney, D., 84, 88, *96*
Marquis, M., 71, *75*
Marsh, T., 186, *195*

Marshall, S. J., 41, *50*, *53*, *54*, 190, *198*, *199*
Marske, A., 71, *74*
Marti, C. N., 188, *200*
Marti, N., 68, *76*
Martin, M., 168, *179*
Martin, S. B., 80, *95*
Martinez, E. E., 127, *133*
Maschette, W., 106, *112*
Mason, M. F., 84, *95*
Matheson, D., 71, *75*
Matz, P. E., *52*
Mayer-Davis, E., 60, *75*, *179*
Mays, R., *199*
Mayville, S. B., 108, *111*
McArthur, L., 84, *96*
McCabe, M. P., 100, *112*
McCarron, P., 7, *13*
McCauley, E., *132*
McClanahan, B., *196*
McCreary, D. R., 108, *111*
McCurley, J., 166, 167, 171, *176*, *177*
McDowell, M. A., 17, *35*, *132*
McDuffie, J., *131*
McEwen, J., 7, *13*
McFadden, M., *52*
McGaghie, W. C., *98*
McGovern, P., 44, *53*
McGowan, B., 20, *35*
McGuire, J. B., 127, *131*, 147, 153, *156*
McGuire, M., 65, *75*
McGuire, M. T., 124, *131*
McIlveen, H., *192*, *197*
McIver, K. L., 40 54
McKay, L., *191*, *198*
McKenzie, T. L., 38, 40, *54*, *55*, 171, *179*, 187, 190, *198*, *199*
McKinlay, S. M., *198*
McKnight, K. M., *133*
McLean, N., 188, *199*
McLeod, H. A., 80, *98*
McMahon, R., *131*
McMillan, T., 194, *196*
McMurray, J., 147, 148, *156*
McMurray, R. G., 38, *54*
McVey, G., 87, *96*
Mei, Z., 4, *13*

Meier, A. M., 118, *134*
Mein, C. A., 29, *34*
Mellin, A. E., 89, *96*, 102, 103, *111*
Mendelson, B. K., 108, *111*
Mendelson, M. J., 108, *111*
Meshefedjian, G., 38, *54*
Messick, S., 147, 153, *157*
Meyer, C., 45, *50*
Meyerhoefer, C., 190, *196*
Meyers, A. M., 56
Meyers, A. W., 173, *178*
Meyers, S., 193, *196*
Meyre, D., 25, 30, *33, 34*
Michel, G., *130*
Miettunen, J., *130*
Miller, C., 69, *75, 76*
Milos, G., *130*
Mirtcheva, D., 191, *199*
Mirza, N. M., 4, *13*
Mitchell, J. E., *129*
Modan, D., *132*
Modi, A. C., 117, *134*
Moffitt, T. E., *132*
Mokdad, A. H., 3, *13*
Monroe, D., 84, *97*
Monti, P. M., 166, *176*
Montuori, J., 146, 152, *157*
Monzavi, R., 161, *178*
Moore, L. V., 192, *199*
Moos, B. S., 144, *156*
Moos, R. H., 144, 147, *156*
Morales, M., 47, *52, 53, 54*
Morgan, C. M., *113*, 123, *131, 134*
Morgan, L., 68, *74*
Morgan, S. B., 88, *94*
Morland, K., 191, 192, 193, *199*
Morrehead, C., 170, *175*
Morrell, J., 38, *51*
Morrison, J., *76*, 138, 143, *156*
Morrow, J. R., Jr., 80, *95*
Morton, G. J., 19, 20, 22, 24, *34*
Mota, J., 194, *199*
Motl, R. W., 155, *156*
Moulton, D., 145, 151, *157*
Moulton, M. M., 123, *131*
Muir, S., *75*
Mulert, S., *96, 111, 132*

Mullan, E., 194, *200*
Muller, B., *130*
Munoz, K. D., 186, *198*
Murdey, I., 41, *50, 53*
Murray, D. M., *55*, 67, *73*, 196, *198, 199*
Murray, L., 38, *51*
Must, A., 6, 8, *12, 13*, 119, 125, *128, 129*, 150, *156*
Mustillo, S., 119, 121, *132*
Mutch, D. M., 25, 26, 27, *34*
Myers, L., 186, *199*
Myers, M. D., 159, *176*
Myers, S., 63, *73*

Nader, P. R., 38, 47, *55, 57*, 171, *179, 198*
Naja, W., *130*
Nanney, M. S., 56
National Center for Health Statistics, 4, *13*
National Heart, Lung, and Blood Institute, *178*
Naumova, E. N., 119, *128*
Nayha, S., 38, *55*
Neale, M. C., 188, *198*
Neary, N. M., 21, 23, 24, *34*
Needham, B. L., 119, *132*
Neel, J. V., 25, 26, *35*
Nelson, M. C., 38, *53*
Nelson-Gray, R. O., 163, *178*
Nemeroff, C., 103, 104, *113*
Nemet, D., 45, *52*
Nestle, M., 69, *74*
Netmeyer, R., 108, *111*
Neumark-Sztainer, D., 62, 63, 64, 65, 66, 70, *72, 74, 75*, 80, 82, 83, 86, 87, 89, 90, *94, 95, 96, 97*, 100, 101, 102, 103, 105, *109, 110, 111, 112*, 120, 123, *128, 129, 130, 132*
Neven, K., 126, *129*
Newhouse, D., 190, *196*
Newman, D. L., 122, *132*
Nguyen, K. P., 186, *198*
Nguyen, T. T., *131*
Niaura, R. S., 146, *155*
Nichols, P. A., 164, *178*

Nicklas, T. A., 44, 46, 47, 50, 52, 53, 54, 185, 186, 195, 196, 199
Nicolopoulos, V., 82, 98
Nieman, D. C., 107, 111
Nissinoff, K. S., 180
Noland, M., 52
Novak, T., 44, 47, 57
Novoa, W., 13

Obarzanek, E., 76, 100, 113, 131
Oberrieder, H., 84, 97
O'Brien, K. S., 83, 97
O'Connell, J., 84, 97
O'Connor, M. E., 130
Oddy, W., 60, 75
O'Donnell, S., 191, 192, 193, 199
Offer, D., 145, 154, 157
Ogden, C. L., 4, 13, 17, 35, 62, 75, 116, 131, 132
Ogden, J., 46, 48, 51, 54
O'Grady, E., 29, 34
O'Hara, N. M., 200
Ohlson, J., 80, 97
Olmstead, M. P., 107, 110, 147, 153, 156
O'Loughlin, J., 38, 54
Olson, C. L., 84, 97
Olson, R., 63, 73
O'Neill, S. J., 107, 110
Onyike, C. U., 118, 132
O'Rahilly, S., 24, 25, 26, 27, 33
Orchard, J., 166, 179
Orvaschel, H., 145, 152, 157
O'Toole, T. P., 69, 75
Overduin, J., 20, 21, 22, 23, 33
Owen, S., 175
Owens, S., 178

Padian, N., 145, 152, 157
Page, A. S., 83, 95
Palmer, M., 13
Paluch, R. A., 43, 56, 126, 129, 170, 171, 172, 173, 176, 177, 180
Pan, D., 199
Pangrazi, R. P., 180
Panter-Brick, C., 47, 51
Paradis, G., 38, 54, 191, 200
Parcel, G. S., 198, 200

Parker, A. W., 170, 178
Parkinson, K. N., 47, 51
Parnaby, O. G., 133
Pate, R. R., 40 54, 64, 76, 200
Patrick, H., 44, 46, 47, 54
Patterson, T. L., 171, 179
Paxton, S. J., 62, 66, 67, 75, 101, 106, 112, 114
Payne, L., 12
Pearce, J. W., 166, 179
Pearce, M. J., 81, 82, 97
Pechiulis, D., 84, 94
Peeters, A., 7, 13
Pencharz, P. B., 180
Penner, B. C., 168, 170, 177
Pepe, M. S., 7, 14
Pereira, M. A., 44, 51
Permutt, M. A., 19, 35
Perrin, E. G., 125, 129
Perrin, J. M., 8, 12, 150, 156
Perrone, L., 33
Perry, A. C., 175
Perry, C. L., 67, 73, 80, 86, 95, 96, 97, 101, 102, 105, 110, 111, 112, 123, 128, 132, 185, 186, 198, 199
Perry, R., 88, 98
Persson, B., 168, 176
Pérusse, L., 17, 19, 33, 35
Pesa, J. A., 86, 97
Petersen, A. C., 145, 154, 157
Peterson, K. E., 53, 69, 72, 197
Peterson, M., 112
Pettersson, K., 45, 56
Pfeiffer, K. A., 40 54
Phelan, S., 137, 157, 180
Phillips, G. A., 55
Phillips, R. G., 81, 97
Pickering, S., 46, 53
Pickett, W., 8, 13, 81, 83, 96, 150, 156
Pietrobelli, A., 52, 128, 162, 177
Pilpel, N., 132
Pine, D. S., 121, 130, 132
Pinhas-Hamiel, O., 126, 132
Pinkerton, B., 72
Piran, N., 87, 97
Pisu, M., 50
Pi-Sunyer, F. X., 22, 35, 179

Platzer, C., 30, *35*
Plomin, R., 48, *56*
Poerier, S., *199*
Polivy, J., 107, *110*
Pollack, H. A., 81, *98*
Pomeroy, C., 138, *156*
Ponza, M., 44, 47, *57*
Popkin, B. M., 38 *53*, 63, *74*
Porteous, L. E., *195*
Porter, J. E., 107, *112*
Post, G. B., 38, *56*
Potrim, L., 191, *200*
Poulton, R., *132*
Powell, K. E., 38, *51*, *198*
Powell, L. M., 191, 192, 193, *199*
Pratt, C., *52*
Pratt, M., 40, *50*
Prentice, A. M., 40 *54*
Presnell, K., 120, *133*
Price, J., 84, *97*
Prinstein, M. J., 81, 82, *97*
Prochaska, J. J., 38, *55*, 64, *75*, 189, *198*,
        199, *200*
Psaltis, K., *114*
Puhl, R. M., 8, *13*, 91–93, *97*, *112*, 162,
        179, 206, 208
Puyau, M. R., 43, *54*
Pyle, R. L., *129*

Quadrel, N. W., 67, *74*
Quintero Johnson, J., *72*

Raczynski, J. M., *199*
Radloff, L., 145, *157*
Raedeke, T. D., 40, *55*
Raether, C., *178*
Raghunathan, T., 63, *76*
Raimondo, P.*35*
Raitakari, O. T., 38, *56*
Ralston, K., 185, *197*
Ramsey, L. T., *198*
Rankinen, T., 17, 18, 25, 26, 27, 31, *35*
Rapoport, L., 48, *56*
Rasmussen, M., 44, *54*
Raustorp, A., *180*
Ravussin, E., 26, 33, 38, *55*
Rawlins, M., 85, *98*

Raymond, N. C., *129*
Raynor, H. A., 159, *176*
Reda, T. K., 22, *35*
Reichman, B., *132*
Reichwald, K., 30, *35*
Reis, A., 28, *35*
Reither, E. N., 118, *134*
Remschmidt, H., *128*
Report of the Second Task Force on
        Blood Pressure Control in Chil-
        dren, 161, *179*
Resiberg, L., 67, *75*
Resnick, M. D., 82, 89, 95, 96, 97, 102,
        103, *109*, *111*, *112*, *130*
Resnicow, K., *196*
Rex, J., 80, *97*
Reynolds, K. D., *199*
Reynolds, R., 48, *54*
Rhea, D. J., 80, *95*
Rhodes, R. E., 40, *53*
Ribeiro, J. C., 194, *199*
Ricciardelli, L. A., 100, *112*
Richards, K. J., 8, *14*, *113*
Richardson, L. P., 120, *132*
Richardson, S. A., 80, *98*
Ricour, C., *134*
Rideout, V. J., 41, *54*, 66, 68, 70, 71, *75*
Rifas-Shiman, S. L., 46, *52*, *55*, 60, 64,
        74, *75*, *76*, *197*
Ringham, R. M., 123, 126, *131*
Rippinger, D., 193, *195*
Ritenbaugh, C., 186, *199*
Robert, D., 66, 68, *75*
Robert, J. J., *134*
Roberts, D. F., 41, 42, *54*
Roberts, H., *12*
Roberts, R. E., 117, *132*
Roberts, S. B., *34*, *178*
Robertson, R. J., 172, *178*
Robins, M., *76*
Robinson, S., 81, *98*
Robinson, T. N., 41, 43, *51*, *54*, 71, *75*,
        118, *129*, 164, 167, *176*, *179*
Rocchini, A. P., 168, 170, 175, *179*
Rock, B. H., *196*
Rockett, H. R., 46, 48, *52*, *54*, *55*, 64,
        73, *74*, *76*, *197*

Rodearmel, S. J., *199*
Rodin, J., 100, 101, *111, 113*
Rodrigo, C. P., *52*
Rodriguez, J., *114*
Rodriguez, M., *114*
Rodriquez, J., *14*
Rodriquez, M., *14*
Roehrig, H. R., 117, *134*
Roemmich, J. N., 43, 56, 172, 173, *176,*
    180
Rogers, B. L., 41, *51*
Rohde, P., *133*
Rosche, C., *13*
Rosen, D., 122, *132*
Rosenberg, D. E., 38, 55
Rosenberg, M., 146, 153, *157*
Rosengard, P., *198*
Rosner, B., *74*
Rosner, B. A., 28, *33*
Ross, C., 119, *132*
Ross, E., 147, 148, *156*
Ross, J., 84, 96
Ross, J. G., *53*
Rossi, J. S., 146, *155*
Roth, D. A., 120, *132*
Rotter, J., 189, *196*
Roux, A. V., 63, *76*
Rowe, D. A., 40, 55
Roysamb, E., 100, *111*
Ruffle, T. M., 146, 152, *155*
Ruschendorf, F., 28, *35*
Rutherford, W. J., *180*

Saar, K., 25, 28, *35*
Sabry, Z., *131*
Saelens, B. E., 40, 41, 42, 43, 55, 95,
    126, 129, 159, 176
Salbe, A. D., 38, 55
Salem, G. J., *179*
Sallinen, B. J., *13*
Sallis, J. F., 38, 39, 40, 41, 47, 54, 55, 57,
    64, *75, 76,* 171, *179,* 189, 190,
    194, *198, 199, 200*
Salmon, J., 190, *200*
Samson, C., 30, 33, *34*
Sanderson, R. S., *95*
Sanderson, S., 48, *56*

Sands, R., 106, *112*
Sandy, J., 127, *131*
Santoro, N., 25, 29, 33, *35*
Santos, P., 194, *199*
Sapochnik, M., *51*
Sarwer, D. B., *180*
Sasaki, J., 170, *179*
Sasse, D. K., 108, *111*
Saunders, R. P., *156*
Sawicki, D., 192, 193, *198*
Sawyer, R., *50*
Scanlon, K. S., *13,* 43, *52*
Schauble, N., 28, *35*
Schechtman, K. B., *56*
Schermer, F., 87, *98*
Schiffer, L., *197*
Schlienger, J., *76*
Schmitz, K. H., 42, 55, 56
School Nutrition Association, 186, *200*
Schreiber, G. B., 76, *100, 113*
Schreiner, P., 122, *133*
Schuftan, C., 169, *177*
Schulenberg, J., 63, *76*
Schulenberg, J. E., 145, 154, *157*
Schuler, R., 107, *112*
Schulz, A. J., 191, 192, 193, *201*
Schumaker, H. D., 84, *97*
Schutz, H., *75*
Schwartz, M. B., 84, 85, 90, *98*
Schwartz, M. W., 19, *34*
Schwarz, G. J., 22, 23, *35*
Schwimmer, J. B., 8, *13,* 126, *133, 150,*
    157
Sebring, N. G., *131*
Seeley, R. J., 18, 19, 20, 22, 23, *35*
Seidel, K. D., 7, *14,* 20
Seifert, S., 44, *53*
Seim, H. C., *129*
Senediak, C., 173, *179*
Serdula, M. K., 6, 7, *12*
Sevenson, S., 188, 192, *197*
Shaffer, A., 192, *200*
Shaibi, G. Q., 170, *179*
Shapiro, J. R., 127, *133*
Shaw, H. E., 68, *76,* 103, 104, *113, 133,*
    188, *200*
Sheard, N. F., *179*

Sheiham, A., *51*
Shenker, I., 107, *109*
Shephard, R. J., 38, *56*
Sherman, C., 106, *112*
Sherman, D. K., 106, *112*
Sherry, B., 43, *52*
Sherwood, N. E., *52, 80, 96, 200*
Sheslow, D., 117, *133, 134*
Shindo, M., 170, *179*
Shipman, S. A., 138, *157*
Shisslak, C. M., 123, *133*
Shore, R. A., 107, *112*
Shroff, H., *14*, 104, *112, 114*
Siegel, J. M., 107, *112*
Siegfried, W., *128*
Sigelman, C. K., 88, *98*
Silink, M., 161, *180*
Silva, P. A., *132*
Silverstein, J. H., *13*
Simon, C., *76*
Simons-Morton, B. G., 40, *50,* 186, *200*
Simonson, D. C., 125, *134*
Sinclair, K. B., *176*
Singer, S., *132*
Sinha, R., 7, *13*
Sinton, M., 67, *76*
Sjostrom, L., *133*
Slater, S., 191, *199*
Smith, A., 48, *54*
Smith, D. E., 122, *133*
Smith, G. D., 7, *13*
Smith, P. R., 138, *157*
Smolak, L., 87, 98, 100, 104, 105, *111, 113, 114, 154, 157*
Snel, J., 38, *56*
Snoek, H., 66, 71, *76*
Snyder, F., 84, *97*
Sobal, J., 82, *98*
Sobol, A. M., 8, *12,* 48, *53, 56,* 150, *156, 197*
Sogaard, A. J., 7, *12*
Solano, H., *13*
Somers, C. L., 101, *111*
Sothern, M. S., 170, *180*
Soubhi, H., 191, *200*
Specker, S. M., *129*
Spence, S. H., 173, *179*

Spielberger, C. D., 146, 152, *157*
Spitzer, R. L., 122, *130, 133*
Spruijt-Metz, D., 61, *76*
Squires, S., 168, *176*
Srinivasan, S. R., 6, 7, *12,* 28, *33*
Staffieri, J. R., 80, *98*
Stallings, V., *73*
Stallings, V. A., *52,* 180
Stamler, J., 7, *12*
Stanley, S., 20, *35*
Stanton, W. R., *132*
Staunton, C. E., 38, *52,* 194, *200*
Stead, M., *195*
Steele, J. R., 171, *178, 180*
Stein, M., 125, *128*
Stein, R. I., *95*
Stephens, M. A. P., *131*
Steptoe, A., 42, *51*
Sterky, G., 168, *176*
Stevens, V., *197*
Stice, E., 68, *76,* 100, 103, 104, 105, *113,* 121, 124, 127, *133,* 188, *200*
Stolley, M. R., *197*
Stone, E. J., *198*
Storey, M., *52*
Stormer, S., 145, 154, *156*
Stormer, S. M., 101, *113*
Story, M., 62, 63, 64, 65, 66, 67, 69, 70, *72, 73, 74, 75, 76,* 80, 82, 83, 86, 87, 89, *94, 95, 96, 97,* 100, 101, 102, 103, *109, 110, 111, 112,* 120, 123, *128, 129, 130, 132,* 185, 186, *197, 198, 199, 200*
Stratton, G., 194, *200*
Strauss, C. C., 81, *98*
Strauss, J., 89, *95*
Strauss, R. S., 8, *13,* 81, 86, *98*
Strawbridge, W. J., 117, *132*
Striegel-Moore, R. H., *74, 76,* 100, *113*
Strien, T., 66, 71, *76*
Strikmiller, P. K., *198*
Strong, W. B., 38, *55*
Stroup, D. F., 3, *13*
Strugell, C., 192, *197*
Stuckey-Ropp, R. C., 194, *200*
Stunkard, A. J., *52, 73,* 81, 96, 118, 122, 126, *133, 134,* 147, 153, *157*

Subbiah, M. T., 17, *35*
Sullivan, M., 118, *133*
Sullivan, P. F., 124, 125, *129*
Summerbell, C. D., 173, *180*
Suskind, R. M., 169, *177, 180*
Sussner, K. M., 39, *53, 198*
Sutton, B. S., *50*
Swallen, K. C., 118, 126, *134*
Swan, D. C., 29, *34*
Syre, T. R., 86, *97*
Szold, A., 7, *11*

Tabak, C. J., 17, *35, 132*
Tajima, N., 161, *180*
Talebizadeh, Z., 115, *134*
Tamar, M., *129*
Tamborland, W. V., 7, *13*
Tammelin, T., 38, *55*
Tan, K., 28, *33*
Tanaka, H., *179*
Tanofsky-Kraff, M., 100, *113*, 123, 124,
    127, *130, 134*
Tantleff-Dunn, S., 99, *114*
Tapper, K., *198*
Taras, H. L., *55*
Tataranni, P. A., 38, *55*
Tauber, M., *33*
Taveras, E. M., 46, *55*, 64, *76*
Taylor, C. B., 67, *74*, 107, *110, 130*
Taylor, C. L., 127, *128*
Taylor, G. L., *199*
Taylor, W., 64, *75, 76*
Taylor, W. C., 38, *55*, 189, *200*
Teachman, B. A., 85, *98*
Teague, B., 7, *13*
Telama, R., 7, *13*, 38, *55, 56*
Tershakovec, A. M., 163, *160, 175*
Testa, M. A., 125, *134*
Teufel-Shone, N. I., *199*
Thakkar, R. R., 40, *56*
Theim, K. R., *130, 134*
Theisen, F., 25, *34*
Thelen, M. H., 100, 102, 103, *114*
Theodoro, M., 115, *134*
Thiel, L., 80, *95*
Thompson, D. I., 185, 188, *195, 196,*
    200

Thompson, J. K., 8, *12, 14*, 99, 100,
    101, 103, 104, 105, 107, 108,
    110, 111, 112, 113, 114, 145,
    151, 154, *156, 157*
Thompson, M. A., 106, *114*
Thorson, C., *178, 180*
Thurfjell, B., 107, *114*
Tibbs, T., 46, 48, *56*
Tiggemann, M., 88, *94*
Tilgner, L., 106, *114*
Timperio, A., 190, *200*
Titus-Ernstoff, L., *72*
Toney, K., 188, *199*
Tounian, A., 30, *34*
Trapl, E., 68, *74*
Tricker, J., 106, *112*
Troped, P. J., 69, *72*
Trost, S. G., 64, *76, 156*, 190, *200*
Trost-Brinkhues, G., *131*
Trowbridge, F. L., *13*
Trudeau, F., 38, *56*
Trueth, M. S., *56*
Tucker, K. L., 41, *51*
Tudor-Locke, C., 41, *56*, 172, *180*
Tulldahl, J., 45, *56*
Turnbull, J. D., 80, *98*
Turner, S., 188, 192, *197*
Tverdal, A., 7, *12*
Tweed, S., 87, *96*
Twisk, J. W. R., 38, *56*
Tybor, D. J., 125, *129*

Udall, J. N., Jr., *180*
Underwood, M. K., 81, *95*
U.S. Department of Agriculture, 193,
    200
U.S. Department of Health and Human
    Services, 7, *14*, 38, *56*

Vallianatos, M., 69, *76*
Valoski, A. M., 166, 167, 170, 171, *176,*
    177
van den Berg, P., 63, 66, *72*, 101, 104,
    108, *110, 111, 114*
Vander Wal, J. S., 100, 102, 103, *114*
Van Horn, L., *197*
van Mechelen, W., 38, *56*

Vara, L. S., 166, 167, *177*

Varady, A., 71, *75*

Varni, J. W., 8, *12*, *13*, 126, *133*, 150, *157*

Vatin, V., 30, *34*

Veijola, J., *130*

Veron-Guidry, S., 106, *114*

Vetrone, G., 108, *110*

Veugelers, P., 189, *201*

Viikari, J., 7, *13*, 38, *56*

Vila, G., 117, 118, *130*, *134*

Vincent, S. D., *180*

Vitousek, K., 125, *134*

Vogel, C., *34*

Vogt, R. A., 164, *177*

Vohra, F. A., 43, *54*

von Almen, T. K., 169, *177*

Voudouris, N. J., 107, *109*

Waclawiw, M., *131*

Wadden, T. A., 95, 118, *134*, 126, 127, *129*, 137, *157*, 163, 164, 165, 168, *175*, *177*, *180*

Wagner, A., 65, *76*

Wake, M., 86, 96, 126, *134*

Walker, R., 84, *97*

Wall, M., 62, *74*, 86, *94*, *112*, 120, *129*

Wallace, W., 117, *133*, *134*

Wallander, J. L., 8, *12*

Waller, J., 101, *114*

Walley, A. J., 22, *33*

Walsh, B. T., *133*

Walts, B., *35*

Wang, G., 7, *14*

Wang, Y., 3, 4, 5, 6, *14*, 63, 71, *75*, *76*

Wang, Y. C., 48, *56*

Wardle, J., 42, 44, 47, 48, *51*, *56*, 101, *114*, 118, 119, *134*, 171, *179*

Warm, D., 192, *201*

Wasson, J., 19, *35*

Waters, E., 86, 96, 126, *134*, *180*

Watkins, G., *201*

Watson, K., 185, 186, *196*, *197*

Watson, L., 84, *94*

Wearing, S. C., 171, *180*

Wechsler, H., 69, 70, *76*

Wehle, C., *131*

Wei, R., *131*

Weicha, J., 69, *72*

Weidner, G., *130*

Weigensberg, M. J., *179*

Weigle, D. S., *33*

Weiner, B., 88, *98*

Weisnagel, S. J., *35*

Weissman, M. M., 121, *132*, 145, 152, *157*

Weizman, A., 47, *53*, 166, *177*

Welch, S. L., *130*

Welk, G. J., 40, *56*

Weltzin, T. E., 125, *129*

Wermter, A. K., 25, 30, *34*, *35*

Wertheim, E. H., *75*, 101, 106, 107, *109*, *114*

Westlake, R. J., 166, *176*

Weyer, C., 38, *55*

Wheeler, M. E., *180*

Whelan, A., 192, *201*

Whelan, E., 38, *51*

Whitaker, R. C., 7, *14*, 42, *51*, 60, *73*, *76*, 120, 121, *130*

White, D. R., 108, *111*

White, M. A., *111*

Whitlock, E. P., 138, *157*

Wiecha, J., *53*, *197*

Wigton, R. S., *98*

Wilfley, D. E., 95, 101, *111*, *113*, 126, *129*, *134*

Willekens, F., *13*

Williams, B. I., *53*

Williams, J. B., 122, 126, *130*, *134*

Williams, S. B., 138, *157*

Williamson, D. A., 106, 108, *111*, *114*

Williamson, S., 42, *51*, 118, 119, *134*

Wilson, G. T., 122, *130*, 173, *180*

Wilson, M. L., *201*

Wind, M., *52*

Wing, R. R., 124, *131*, *133*, 163, 165, 166, 167, 168, 170, 171, 172, 173, *176*, *177*, *178*, *180*

Wing, S., 191, *199*

Wisniewski, L., 123, 126, *131*, 166, 167, *177*

Wolach, B., 45, *52*

Wolf, A. M., 7, *14*, *54*

Wolk, S., 121, *132*
Wolke, D., 83, *95*
Womble, L. G., *180*
Wood, K. C., 107, *114*
Woodall, K., 170, 173, *177*
Woodfield, L. A., 107, *112*
Woods, S. C., 18, 19, 20, 22, 23, *35*
Woolgar, M., 38, *51*
Woolner, J., *198*
Woolson, S. L., *133*
Worthman, C., *132*
Wright, C. M., 47, *51*
Wright, D., *76*
Wright, J. A., 7, *14*
Wrigley, N., 192, *201*
Wrotniak, B. H., 43, *56*, 172, 173, *180, 181*
Wu, Y., 171, *177*
Wyatt, H. R., *199*
Wylie-Rosett, J., 147, 148, *156*
Wynne, K., 20, 21, 23, 24, *35*

Xu, J., 84, *95*

Yamamiya, Y., 8, *14*, 104, *114*
Yancey, A. J., 107, *112*
Yang, M., *198*

Yang, S., 63, *76*
Yang, S. J., *53*
Yang, W., 25, *35*
Yang, X., 7, *13*, 38, *55, 56*
Yanover, T., 104, *114*
Yanovski, J. A., *13*, 113, *134*
Yanovski, S. Z., *113, 130, 131, 134*
Yassouridis, A., *131*
Yawn, B. P., 84, *97*
Yip, R., *13*

Zabinski, M. F., *95*
Zakeri, I. F., *52*, 185, 186, 194, *195, 196, 197, 198, 200*
Zavela, K., *130*
Zeller, M. H., 117, 118, *134*
Zenk, S. N., 191, 192, 193, *201*
Zhang, Q., 63, *76*
Zhou, L., 60, *75*
Zhou, X. H., 161, *176*
Ziegler, A., 28, *35, 128*
Ziegler, P., 47, *57*
Zimmet, P., 161, *180*
Zipper, E., *134*
Zive, M. M., 47, *57*
Ziyadeh, N., *72*
Zuberi, A., *35*

SUBJECT INDEX

Accelerometers
    in measurement of early physical
        activity, 40
    in measurement of sedentary behavior,
        43
Activity, 146, 149
Adipocytes, 20
Adiposity signals, 19
    criteria for, 19–20
Adjustment difficulty, history of, 151
Adjustment disorder, assessment for,
    152
Advertising, unhealthy food choices
    and, 68. *See also* Television
    advertising
Advocacy for obesity support, 206–207
Aerobic exercise, 170
African American households, fruits
    and vegetables in *vs.* White
    households, 44
African American neighborhoods, food
    accessibility in, 192
Age
    child, dietary patterns and, 44
    gene expression and, 32
    gene interactions and, 204
    teasing and, 101
Aging, gene activity and, 25
Agouti-related protein (AGRP)
    effects of, 23–24
    promotion of food intake and energy
        expenditure, 22–23
Albright hereditary osteodystrophy
    (AHO), 27
American Academy of Pediatrics
    policy statement on obesity, 205

Council on Sports Medicine and Fit-
    ness and Council on School
    Health, recommendations of,
    205–206
Amylin, nutrient control and, 22
Anthropometric assessment, 139–140
    of feelings regarding visit, 141
    interviews in, 140–141
    of reason for visit in, 141
    weight history in, 141–142
Antifat biases, 84
Anxiety disorders and obesity, 119
    assessment of, 146, 152
    loss of control and, 123
    in overweight children, 118
Appetite, ghrelin and, 22
Appetite control, brain centers in, 22, 23
Appetite reduction, 168
Appliance-monitoring devices and
    measurement of sedentary time,
    43
Arcuate nucleus in energy physiology,
    22–23
Asking skills in mediation of dietary
    change, 187
Assessment
    anthropometric, 139–140
    behavioral, 137, 138–142 (*See also*
        Behavioral assessment)
    goals of, 137
    medical, 138–139
    parental inclusion in, 137
    psychometric, 143–154 (*See also* Psy-
        chometric assessment)
Association studies of polygenic obesity,
    29
Asthma and adiposity in children, 6

At risk for overweight, defined, 116
Attention-deficit/hyperactivity disorder
        (ADHD), 152
    relationship to obesity, 125
Attitudes
    toward overweight peer, attribution
        theory and, 88–89
    weight-related, among teachers and
        school health workers, 83
Attribution theory, controllability of
        obesity and, 88–89

Bardet-Biedl syndrome (BBS), 27
Behavioral assessment
    anthropometric assessment in,
        139–140
    review of medical assessment in,
        138–139
Behavioral contracting, 167–168
Behavioral problems in overweight chil-
        dren, 118
Behavioral treatment, family-based
    efficacy of, 173
    future research in, 174
Behavior change vs. weight change, 95
Behavior modification
    family, 173
    family role in, 165–168
    feedback in, 165
    functional analysis of behavior in,
        163–164
    goal setting in, 164
    self-monitoring in, 162–163
    social support, 165
    stimulus control in, 164–165
Binge eating
    assessment of, 124, 153
    binge eating–depression–obesity
        interrelationship, 120,
        123–124
    body dissatisfaction-related, 100
    childhood obesity and, 123–124
    in children, 122
    defined, 122
    depression and obesity and, 120, 123
    loss of control, obesity-associated,
        and 122

risk factors for, 103
    symptoms of, assessment for, 140
    teasing-related, 102
    weight loss programs and, 127
Binge eating disorder (BED), 122
    behaviors in, 153
    criteria for children under 14 years,
        127
    and overweight in adults, 122
    research criteria for, 152
    symptomatic behaviors for, 149
Biological factors. See also named factor
    gastrointestinal peptides, 20–22
    neuropeptides, 22–24
    peripheral hormones, 19–20
Body dissatisfaction, 100, 204. See also
        Body image dissatisfaction
    loss of control and, 123
    in overweight vs. normal weight girls
        and boys, 100
    parental weight control behaviors
        and, 66
    research on, 207
    teasing and, 101
Body image, 162
    assessment of, 145, 154
    defined, 99
    enhancing, and weight loss strategies,
        109
    measures of, 105, 106–108
    mediation between appearance-
        related teasing and eating dis-
        turbance, 101
    problems, weight-based teasing and,
        101
    teasing and, 100–101
    unhealthy weight control behaviors
        and, 102–103
Body image dissatisfaction, 80, 154. See
        also Body image disturbance
    behavioral effects of, 154
    dual pathway model of, 103–104
    loss of control and, 123
    in overweight vs. normal weight girls
        and boys, 100
    parental weight control behaviors
        and, 66

research on, 207
teasing and, 101
tripartite influence model, 104
Body image disturbance
assessment measures for, 104, 106–108
risk factor models of, 103–104
treatment of, 104–105
victimization and, 8
Body mass index (BMI)
depression and, 119
overweight and, 3
percentiles, 140
in screening for treatment, 160–161
Breast-feeding
and decreased risk for overweight, 60
diaries of, 47
eating behaviors and, 45
Bulimia nervosa, 122
assessment of, 124
dual pathway model of, 103
in high school and college females,
103
Bulimic symptoms, risk factors for,
103–104
Bullying. *See also* Victimization
assessment of, 150–151
obese perpetrators of, 83
by overweight child, 131
by peers, 81
response to, 150–151

Cardiovascular risk factors
child obesity and, 6
characterization of, 41
Child-care setting, healthy diet and, 47
Childhood obesity (ages 8 through 18)
attention deficit/hyperactivity disorder and, 125
depression and, 116–121
eating disorders and, 122–125
lifestyle interventions for, 126–128
in Prader-Willi syndrome, 115
quality of life and, 125–126
Childhood obesity–depression
relationship
cross-sectional studies of, 117, 118,
119–120

factors in, 119–120
longitudinal relationships between,
120–121
Child Nutrition Improvement and
Integrity Act of 2004, mandates
of, 186
Cholecystokinin (CCK), 21
Cocaine- and amphetamine-related
transcript (CART) neuropeptide,
suppression of food intake by, 23,
24
Comorbidity in obesity
depression, 116–121
eating disorders, 122–125
Conduct disorders and development of
overweight, 121
Conflict over food, 148–149
Coping strategies, 151
definition of, 41

Depression, 204
assessment of, 145–146, 151–152
binge eating and, 123
in children, factors in, 117
in clinical *vs.* community samples of
obese children, 117–118
and development of obesity,
120–121
family-based behavioral weight management, 127
improvement with weight loss programs, 126–127
in obese, treatment-seeking children,
117–118
and overweight, reciprocal relationship, 117
in overweight adults, 116–117
as cause and consequence of overweight, 117, 121
as risk factor for development of
overweight, 121
severity of obesity and, 118–119
victimization and, 8
weight-based teasing and, 101
Depressive symptoms
assessment of, 124, 141
body dissatisfaction-related, 100

Depressive symptoms, *continued*
   interventions for, 127
   loss of control and, 123
   teasing and, 86, 87
Diet, in weight history, 142
Dietary behaviors. *See also* Eating
      behaviors, etiology of
   etiology of, 43–47
   measurement of dietary intake, 47–48
   recommendations for, 49
   TV influence on, 47
Dietary change
   family involvement in, 188
   mediators of, 187
Dietary intake
   home food availability and, 188
   meal structure and, 189
   measurement of, 47–48
   parental influence on, 188–189
   developmental differences in, 189
   parent report, 47
   social context and, 189
Dietary modification, 168–169
Dietary patterns
   assessment of, 147, 148–149
   in childhood, 7–8
   economy and, 191
   environment and, 191
   in etiology of weight problems, 8
   mediating variable model and,
      183–184
Dietary recommendations, children
      meeting, 43
Dietary restraint
   assessment of, 153
   thin ideal and, 103
Dietary restriction and decrease in
      bulimic symptoms, 127
Dieticians, negative attitudes and
      stereotypes toward obese individ-
      uals, 84
Dieting, 102
   assessment of, 124
   social norms and, 67
   teasing-related, 102
   weight gain with, 66
Diet pills, 102

Diet records, 47
Discipline, assessment of, 144
Disordered eating behaviors
   body dissatisfaction-related, 100
   teasing-related, 102
   weight-based teasing and, 101
Displacement, positive reinforcement
      and, 165
Dissonance induction program in pre-
      vention of eating disorders, 105

Early childhood, familial influences in,
      60–61
Early physical activity. *See also* Physical
      activity; Sedentary behavior
   diet and, 39
   etiology of, 39–40
   measurement of, 40
   parental correlates, 39, 40
   physical environment and, 39
   psychological correlates, 39
   psychological variables in, 39
Eating attitudes, assessment of, 124
Eating behaviors
   breast-feeding and, 45
   demographic factors in, 44
   etiology of, 43–47
   food restriction and parental control,
      45–46
   genetic factors in, 44
   meal time structure, 46
   modeling, 46
   New Moves (school-based program)
      and, 90
   parental modeling and, 46, 62–63
   parent factors in, 44–45
   physical context and, 46–47
   social context, 46–47
   stigma and, 92
   television viewing and, 47
Eating disorders, 109
   assessment of, 147, 152–153
      in childhood obesity, 124
      interview in, 124
      self-report in, 124
   loss of control and, 123
   measures for, 106, 107

prevention programs for children and adolescents at risk, 105

risk factors for, 103

screening questionnaires for, 127

Eating disturbance

risk factor models of, 103–104

weight-based teasing and, 101

Eating habits

lifestyle approach to changing, 169

self-monitoring for awareness of, 169

Economic burden of obesity, 7

Ectonucleotide pyrophosphatase/phosphodiesterase 1 (ENPPI) gene polymorphisms

in obesity, 30

Educational settings, effectiveness of, 88

Educators

negative attitudes regarding obesity, 83

of obese children, suggested changes for, 85

Elementary school children

body dissatisfaction in, 100

moderate to vigorous physical activity in, 187

teasing and weight in, 83

Energy balance

arms of (physical activity and diet), 9–10

energy balance equation, 18

energy gap in weight gain in children, 48

energy imbalance, 9

Energy metabolism

hypothalamus in, 22

neuropeptides and, 22, 23

Energy regulation, biochemical pathways in, 19

Environment

dietary patterns and, 191

food deserts, 192

locational disparities in, 192–193

obesigenic, 26

and prevalence, 204

youth physical activity and, 193–194

Environmental changes, identification through analysis of behavior, 163–164

Epidemiology, molecular, 19

Ethnicity

food store accessibility and, 192

moderation of obesity–depression relationship in adults and, 119

parent, dietary patterns and, 44

prevalence trends and, 4–6

TV viewing and, 42

Etiology

research in human obesity gene map and, 203–204

of weight problems, 8

of sedentary behavior, 41–42

Exercise

aerobic, 170

resistance training, 170

in weight history, 142

Exercise patterns in etiology of weight problems, 8

Familial influences

on eating behavior, 62–64

in infancy and early childhood, 60–62

on physical activity, 64–65

in preadolescence and adolescence, 62

on sedentary behavior, 65–66

on weight concerns, 66

on weight control behaviors, 66

Family

assessment of, 144, 147

dietary intake and, 188–189

educating on healthy behaviors, 171–172

physical activity and, 189–190

conceptual models of, 190–191

intervention in, 190

obesity prevention in, 189–190

in obesity prevention, 188

Family-based treatment programs, 207

Family history

family medical history, 139

family routine in, 143–144

mental health history in, 144

psychosocial issues in patient's life, 143

validated, written assessment measures of, 144, 147

Family meals
    eating behavior and, 63
    socioeconomic status and, 63–64
Family Relationship Inventory, 144, 147
Family Ritual Questionnaire: Dinner
        Time, 144, 147
Family support
    for coping with stigmatization, 89
    for weight control, 166, 167–168
Fast foods
    and higher childhood BMI, 43
    in school lunches, 69
Fatty taste preference, 44
Feedback, 165
    negative, 204
    through self-monitoring, 162
Food access
    locational disparities in, 191, 192–193
    price disparities in, 191, 193
Food deserts, 192
Food intake
    3-day food record, 148
    24-hour recall, 47, 148
    parental influence on, 188–189
    patient behaviors concerning, 148
Food preferences
    modeling and, 189
    parental influence on, 188–189
Food restriction, parental, eating behav-
        iors and, 45–46
Fruit and vegetable consumption
    family meals and, 63
    school-based interventions for,
        185–187
    in school cafeteria, 185

Gastrointestinal peptides
    satiation peptides, 21
    satiation signals, 20–21
    summary of obesity-related, 21
Gender
    depressive symptoms and, 124
    dietary patterns and, 44
    dieting and, 102–103
    moderation of obesity-depression in
        adults, 119
    obesity and anxiety and, 119
    overweight/obesity prevalence, 4–5

parental feeding practices, 45
parental modeling and, 62–63
prevalence trends and, 4–6
television viewing and, 42
Gender differences in dating and obesity,
        82
Gene–behavior interactions, 31, 32
Gene–diet interactions, 31, 32
Gene–environment interactions, 31, 32
Genetic factors, 17–18
    and binge eating–depression–obesity
        interrelationship, 124
    in eating behaviors, 44
    in monogenic obesity, 26
    obesity susceptibility loci, 24
    in polygenic obesity, 27–30
    in syndromic obesity, 26–27
    "thrifty genome" of ancestors, 25–26
    in weight history, 142
Genomic alterations, summary of obe-
        sity-related, 25
Ghrelin (hormone), 22
    gene for, 29
Global screen time, 149. See also TV
        viewing
Glucagon-like-peptide-1 (GLP-1), 21
Glycemic index (GI)
    carbohydrate intake and, 18
    diet and, 169–170
    physiological response to, 18
Goals
    in behavior modification, 164
    reappraisal of, 164

Health care costs of pediatric obesity,
        comorbidities and, 7
Health care professionals
    antifat bias of, 84
    negative attitudes and stereotypes
        toward obese individuals, 83, 84
    of obese children, suggested changes
        for, 85
    negative attitudes and stereotypes
        toward obese individuals, 84
    strategies for behavioral change vs.
        weight change, 95
    support for overweight patients and
        students, 90

Health care settings, stigmatization in, 83–85
Health-promoting family model, 190
Health-related quality of life. *See also* Quality of life
    in overweight youth, 8
    peer victimization and, 8
Healthy lifestyle choices, family support of, 89
Hispanic neighborhoods, food store accessibility in, 192
Home-based interventions to promote health, 89
Hunger cues, response to, 46
Hypothalamus, 22, 23

Impaired glucose tolerance and adiposity in children, 6
Impulsivity, overeating and, 125
Individualized education program (IEP), 150
Infancy, familial influences in, 60–61
Insulin, 20
Insulin resistance and adiposity in children, 6
Interventions, long-term, 207
Interviews
    adolescent, 140
    parent-and-child vs. child-only, 140
    semistructured, 140–141

Laxative use, 102. *See also* Purging
    gender and, 103
Leptin, 20, 29
Lifestyle interventions
    behavioral, 126
    to changing eating habits, 169
    to integrate physical activity into daily activities, 170
    weight loss programs, 126
Linkage analysis, heritability and variance components in obesity, 28–29
Loss of control
    binge eating and, 122
    psychological symptomology associated with, 123

Low self-esteem
    victimization and, 8
    weight-based teasing and, 101

Market environment
    locational disparities in, 191, 192–193
    price disparities in, 191, 193
MCH receptor Type 1 (MCHR 1) gene and extreme obesity, 30
MC4R mutations
    in childhood obesity, 29
    measurement of, 42–43
Media. *See also* TV advertising
Media influence, body dissatisfaction and eating disturbance and, 104
Medical assessment, 138–139
Medical morbidity and obesity, 6–8
Melanocortin-4 receptor (MC4R) mutations
    gene in childhood obesity, 29
    gene in monogenic obesity, 26
    measurement of, 42–43
Mental health history, 133
Mental illness, history of, 151
Metabolic syndrome
    adiposity in children, 6
    criteria for, 161–162
Modeling
    eating behaviors and, 46
    food preferences and, 188
    parental (*See* Parental modeling)
Molecular biology
    implications for clinical practice, 30–31
    implications for research, 30–31
Mood disorders, 152
Morbidity
    medical, 6–8
    psychological, 8
Mortality, obesity as risk factor for, 7
Mothers, overweight and obese
    breast-feeding and, 60
    and child risk for overweight, 60
Motivation, 207

Negative affect, bulimic symptoms and, 103
Negative feedback, consequences of, 8

Negative feedback system, peripheral
hormones in, 19
Neighborhood, healthy diet and, 47
Neophobia, 188–189
Neuropeptides, 22–24
summary of obesity-related, 23
Neuropeptide Y (NPY)
in arcuate nucleus, 22, 23
promotion of food intake and energy
expenditure, 22–23
New Moves program
for body image issues and eating
behaviors, 105
for overweight or at risk for overweight girls, 90–91
Nurses, negative attitudes and stereotypes toward obese individuals,
84
Nutritional genomic studies, 31
Nutrition education in schools, 185
Nutrition interventions
curriculum and cafeteria modifications, 186
environmental, 186
high school, 186
middle school, 185–186
National School Lunch Program and
wellness policy, 186
Planet Health, 185
school-based, 185–187
social marketing, 186

Obesigenic lifestyle, gene interaction
and, 18
Obesity. *See also under named influence*
attributions about causes of, 207
definitions of, 203
genetic factors in, 26–30
hormonal factors in, 19–20
influences on
familial, 59–66
peer, 66–68
societal, 68–71
medical morbidity and, 6–8
metabolic factors in, 20–22
neuronal factors in, 22–24
pediatric, obesity link to, 7–8

psychological consequences of, 85–86
and quality of life, 126
Obesity–binge eating reciprocal rela-
tionship, 124
Obesity classification, genome-based, 31
Obesity risk management, geneticists in,
32
Obesity-susceptible genes, 26
Observation, direct, in early physical
activity measurement, 40
Observational measures of dietary pat-
terns, 47, 48
Oppositional behavior, 152
Oppositional defiant disorder, over-
weight and, 121
Overweight, defined, 116. *See also* At
risk for overweight

Parental control, eating behaviors and,
46
Parental encouragement of physical
activity, 64, 65
Parental influence
body dissatisfaction and eating disturbance and, 104
on food preference and intake,
188–189
Parental modeling. *See also* Modeling
eating behaviors and, 46, 62–63
influence on dietary practices of children, 63
of physical activity, 64
physical activity changes and, 173
Parental support for physical activity,
190–191
Parent education, dietary patterns and,
44
Parent factors in eating behaviors, 44–45
Parent report
of dietary intake, 47
of early physical activity, 40
in measurement of sedentary behavior, 42–43
Parents
early physical activity and, 39, 40
guidelines for obesity prevention and
healthful behavior promotion,
49

24-hour food recall interviews, 47
    involvement in exercise and physical
        activity, 172–173
Pediatrician, collaboration with, 138
Pedometers
    in measurement of early physical
        activity, 40
    in measurement of physical activity,
        172
Peer difficulties, 150–151
Peer influence
    body dissatisfaction and eating dis-
        turbance and, 104
    effect on health and risky behavior,
        67
    peer role models of healthy diet, 67
    during preadolescence and adoles-
        cence, 66
    on preadolescents and adolescents,
        62
Peer modeling, eating behaviors and, 46
Peer relations, 162
Peptide YY (PYY), 21–22
Peripheral hormones
    signals in negative feedback system,
        19
    summary of obesity-related, 20
Peroxisome proliferator-activated recep-
        tor gamma 2 (PPAR gamma-2),
        variants and obesity-related Type
        2 diabetes and, 30
Pharmacotherapy, adjunctive to behav-
        ioral modification, 168
Physical activity, 146, 149, 170. See also
        Early physical activity; Sedentary
        activity
    aerobic exercise, 170
    after school programs, 70
    assessment of, 149–150
    in childhood, 7–8
    decrease in opportunities for, 48
    defined, 38
    early (See Early physical activity)
    exercise goals, 172–173
    family and, 189–190
        conceptual models and, 190–191
        intervention in, 190

prevention in, 189–190
    promotion of and involvement
        in, 171–173
    promotion of opportunities for, 89
    goals for, 172, 173
    home equipment, 194
    medical benefits of, 171
    New Moves (school-based program)
        and, 90
    outdoor, enhancement of, 205
    parental influence on, 64–65, 189–190
    parental support of, 190–191
    pedometer measurement of, 172
    peer influence in decline of, 67–68
    physical education classes, reduction
        of, 70
    play structures and playgrounds, 194
    recommendations for, 49
    resistance training, 170
    transportation effect on, 190
    walk-to-school initiatives, 194
Physical activity patterns, mediating
        variable model and, 183–184
Physical context, eating behaviors and,
        46–47
Physical education
    American Academy of Pediatrics'
        Council on Sports Medicine
        and Fitness and Council on
        School Health recommenda-
        tion, 206
    changing lessons in, 187–188
    Child and Adolescent Trial for Car-
        diovascular Health (CATCH)
        and, 187
    Middle School Physical Activity &
        Nutrition study, 187
    reduction of schools classes for, 70
    negative prejudices toward obesity,
        84
Physical education staff, antifat biases
        among, 84
Physical examination, 139
Physical health, effect of weight stigma
        on, 93
Physicians, level of care for overweight
        men, 84

Polygenic (common) obesity, 27–28
  association studies of, 29–30
  linkage studies of, 28–29
Positive parenting techniques, 165
Positive reinforcement, 165
Pouring rights contracts in schools, 68,
  69
Poverty, overweight/obesity and, 4
Prader-Willi syndrome (PWS), 27
Preadolescence, familial influences in, 62
Prevalence of overweight/obesity
  factors in, 204
  of adolescent, 62
  of pediatric, 3
  socioeconomic status and, 4–6
  trends in
    ethnicity and, 4, 5
    gender and, 4–5
Prevention of obesity
  economy in, 191–193
  environment in, 191–193
  families in, 188–191
  of pediatric obesity, 7
  schools in, 185–188
Price disparities, 193
Propriomelanocortin (POMC)
  hypothalamic, 24
  coding, mutation screening in, 29
  gene, insertion in and insulin levels,
    29–30
  neurons
  coexpression of and CART, 24
  suppression of food intake, 23
Psychometric assessment
  dietary patterns of, 148–149
  eating disorders of, 152–154
  family history of, 143–147
  physical and sedentary activities of,
    150–151
  psychopathology of, 152–152
Psychosocial consequences of stigma, 92
Psychosocial functioning, assessment of,
  153–155
Psychosocial issues in treatment screening, 162
Psychosocial stressors, assessment for,
  140, 142

Purging behaviors. *See also* Laxative use
  assessment of, 153
  weight loss programs and, 127

Quality of life. *See also* Health-related
    quality of life
  defined, 125
  in obese children, 126
  school-related, 150

Race
  locational disparities in food stores,
    192–193
  physical activity and, 65
  prevalence trends and, 4–6
  television viewing and, 42
Recreational infrastructure, youth phys-
    ical activity and, 194
Resistance training, 170
Restricting behaviors, 102
Restrictive eating, weight gain and,
    61–62
Restrictive feeding style
  maternal, 61
  parental, 61
Romantic relationships, overweight
    adolescents and, 82
Routine
  family, 143–144
  patient, 144

Salty taste preference, 44
Satiety cues, response to, 46
School performance, deficits in, 150
Schools
  food environments in, 185
  food options in, 68–69, 68–70
  healthy diet and, 47
  increasing physical education in,
    187–188
  influence on obesity, 68–70
  nutrition interventions in, 185–187
  open campus lunch policies, 68–69
  physical activity and, 70
  physical education changes in,
    187–188
  vending machines in, 68, 69

Sedentary activity. *See also* Early physi-
    cal activity; Physical activity
    assessment of, 149–150
    chronic health problems from, 171
    reducing, 172
Sedentary behavior
    characterization of, 41
    definition of, 41
    etiology of, 41–42
    measurement of, 42–43
    television watching as, 41
Self-efficacy
    assessment of, 154–155
    mediation of dietary change, 187
    research on, 207
    V.I.K. program and, 105
    Weight Efficacy Life-Style Question-
        naire, 146, 154–155
Self-esteem, 85
    assessment of, 146–153, 153–154
    child, maternal weight concerns and,
        61
    negative association of weight with,
        in elementary school children,
        86
    in obese children and adolescents, 86
    obesity diminishment of, 86
    teasing effect on, 86–87, 101
    victimization and, 8
Self-induced vomiting, 102. *See also*
        Purging behaviors
    gender and, 103
Self-monitoring
    of eating habits, 169
    purpose of, 162
    for situational circumstances of
        behavior, 163
    tools for, 163
Self-report measures of diet-related vari-
        ables, 47
Sibutramine, 168
Snacks, 148
snack bars in schools, 68
snack food intake, restriction to food
        access and, 61
snack foods and higher childhood BMI,
        43

snacking, television viewing and, 71
snack vending machines, effect of, 185
Social environment, eating behaviors
        and, 46–47
Social isolation
    of overweight adolescents, 81
    by peers, 81
Social marginalization
    by adolescents, 81, 82
    by children, 81
    defined, 81
    by peers, 81
Social norms, dieting and, 67
Socioeconomic status and moderation
        of obesity-depression in adults, 119
Socioeconomic status outcomes of
        stigma, 92
Soft drinks
    and higher childhood BMI, 43
    in schools, 68, 69, 70
Sport and recreation programs, commu-
        nity, 206
Stature, assessment of, 139
Stereotyping of obesity, 80
Stigmatization
    academic outcomes of, 92
    increase in, by children, 80–81
    decreasing, 87–89
    within educational and health care
        settings, 83–85
    by peers, 80–83
    psychological consequences of,
        86–87
    psychosocial consequences of, 92
    reduction, research in, 93
    school-based intervention for, 87
    sources of, 92
    support for overweight individuals,
        89–91
Stimulus control, 164–165
    home environment in, 168
    limiting TV access, 164
StopLight Diet, 168
Substitution, positive reinforcement
        and, 165
Successive approximation, goal setting
        and, 164

Suicide attempts, teasing and, 86, 87
Suicide ideation, 204
    teasing and, 86, 87
    weight-based teasing and, 101
Support for overweight individuals,
        89–91
Sweet taste preference, 44

Teachers, support for overweight
        patients and students, 90
Teasing, 80, 100
    age of onset and, 101
    assessment of, 145, 151
    association with depression and
        overweight, 120
    and body image dissatisfaction,
        100–101
    history, 162
    by peers, 81, 82–83
    response to, 150–151
    strategies for dealing with, 87
    types of childhood, 101
    V.I.K. program for, 105
Television advertising. See also
        Advertising
    of calorie-dense, low-nutrient foods
        and beverages, 71
    food choices and, 41
    influence on dietary behaviors, 47
Television sets, number and placement
        of and promotion of sedentary
        behavior, 65–66
Television viewing. See also Global
        screen time
    correlates of, 42
    correlation of time and weight gain
        and obesity, 71
    diet and, 48
    minority ethnic and racial back-
        grounds, 42
    as obesity risk, 41
    recommendations for, 49
    unsafe neighborhood and, 42
Thin-ideal internalization
    body dissatisfaction and dietary
        restraint, 103

body dissatisfaction and eating dis-
        turbance and, 104
    consequences of, 103
Thin-oriented society, effect of, 90
Thought disorder, 152
Thrifty Food Plan (TFP), store price dis-
        parities for, 193
Transport, youth physical activity and,
        194
Trauma, history of, 151
Treatment, screening for
    body mass index in, 159–160
    domains in, recommended medical
        assessment for, 161
    guidelines for children and adoles-
        cents, 160
    metabolic syndrome in, 161–162
    psychosocial issues in, 162
TV viewing. See Television viewing
Type 2 diabetes mellitus and adiposity
        in children, 6

Unhealthy weight control behaviors,
        102–103
    body dissatisfaction-related, 100,
        102–103
    in puberty and adolescence, 67
    teasing-related, 102

Vending machines, access to in schools,
        68, 69
Very Important Kids (V.I.K.) interven-
        tion, 204
    components of, 87–88
    effectiveness of, 88
    family component of, 88
    promotion of healthy body image
        and weight-related behaviors,
        87–88
    school-based, to prevent stigmatiza-
        tion, 87
Victimization. See also Bullying
    by bullies, 150
    psychological and psychosocial
        effects of, 8
    relational, 81
    weight-based, 207

Walk-to-school initiatives, 194
Weight, assessment of, 139–140
Weight-based teasing. *See* Teasing
Weight bias, 206, 207
    negative social feedback and, 8
Weight control
    behavior modification for, 162–168
        (*See also* Behavior modification)
      efficacy of, 173–174
    dietary components of, 168–170
    physical activity in, 170–173
Weight control behaviors
    parental modeling of, 66
    social norms and, 67
    unhealthy, 90

Weight discrimination, 162
Weight history, 141–142
    parent report of, 141
    past weight loss attempts, 142
Weight-related prejudice, exploring
      with school staff, 83
Weight-related teasing. *See* Teasing
Weight stigma, 206, 207
    research areas needed, 91–93
Weight teasing. *See* Teasing
Wellness
    school council for, 206
    school policy, 186

z scores for overweight, 3

ABOUT THE EDITORS

Leslie J. Heinberg, PhD, is an associate professor of medicine for the Cleveland Clinic Lerner College of Medicine of Case Western Reserve University, Cleveland, Ohio, and director of behavioral services for the Bariatric and Metabolic Institute at the Cleveland Clinic Foundation, Cleveland, Ohio. She previously served as clinical director of Healthy Kids/Healthy Weight, a comprehensive, multidisciplinary evaluation and intervention pediatric obesity program at Rainbow Babies and Children's Hospital, Cleveland, Ohio. Dr. Heinberg coauthored (with J. Kevin Thompson) the book *Exacting Beauty: Theory, Assessment, and Treatment of Body Image Disturbance* (American Psychological Association, 1998) and has published more than three dozen articles related to body image, eating disorders, and obesity. She has also served as a coinvestigator on six federally funded studies of obesity prevention and treatment or body image.

J. Kevin Thompson, PhD, is a professor in the Department of Psychology, University of South Florida, Tampa. He has written, edited, or coedited five books on the topics of obesity, eating disorders, and body image: *Body Image, Eating Disorders and Obesity: An Integrative Guide for Assessment, and Treatment* (American Psychological Association [APA], 1996), *Exacting Beauty: Theory, Assessment, and Treatment of Body Image Disturbance* (APA, 1998); *Body Image, Eating Disorders, and Obesity in Youth: Assessment, Prevention, and Treatment* (two editions; APA, 2001, 2009); and *The Muscular Ideal: Psychological, Social, and Medical Perspectives* (APA, 2007).